Pediatric History and Physical Diagnosis for Nurses

Library of Congress Cataloging in Publication Data

Alexander, Mary Merkel.
    Pediatric history taking and physical diagnosis for
nurses.

    First ed. published in 1974 under title: Pediatric
physical diagnosis for nurses.
    Includes bibliographies and index.
    1.   Children—Medical examinations.   2.   Physical
diagnosis.   3.   Medical history taking.   4.   Pediatric
nursing.   I.   Brown, Marie Scott, joint author.
II.   Title.   [DNLM: 1.   Pediatrics—Nursing texts.
2.   Physical examination—In infancy and childhood—
Nursing texts.   3.   Medical records—Nursing texts.
WY159 A377p]
RJ50.A4 1979   618.9'2007'54   78-9679
ISBN 0-07-001019-6
ISBN 0-07-001018-8 pbk.

This book was set in English Times by Allen Wayne Technical Corp.
The editor was Mary Ann Richter
and the production supervisor was Milton J. Heiberg.
R.R. Donnelley & Sons Company was printer and binder.
The line drawings were done by Dorothy Markel Alexander, B.S.J.M.A.

NOTICE

Medicine is an ever-changing science. As new research and
clinical experience broaden our knowledge, changes in treatment and drug therapy are required. The editors and the
publisher of this work have made every effort to ensure that
the drug dosage schedules herein are accurate and in accord
with the standards accepted at the time of publication.
Readers are advised, however, to check the product information sheet included in the package of each drug they plan to
administer to be certain that changes have not been made in
the recommended dose or in the contraindications for administration. This recommendation is of particular importance in
regard to new or infrequently used drugs.

Pediatric History Taking and Physical Diagnosis for Nurses

Second Edition

Mary M. Alexander

Instructor, Department of Pediatrics
School of Medicine
University of Colorado

Marie Scott Brown

Associate Professor of Parent-Child Nursing
University of Colorado

McGraw-Hill Book Company

New York   St. Louis   San Francisco   Auckland   Bogotá   Düsseldorf
Johannesburg   London   Madrid   Mexico   Montreal   New Delhi
Panama   Paris   São Paulo   Singapore   Sydney   Tokyo   Toronto

Contents

Preface

Since the first edition of *Pediatric Physical Diagnosis for Nurses,* marked progress has been made in the nursing profession in expanding the role of all nurses in relation to the use of physical diagnostic skills. Few nurses continue to feel that these skills are only in the purview of the physician and, according to a poll conducted by the University of Colorado, over 95 percent of the accredited baccalaureate programs are now incorporating physical assessment skills. Sometimes, these skills are taught only in relation to the adult client, but it is hoped that this attitude will change, and that nurses will begin to appreciate the age-specific differences in the assessment of children. We hope this book will be helpful in promoting this appreciation.

The book has been greatly expanded since the last edition. In addition to physical assessment skills, we are also including two other major areas of data collection: history taking and screening tests. These chapters were originally published in *Ambulatory Pediatrics for Nurses,* the sequel to *Pediatric Physical Diagnosis for Nurses.* That book will still serve as a sequel, but will be further expanded to deal with common illnesses in children.

The chapters on physical diagnosis itself have also been significantly updated—the pelvic exam is now included in the female genitalia; some of the newer information in the skeletal section reflects the growing body of knowledge in the field of sports medicine.

We hope that this contribution to the literature of pediatric nursing will help the nursing profession to give more holistic care to the children for whom they care.

We would like to express appreciation to all of the many readers who have offered suggestions and particularly to Dr. Helen Britton, Ms. Judy Igoe, and Dr. Jerry Northern for their painstaking critique of the book.

Mary M. Alexander
Marie Scott Brown

Pediatric History Taking and Physical Diagnosis for Nurses

Chapter 1

The History-Taking Interview: Its Purpose and Place in the Assessment Process

A very important part of the well-child visit is the history-taking interview. Most clinicians feel that about 80 percent of the information the nurse will use in the assessment process will be discovered during the history taking (15 percent will come through physical examination and five percent through laboratory test results). It is important to remember, however, that assessment is only one of the four goals of history taking. Assessment relates to the communication from the family to the nurse, but information must also go from the nurse to the family in the form of education and counseling. The four goals of the history-taking process, then, are:

1 Establishing rapport between the family and the examiner
2 Assessment (from family to nurse)
3 Education (from nurse to family)
4 Counseling (from nurse to family)

Assessment of a child includes four basic components: subjective data (history taking), objective data (the physical examination and laboratory

1

testing), assessment (the interpretation of subjective and objective data), and a plan (the action taken). Although these four categories can be discussed separately, they are, in reality, closely related. The examiner, may begin to take some history, but stop to talk about a problem the parent or child wants to discuss immediately. During the physical examination questions may also arise that need an immediate answer. It is impossible to postpone all the counseling and education until the end of the visit.

Although every workup includes all components, certain types of assessments may place heavier emphasis on certain components. It is a mistake, however, to omit any of them entirely. For example, when a nurse does only a physical examination and the child presents with a bump on the leg, certain questions will remain unanswered, such as: Does it hurt? When did it appear? Have you ever had one before? Does anyone else in the family have one? Without this kind of information it is hard to reach an accurate conclusion. On the other hand, if during the history taking the mother mentions that the child has a pain in his big toe, after the examiner has asked some further questions about the pain, it is important to then actually examine the toe before reaching any conclusions or offering any suggestions. Often, after performing one part of the workup, the examiner thinks he or she has a good idea of what is going on, only to have the entire picture change as more information is gathered.

Good history taking involves the ability to question each parent and child individually. The way the questions are asked, which questions are asked, and the examiner's facial expressions, body gestures, and relaxed attitude all aid in obtaining the total picture of what is happening to the child.

KINDS OF INTERVIEWS

There are several kinds of interviews, each appropriate for different times, places, and needs. The *well-child interview* is the one most frequently done by nurses working in ambulatory pediatrics. Initially it usually includes a complete history; at subsequent visits an interim history is obtained. Appropriate counseling and education is a vital part of this interview.

The *problem interview* is also common. In this interview the child is brought to the clinic because of some immediate problem (either physical or emotional) and the entire visit may be limited to factors relating to that problem. With this situation the nurse has several alternatives: (1) take a brief history and decide that the problem is so severe that the child needs to see a physician immediately, (2) take a brief history and decide that the problem is something that can be handled without a complete workup, or (3) take a brief history and decide that the child also needs a complete workup and proceed to handle the problem after finishing this workup. Whether the nurse handles the problem or makes a referral, it is important that he or she check to see where the child is getting regular care and make appropriate arrangements for some continued care. It is important not only to treat the presenting symptom but to provide for the total care needed by the child. Occasionally what the child is presenting is not the most important problem, but only the excuse for seeking help for something else. If the interviewer does not take time to elicit the real problem, the family may return again and again with some minor complaint or give up using the health system entirely.

Once a problem has been identified, the nurse may hold a *therapeutic interview.* Sometimes the value of talking is underestimated. If previous visits have isolated the problem, the nurse and parents, or nurse and child, or all three may need some time to discuss what is happening and why the family thinks it is happening and to explore some possible solutions. These are frequently the problems for which there is no fast, simple cure. There is often a tendency to refer all complicated or long-term problems to someone else, and in severe situations this is necessary, but often the nurse, with the help of a consultant, is in a better position to handle the situation herself.

There are also *information-getting* and *information-giving interviews.* It should be remembered that every question asked during the history should have some purpose in the child's care—for either the present or future use. For example, it may be important to know the financial status of the family if the nurse thinks the child may need an expensive allergenic diet. Or it may be important to ask about the number of bedrooms the family has before suggesting that the parents move the newborn out of their bedroom. The information-giving interview is also important. It is sometimes easy to avoid giving advice, but if the family asks a question, they deserve an answer. If the nurse cannot answer the question until more information is obtained from the history and physical, the examiner must tell the parent that more information is needed and then come back to the question later in the interview. If the examiner does not know the answer to the question, it is best to tell the family that she does not know but will find out. Sometimes during the visit the nurse simply looks up the information or asks the appropriate person and returns to the examining room with the answer. Other times, the answer requires more time and must be put off until the next visit or a telephone call at a later date. But it is extremely important never to make up an answer; this will destroy any trust.

APPROACH TO THE HISTORY-TAKING INTERVIEW

The entire history should be considered from the viewpoint of both the interviewer and the interviewee. If the interviewer is relaxed and unhurried, the family will generally relax and become more comfortable. Privacy should be provided for the session. Note taking should be as casual as possible. The examiner must be warm, friendly, nonjudgmental, responsive, and courteous. The nonverbal communication displayed by facial expressions may serve as a clue influencing the parents or child to change their story to please the nurse. It is important for the examiner to know what the family thinks was said, rather than what was actually said.

The arrangement for the interview will depend on the age of the child. An infant is usually content to sit on his parent's lap while the examiner talks with the parent. The toddler may wish to sit on the parent's lap or play with a few toys on the floor. The school-age child needs his own chair to sit on, and the examiner may take some history from the parent and some from the child. The nurse should be spontaneous, enthusiastic, and friendly, using simple words that the child can understand. The examining room should contain some furniture to fit the child's size: a small chair, steps to the examining table, etc. Bright colors, pictures, and mobiles also help. Some durable colorful toys may help the child to relax and can give the examiner a great deal of information about the child's coordination and motor activity.

METHODS OF INTERVIEWING

There are several ways of obtaining information from the family. A printed form may be handed to the parent (see Examples 3, 4, and 5 at the end of this chapter) with instructions to fill in the blanks. This is limited and can give a stereotyped and often inaccurate view of the family. The examiner, when using direct questioning, can expect direct, short answers in return. Examples of direct questions would be: "How old are you?" "Did you eat an egg for breakfast this morning?" "Did you have prenatal care?" The most effective, but most difficult and time-consuming way to obtain the information is to ask how the parent or child sees the situation. This is an indirect method of questioning. The nurse simply fills in the gaps and gives gentle direction to obtain the information needed. Such phrases as "Tell me about. . .," "What do you remember about. . .," and "How was your . . ." leave the family free to tell the situation from their viewpoint. Most interviews are combinations of all three methods. The family may be presented with a printed form, which the nurse reviews when he or she asks more direct questions and, when appropriate, elicits more information through a more specific detailed personal account of the problems.

RECORDING

The information gathered from the history-taking interview must be written into some organized form that can be used later by the same examiner or understood by others. Everyone develops a personal method of recording, but a write-up should never be as short as "11/12/78—bean in, bean out" for the child who had a bean removed from the external ear canal, or as long as the 10- to 15-page write-ups that beginning medical and nurse-practitioner students do when they are first learning. Some practitioners feel that nothing should be written during the workups—the nurse talks with the parent and child, does the examination and any indicated counseling, and does the charting only after the family has left. Others feel they need to begin the recording during the interview partly because of the time pressure and partly so that they will not forget important information. A stack of unfinished charts at the end of the day will not be recorded correctly. Probably a combination of some writing during the interview and some afterward is the most comfortable and efficient. Note taking should not be so vigorous as to make the family uncomfortable or so long that the flow of conversation is stopped. With practice the nurse learns to judge how much space to leave for more detail later and which words to jot down as he or she goes. A history is not written out in complete sentences and paragraphs, but in outline form with headings, short phrases, and key words.

The information gathered during the workup is organized and written up according to the problem-oriented system. This system, which was developed by Dr. Lawrence L. Weed, uses several categories of information and divides the information into four large categories: subjective data, objective data, analysis, and plan. This sometimes is referred to as S.O.A.P. Some of the subcategories within these major categories are similar to those used in the older standard method. The record includes a problem list that changes as old problems are solved and new ones added. Examples of the problem-oriented system are given at the end of this chapter.

PROBLEMS

Not every interview runs smoothly. A variety of problems can occur. Frequently there is a language barrier; sometimes it is the difficulty of two different languages, but more often the barrier is more subtle, and although both the nurse and the family speak English, there is faulty communication. Many families are eager to please in the nurse's office and will nod and smile appropriately even when they do not understand the instructions being given. Very few families will admit that what the nurse is saying does not make any sense to them. Clarification of words may be necessary for both parties to understand one another. For instance, does the parent really know what "decongestant" means, and what does the parent mean when describing the child as "spoiled?" The nurse also needs to gauge the reliability of the informant. The history of an infant brought in by a baby-sitter, aunt, or grandmother is very difficult to evaluate. On the other hand, the parent who works all day may not have some of the necessary information either.

Sometimes the problems in the history-taking interview are caused by the family; other times it is the fault of the examiner. Most often it is due to a poor interaction between the two. The nurse may be tired, and not as observant and careful as usual. Sometimes a nurse just does not get along with a particular family. If the nurse knows that good care cannot be given to a family because of a personality conflict, it is important that someone else be asked to see the child. Often cues are missed and important questions skipped because of a poor relationship. The mother who states, "Oh, I don't think I can stand this anymore," may not be joking and certainly does not need the answer, "You're doing just fine." Sometimes the nurse meets her own objectives, but fails to meet the child's or parent's. If this is discovered early, there may be time for correction; if not, the family may give up trying to get help from the health care system. Fortunately most of these problems of communication can be corrected with time. Some families may come only once, but if the parent and child know the nurse is concerned, often they will return, and with time and a growing relationship, some of the initial problems may be resolved.

HISTORY TAKING

INFORMATION TO BE INCLUDED IN THE HISTORY

The following is an outline of the specific information needed for a health history. The following headings and questions are those traditionally used.

Chief Complaint

Why is the child attending clinic today? (Generally the answer is a simple statement in the parent's own words, e.g., "well-child care," "cold," "earache.")

Present Illness

What signs and symptoms of illness is the child showing? (It is best to list the symptoms in order of appearance. Sometimes specific questions must be asked, e.g., Is the child coughing? When? What kind? How much? Does the child have diarrhea? When? What kind? How much? For how long?) How is the child acting otherwise? (How is his or her appetite? Bowels? Fluid intake? Sleep? Activity?) Has the child been exposed to others with illness? (Anyone in the family? Relatives? Friends? School? What type of illness was it?) What kind of treatment has the mother been giving? (Has she sought medical care before? Any medications? Any procedures?)

Past History

Birth

Prenatal How was the mother's health during her pregnancy with this child? Where did she receive her prenatal care and for how many months of the pregnancy? Did she have any infections? During what month? Did she have any illnesses? During which month, and how were they treated? Did she have any accidents? When and how was she treated? Was she taking medications during the pregnancy? What kind and why? At what point during pregnancy? What is her blood type? What is the child's father's blood type? Does she know the child's blood type? Did she have any x-rays during her pregnancy? Was she on any special diet during the pregnancy? How nutritional was her diet? Was she hospitalized during her pregnancy? When and for what reasons? How many living children does she have? Was either she or her doctor worried about this pregnancy for any reason? Did the pregnancy last 9 months? (A report of the baby coming less than 2 weeks early or late is usually not significant unless accompanied by a history of low birth weight or neonatal problems.)

Natal How long was the labor and were there any problems? What type of delivery was it? What kind of anesthesia was used and were there any problems? (Such questions as: Did the baby come headfirst? Did the doctor use forceps? are often helpful in eliciting this information.) Where was the baby born? What was the baby's birth weight? What was the baby's condition at birth? Did the baby cry? Was the baby blue? Did the baby need oxygen?

Postnatal Did the baby have any problems during the stay in the nursery? What was the length of the baby's hospital stay? Did the mother and infant come home together? Did the baby have jaundice? Was the baby ever cyanotic or blue? Were there any feeding problems during the hospitalization? Did the baby develop any rashes? How much weight did the baby lose?

Allergies Is the child allergic to any foods? To any medications? To any insects? To any animals? At any seasons? If so, describe what happens with these allergies. Does the child ever break out in rashes? Does the mother know why?

Accidents Has the child ever had an accident? If so, was it in the car? At home? At school? At the babysitter's? Can the mother describe what happened? What was the treatment? Where was the child treated? What was the child's reaction? Any residual?

Illnesses Has the child had any infections? When? Where? What treatment? What follow-up? Has the child had any childhood diseases? Measles? Rubella? Roseola? Mumps? Chickenpox? Whooping cough?

Operations Has the child ever had any operations? When? For what condition? Where? What was the outcome?

Hospitalizations Has the child ever spent any time in a hospital? For what reason? Where? Is this condition resolved? Any residual?

Immunizations Has the child had any immunizations? Which kinds? Any reactions? Any boosters? (Usually a written record is the most accurate source of this information.) Has the child been tested for tuberculosis? How? When? What was the result? Has the child ever had x-rays?

Family History

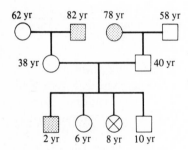

Family Members What is the mother's age and state of health? What is the father's age and state of health? Are there any siblings? What ages and what sex? State of health? (A diagram is often used to show this. A circle indicates a female and a square indicates a male; a horizontal line indicates a marriage, and a vertical line indicates a descendant. A blackened circle or square indicates that the individual is deceased. An X indicates the child with whom this particular history is concerned. The diagram on page 000 shows a maternal grandfather who died at age 82 and paternal grandmother who died at age 78, a 62-year-old maternal grandmother and a 58-year-old paternal grandfather alive, two parents alive, a 38-year-old mother and 40-year-old father, one 10-year-old brother, and one 6-year-old sister alive, and one brother who died at 2 years of age; the child about whom the history is taken is an 8-year-old girl.)

Family Diseases Within the immediate family, including both sets of grandparents and first aunts and uncles, are any of the following conditions present?

Eyes, Ears, Nose, and Throat Are there any nosebleeds? Sinus problems? Glaucoma? Cataracts? Myopia? Strabismus? Any other problems with their eyes, ears, nose, or throat?

Cardiorespiratory Is there any tuberculosis? Asthma? Hay fever? Hypertension? Heart murmurs? Heart attacks? Strokes? Anemia? Rheumatic fever? Leukemia? Pneumonia? Emphysema? Any other problems with heart or lungs?

Gastrointestinal Does anyone have ulcers? Colitis? Any other problems with stomach or intestines? Does anyone have kidney infections? Bladder infections?

Musculoskeletal Are there any congenital dislocated hips? Muscular dystrophy? Arthritis? Club feet? Any other problems with bones or muscles?

Neurological Does anyone have convulsions? Mental retardation? Mental problems? Comas? Epilepsy?

Special Senses Is anyone deaf? Blind?

Chronic Does anyone have diabetes? Congenital anomalies? Cancer? Tumors? Thyroid problems?

General Are there any other medical problems in the family that the patient thinks are important?

Social Where does the family live? In a house? Apartment? Room? How large? Is there a yard? Are there stairs? Does anyone live with the family? Grandparents? Aunts? Uncles? Friends? What is the financial situation of the family? Does the father work? Does the mother work? What are their occupations? If no one works, how are they living? Is there any outside help? Baby-sitters? Day-care centers? Schools? What is the general relationship of the family members? Do they seem to be a happy family? Chaotic family? Sad family? Depressed family? Violent family?

Review of Systems

Eyes, Ears, Nose, and Throat Does this child have persistent nosebleeds? Frequent streptococcal sore throats? Frequent colds (more than four a year)? Pneumonia? Frequent earaches? Do the child's eyes ever cross? Do they tear excessively?

Cardiorespiratory Does the child have any trouble breathing? Running? Finishing a 3- to 4-oz bottle without tiring? Does the child turn blue?

Gastrointestinal   Does the child have any problems with diarrhea? Constipation? Bleeding around the rectum? Bloody stools? Pain? Vomiting?

Genitourinary   Does the child have a straight, strong urinary stream, or does the urine just dribble out? Urinary frequency? Is there any pain? Bleeding? If an older girl, does she menstruate? How often? Any problems?

Neurological   Has the child ever had a convulsion? A fainting spell? Tremors? Twitches? Blackouts? Dizzy spells? Frequent headaches?

Musculoskeletal   Has the child ever broken any bones? Had any sprains? Complained of pain in the joints, swelling, or redness around the joints?

Special Senses   Does the child see well? Hear well? Does the child seem clumsy? Can the child see the blackboard from where he or she sits in the classroom? Is the child always falling or walking into doors?

Chronic   Any long-term diseases?

General   Any other problems?

Habits

Eating   Is the child's appetite good? Poor? Varied? If on formula, what kind, how much, how is it mixed, and how frequently? How much does the child take in a 24-hour period? What kinds of foods does the child eat? Meat? Fruits? Vegetables? Cereals? Juices? Eggs? Sweets? Milk? Snacks? How often? What size portions? How many times a week or day does the child eat each of these? Does the child feed herself or himself? Does the child use a cup? Spoon? Knife? Fork? Is the child messy? Does the child sit with the rest of the family? Does the child take vitamins? What kind? How often? How much? What is the family attitude toward food? Is it used as a symbol of love? A bribe? A reward? What is the emotional climate of the meals? Relaxed? Tired? Rushed? Tense?

Bowels   What are the child's bowel patterns? Frequency? Consistency? Color? Any discomfort? Is the child toilet trained? Is toilet training planned? When? Any problems? If the child is toilet trained, does he or she have accidents? If so, are they during the day or night? How often? Are they frequently associated with emotional upsets?

Sleep   When does the child go to bed? Wake up? Does the child awaken during the night? How often? What happens? What does the parent do? Any nightmares? Night terrors? Does the child take naps? When? For how long? Where does the child sleep? How many hours does the child sleep in a 24-hour period? When awake, is the child alert? Or does the child seem to need more sleep than he or she is getting?

Development How does the child compare with his or her siblings? Quicker to learn? Slower to learn? When did the child first sit? Stand? Roll over? Talk? Walk? What kinds of activities does the child do now? What is the child doing that is new since the last visit? What grade is the child in? Does the child like school? Does the child have playmates? What does the child like to do in school? What does the child like to play?

Exercise/Play What types of play or games does the child engage in and how often? Does the older child engage in sports? Team activities? For the adolescent, do they do regular exercises? How much walking, running, or other large motor activities are involved in their daily living patterns?

Personality What kind of personality does this child have? Is he or she quiet? Outgoing? Does the child have a temper? How does the child cope with stress? By withdrawal? By aggression? By decompensation? By symptoms of illness? How does the child handle emotions like anger, fear, jealousy, or others? Is the child able to relax well?

Family Relations How do the members of the family get along? How do they handle disagreements within the family? How do they handle external stress? What things do they do together? How often? Do they enjoy them?

Sexuality How much does the younger child ask about sexuality and what is the child told about it? What is the child's attitude toward it and what is the attitude of those around the child? Does the child masturbate? How is this handled by the rest of the family? What are the child's own feelings about it? What is the child's attitude and those of the family toward nudity in the home? What does the child know about the changes beginning in his or her body: early breast development, penile and testicular enlargement, pubic hair, axillary and facial hair, changes in body proportions, voice changes, menstruation, and noctural emissions?

Some of the questions asked when taking a complete history need to be modified for specific ages, and some areas need more detailed information if problems are encountered. But generally if the nurse covers these six areas, he or she has a good idea about which topics may need more information. The nurse must also decide which of these areas need to be discussed at every visit, which must be investigated at regular intervals, and which need to be discussed only once. Certainly once the birth history has been taken and no problems appear, there is no reason to repeat that material at every visit. However, the habits of the child change from visit to visit, sometimes from day to day, and this may be an important area to include in every history. The review of systems can easily change, but usually it will take a longer period of time for significant change to appear. The nurse may decide to routinely take a review of systems once a year rather than monthly or weekly. The nurse must go through each category and make a decision about how frequently it will be discussed.

HISTORY OF AN ILLNESS

When dealing with sick children, the nurse enters an often undefined area binding nursing and medicine. There are some very definite limits within this area, but they are often difficult to determine. Every state legally defines the activity of nursing, and institutions employing nurses define these activities more specifically. Generally nurses may not write prescriptions or perform certain procedures (e.g., surgery, spinal taps) on their own. There are some things nurses can do independently, and additional activities they can do in conjunction with and under the supervision of a physician. When dealing with sickness nurses should develop a specific set of protocols for their area. These should be agreed upon by the nurse and the physician. Furthermore nurses must know their limits, the expectation of the employing agency, resources, and referral sources.

Another problem encountered when dealing with pathology is the *differential diagnosis* approach versus the *list of symptoms* approach; these represent two entirely different thinking processes. Until the last few years physicians worked diligently at finding the proper label for every disease. It was important to define the condition in one word: diabetes, hypertension, hepatitis, etc. But with the newer methods of recording which emphasize the symptom and dealing with each symptom, the single label may become less important.

In most clinic settings the nurse will work out some procedures with the physician for handling sick children. There should be some agreement on what are minor illnesses, how they can be treated, and when or if the physician should see each ill child. There will always be children who come in for well care but are found to be ill. But if the nurse has a good working relationship with the physician, problems should be minimal and the child should receive very good, comprehensive care.

In eliciting information in the category "Present Illness" some questions need to be asked generally, and other questions should be asked in specific situations. In general there are five areas to gather information about: (1) how long ago the child was entirely well, (2) symptoms of this condition, (3) habits found with this condition, (4) exposures, and (5) treatment.

It is important to know when the child was well last to ascertain whether the present illness is a slow, chronic process or a sudden, acute episode. The information should be recorded as 3 days ago or 1 week ago, not as Thursday or Monday or Tuesday since the next person reading the chart will not know on what day of the week the chart was written.

The progress of the condition is recorded as a progression of symptoms. Some parents can tell this progression in an orderly, detailed way; others need some guidance and prodding. The examiner should ask about the child's condition 3 days ago, 2 days ago, yesterday, today, this morning, and this afternoon. The examiner may have to ask whether certain conditions were present—coughing, diarrhea, constipation, vomiting, earache, stomachache, pain, etc.—and what is bothering the child or parent the most—the coughing at night, the pain, the noneating.

It is important to find out about the child's general habits since the condition appeared. How is the child's appetite? How are the child's bowels? Is the child sleeping? What is his or her level of activity? The child who is eating as usual, having no bowel problems, sleeping through the night, and playing or going to school as usual is probably not as ill as the one who is not eating, is having diarrhea, is waking at night with a cough, and is refusing to go to school.

Exposures can be another important factor. The examiner should ask whether the child has recently been exposed to anyone showing similar symptoms or streptococcal infections, childhood diseases (measles, mumps, chickenpox, etc.), viral infections, etc. Is anyone else in the immediate family or neighborhood ill, and if so, how are they ill? Are those members having the same symptoms or the same progression of illness, and what has been the outcome?

It is important to find out what kind of treatment the child has received so far. What has the mother been doing for the condition? Has the child been seen by another nurse or doctor? How much and how often has the child been taking any medications and have they seemed to work? It is important to include questions about both the traditional medications and home remedies or nontraditional treatments.

The questions asked when seeing a sick child will vary with some conditions such as rashes, pain, diarrhea, and colds. The American Academy of Pediatrics has made up a list of such questions to fit certain situations (see Table 1-1).

Table 1-1 Suggested Questions for Interviewing

Identification of problem	To be seen by M.D. if:	Home treatment and follow-up
Specific guidelines for medical factors applicable to abdominal pain		
Where is the pain? How does the child react to the pain? 1. Is it constant or does it come and go? 2. Is it related to feeding? 3. Does it interrupt sleep? 4. Does it cause him to cry out? 5. Does he favor any one position? 6. Is he walking and standing normally? How does the child describe the pain? Is he constipated, having diarrhea, or passing a lot of gas? Has he vomited? Does he have a sore throat, cold, or cough? Is he urinating normally? Does he have a fever? Does his abdomen feel tense or rigid? Has he been hit in the abdomen? Could he have strained abdominal muscles? Has he been upset or anxious about anything recently?	Child is under 4 years and has no symptoms of an infection. Pain is severe, constant, localized, and causing child to cry out or double up. Abdomen feels tense and rigid. There are any urinary problems. There is abdominal pain following trauma to the abdomen.	Nothing by mouth except ginger ale or Seven-Up. Warm tub bath. If suspicious of "pain" on a "tension" basis, talk with mother to try to identify the problem. Plan follow-up call in a few hours. Observe for signs of change; instruct mother to call back immediately if child's condition worsens.
Specific guidelines for medical factors applicable to colds and coughs		
Cough? 1. Is it dry or loose? 2. When does child cough most? 3. Does it wake him from sleep? Is child breathing any differently than normally? 1. faster? 2. harder?	Afebrile with cold, then fever 3–4 days later. Cough wakes child when asleep. Significant changes in breathing pattern. Child less than 3 years with cold and temperature for 2–3 days without improvement.	Nose drops with instructions for use as specified by M.D. Decongestants (dosage as specified by M.D.) Cough syrup (type and dosage, specified by M.D.) Vaporizer or cool steam or shower.

Table 1-1 Suggested Questions for Interviewing *(Continued)*

Identification of problem	To be seen by M.D. if:	Home treatment and follow-up
Specific guidelines for medical factors applicable to colds and coughs (Continued)		
3. shallower? 4. retracting? 5. noisy? 6. grunting? Any signs of earache or sore throat? What does the nasal discharge look like? How is child sucking (if infant)? Does child have a fever? Does child have any allergies?	Thick, foul-smelling, or bloody-colored nasal discharge.	Ear bulb syringe to clear infant's nose before feeding. Postural drainage (nasal discharge). Elevate head of bed with books or blocks (for breathing). Position infant on stomach to increase drainage from nose. Be sure house is not too warm and/or dry. If allergy suspected, follow up with mother and plan medical follow-up with M.D. If child is less than 3–4 years, plan telephone follow-up with mother because of the incidence of colds as presenting signs of streptococcal infection in this age group. Give mother specific changes in condition which should be reported immediately.
Specific guidelines for medical factors applicable to diarrhea		
If infant, review feeding practices. When did diarrhea start? What does it look like? How many stools in 24 hours? How large are they? Does he have cramps? Does he have a fever? Has he vomited? What has he had to eat and drink? Is she urinating normally?	There is blood in the stools. More than 12–15 diarrhea stools per day, or smaller number but large quantity (in infant). Signs of dehydration (skin, tongue, eyes, thirst, scant urine). Diarrhea for more than 48 hours, with no improvement.	If related to infant feeding, review practices. Nothing by mouth for 2–4 hours. Then, ginger ale or Seven-Up until diarrhea stops. Progress diet slowly. Antispasmodics (as prescribed by M.D.). Watch for dehydration.

Table 1-1 Suggested Questions for Interviewing *(Continued)*

Identification of problem	To be seen by M.D. if:	Home treatment and follow-up
	Specific guidelines for medical factors applicable to diarrhea *(Continued)*	
Does skin or tongue look dry? Eyes sunken? Is she thirsty? Drinking fluids well?		If actually only "loose" stools: 1. Give no fruit. 2. Reduce bulk. 3. Give cottage cheese. 4. Keep diet bland. Have mother report back if diarrhea fails to improve in 48 hours or if it recurs. If other problems, see specific problem guideline.
	Specific guidelines for medical factors applicable to earache	
Does he have a fever? Does he have a cold or sore throat? Has he had one in the past week? Is there or has there been any drainage from the ear? What does it look like? How much does the ear hurt? Constantly? On and off? Associated with swallowing? Is there any itchiness and/or a burning sensation associated with the discomfort? Has he been doing a lot of swimming? Does he complain when you touch the ear? Is there any swelling around the ear? Exposure to mumps?	Suspicion of otitis media: 1. Sudden, acute, severe discomfort 2. Drainage from ear 3. Discomfort when the ear is touched 4. Mild complaints of ear discomfort associated with temperature over $101°F$ for 24 hours. Suspicion of external otitis: 1. Presence of itching and/or a burning sensation. 2. Discomfort when ear is touched. 3. Child has been doing a lot of swimming.	External heat. Aspirin or similar compound at dosage for age specified by M.D. Decongestant at dosage for age specified by M.D. Exempt, narcotic codeine-containing cough mixtures at dosage for age specified by M.D. No swimming. Watch temperature. If other problems, refer to specific problem guidelines.
	Specific guidelines for medical factors applicable to fever	
How long has he had fever? How much? Constant or periodic? Does he have an earache or is he rubbing or pulling at his ear?	There is fever of $101–102°F$ for 3 days without explanation. Neck is stiff. Low grade, but unexplained, fever for 5 days.	Aspirin or similar compound at dosage for age specified by M.D. Keep child in cool environment. Push fluids.

Table 1-1 Suggested Questions for Interviewing *(Continued)*

Identification of problem	To be seen by M.D. if:	Home treatment and follow-up
	Specific guidelines for medical factors applicable to fever (Continued)	
Does he have a sore throat, cold, or cough? Is he nauseated or has he vomited? Does he have a stiff neck? Can he bend his chin to his chest? Is he urinating normally? Any burning or pain? Has he had any diarrhea? Does he have any rash? Has he ever had a febrile convulsion?		Sponge for temperature over 103°F. Phenobarbital if the child has had a previous convulsion at dosage specified by M.D. Watch for change. Report back. If problem is more specific, refer to applicable problem guideline.
	Specific guidelines for medical factors applicable to rashes	
Where did it first occur? Has it spread? To where? What does it look like? 1. Color? 2. Flat or raised, blisterlike? 3. Is it weeping? 4. Is it crusted? 5. Is it scabbed? Does it itch? Does child have a fever? Does he have enlarged glands? Does he have a sore throat? Does he have any other signs of illness? Is he allergic to anything? 1. Any new clothes? 2. Any new foods? 3. Any new detergent, bleach, or rinse agent being used? 4. Has he been playing in the woods? Is his neck stiff? Can he touch his chin to his chest? Has he ever had a rash like this before?	Presence of stiff neck. Presence of enlarged glands and/or sore throat. Rash is present and child sounds "really sick." Rash sounds like a childhood disease and mother wants definite diagnosis.	If common communicable disease, teach management, complications to watch for, incubation period, and follow with mother. If allergy is suspected: 1. Remove allergen. 2. Give antihistamine (dosage specified by M.D.). 3. Give baths with soothing agent, e.g., baking soda, corn starch. 4. Apply external lotion, e.g., calamine lotion, to suppress itch. 5. Follow-up as indicated for further workup. If child seems well except for rash, have mother call back next day.

Table 1-1 Suggested Questions for Interviewing *(Continued)*

Identification of problem	To be seen by M.D. if:	Home treatment and follow-up

Specific guidelines for medical factors applicable to sore throat

Does he have a fever? Are the glands in his neck enlarged and/or tender? Have you looked at his throat? Any white patches? Is his throat sore just in the morning or continuously? How much is his appetite affected? Any liquids or foods in particular he is refusing? Does he have a cold? Earache? Coughs? Does he have a stomach-ache? Has he had any nausea or vomiting? Diarrhea? Has he had a lot of sore throats? Streptococcal infections? Does he have any rash? Does he have any open sores?	Suspicion of streptococcal throat: 1. Severe sore throat causing decrease in appetite. 2. Enlarged lymph glands. 3. Presence of white patches in throat or petechiae on palate. 4. Temperature over 102° F. 5. Child acts "miserable." 6. Indication of rash on body. 7. Indications of skin infection. History of susceptibility to sore throats, even if symptoms are mild.	Push bland fluids, e.g., tonic, water, popsicles, gelatin desserts. Soothing, coating substance, e.g., syrup, honey. Add humidity to room and keep room cool but comfortable. If other problems, refer to specific problem guidelines.

Specific guidelines for medical factors applicable to vomiting

When has child vomited? How much? How often? Type and color of vomitus? Is vomiting forceful? If infant, review feeding practices. Is child nauseated? Retching? Is child coughing? Breathing normally? What did he eat or drink before this started? Have you made any recent changes in his diet? Could he have eaten any poisonous substance or any medicines? Does he have gas? Diarrhea? Stomach pains?	Forceful vomiting in infant under 3 months. Signs of dehydration (skin, tongue, eyes, thirst, scant urine). Ingestion of poison or medication. Blood in vomitus. Associated, severe abdominal pain. Frequent and constant vomiting. Duration of more than 24 hours with no improvement.	If related to infant feeding, review practices. No fluids or solids for 2–4 hours. Coca-Cola syrup every 15 minutes six times. Ginger ale or Seven-Up in small quantities frequently. No solids or milk for 24 hours. Start progressing diet 24 hours after last vomiting. If medication is indicated, consider suppository. Watch for dehydration. Antiemetic (as prescribed by M.D.). Have mother call back if no progress in 2–4 hours.

Table 1-1 Suggested Questions for Interviewing *(Continued)*

Identification of problem	To be seen by M.D. if:	Home treatment and follow-up
Specific guidelines for medical factors applicable to vomiting *(Continued)*		
Does he have a fever? Is he urinating normally? Is he very thirsty? Irritable? Twitchy? Do skin or tongue look dry? Are eyes sunken?		Have mother call in daily for instructions if vomiting is of concern. Give mother specific guideline of change in condition which should be reported immediately. If other problems, refer to specific problem guideline.

Printed by permission of the American Academy of Pediatrics, *Standards of Child Health Care*, Evanston, Ill.: American Academy of Pediatrics, 1972, pp. 47–54.

The following two examples show a complete written history on a well-child visit (Example 1) and a history of a child with an illness (Example 2). Both examples are written according to the problem-oriented method.

Example 1 Complete History Recorded According to the Problem-Oriented System

PROBLEM 1 Well-child care (first visit)

SUBJECTIVE

Data Base 4-year-old girl

Past History

Birth

Prenatal Mother's second pregnancy. From her third to ninth month she was followed at Denver General Hospital Clinic. She had a kidney infection during the pregnancy. Her doctor placed her on vitamins and iron tablets for the entire pregnancy. Both she and the baby's father have Rh positive blood types. She followed her normal diet except for slight sodium restrictions during the final trimester. She has had no abortions or miscarriages.

Natal Labor lasted 5 hours. Her husband was able to be with her most of the time. She received a caudal anesthetic and the baby was delivered by vertex. Baby born at DGH. Birth weight 7 lb , 5 oz. She cried spontaneously and did not need oxygen.

Postnatal Nursery stay uneventful with mother and infant going home after 3 days. Infant exhibited slight jaundice on third and fourth days, but no cyanosis or rashes. She lost 3 oz during first week. Breast feeding was initiated in hospital and went well; baby was hungry and sucked well.

Allergies No allergic reactions to medications, insects, animals, or seasons. Breaks out in fine, macular, itchy rash 12 hours after eating tomatoes.

Accidents None.

Illnesses Chickenpox at $2\frac{1}{2}$ years. Rubella at 3 years.

Operations Tonsils removed at $3\frac{1}{2}$ years. Stayed in hospital 1 night; no adverse reactions.

Immunizations DPT 1—1/1969, DPT 2—3/1969, and DPT 3—5/1969 (given by private pediatrician in Kansas City). DPT booster—5/1970 (given at Colorado General Hospital clinic). Trivalent polio—1/1969, trivalent polio—2/1969, and trivalent polio—4/1969 (given by private pediatrician in Kansas City). Trivalent polio booster—5/1970. Tine test—7/1969 (negative; given at Colorado General Hospital clinic). Measles-rubella-mumps vaccine—6/1972.

Family History

Family Members Mother—30 years, good health; father—35 years, back problems treated at work clinic. Siblings: Jane—3 years, good health; John—6 years, partially deaf, attends special school.

Family Diseases (Review of systems)

Eyes, Ears, Nose, and Throat No nosebleeds, sinus problems, glaucoma, or cataracts.

Cardiorespiratory No tuberculosis, hypertension, heart murmurs, strokes, anemia, rheumatic fever, asthma, leukemia, or pneumonia. Mother has hay fever in springtime.

Gastrointestinal No ulcers or colitis.

Genitourninary Mother had kidney infections with each pregnancy and is still being seen in UTI clinic for recurring problem.

Musculoskeletal No arthritis, club feet, or congenitally dislocated hips.

Neurological No convulsions, mental retardation, mental problems, comas, or epilepsy.

Chronic No diabetes, cancer, or tumors.

General (including special senses) Older sibling partially deaf; maternal aunt totally deaf from birth.

Social Family of five live in small, two-bedroom house with no basement and tiny yard. Father works nights as trainman and sleeps during day. Mother home with children. Family struggles to keep within a budget; recreational activities limited. Father becoming more interested in helping with children as they get older.

Review of Systems (of child)

Eyes, Ears, Nose, and Throat No persistent nosebleeds, frequent colds, or earaches. Had five streptococcal throat infections year of tonsillectomy.

Cardiorespiratory No trouble breathing, no turning blue, and no choking. Keeps up with other children; runs stairs.

Gastrointestinal No problems with diarrhea, constipation, bleeding, bloody stools, pain, vomiting, encopresis.

Genitourinary No problems with frequency, pain, bleeding, enuresis.

Neurological No convulsions, fits, seizures, blackouts, dizzy spells, epilepsy.

Musculoskeletal Broke right middle finger in fall from tricycle in 1970. No complaints of joint pain or swelling.

Senses Mother feels she hears and sees; no vision or hearing testing ever done.

Habits

Eating Good appetite; eats most foods: cereal, milk, fruit, vegetables, and meat daily; eggs four to five times per week. Likes snacks of fruit, cookies, juices, candy.

Sleeping Generally in bed by 8:00 and 9:00 and up by 6:30 or 7:00. Will sometimes take short nap in afternoon. Sleeps in top bunk bed in children's bedroom. No problems with nightmares or night terrors.

Elimination Mother unsure of pattern since child goes by herself and rarely complains of problems. No recent diarrhea or constipation. Toilet trained since early in third year.

Development Friendly, outgoing little girl who gets along well with most people. Has several girl friends on block. Knows her name, can dress herself, can count to 5, and is looking forward to school next year.

OBJECTIVE

Measurements Weight, 36 lb; height, 41 in.

Physical Examination (Total explanation of physical findings would be written into this area.)

ASSESSMENT Normal 4-year-old

PLAN

Therapeutic   DPT booster and polio booster given. DDST done. Hct done. Urinalysis done. Vision tested normal. Hearing tested normal.

Education

1. Discussed eating and snacking; limit candy intake and watch tooth brushing.

2. Discussed getting ready to go to school, learning to cross streets, tie own shoes, knowing home address, and phone number, etc.

3. Return to clinic in 1 year for health check; all screening, check on school readiness.

Example 2   History of an Illness Recorded According to the Problem-Oriented System

PROBLEM 2   Cold and fever

SUBJECTIVE

Data Base   5-year-old boy

Present Illness   Child well until 3 days ago, then began sneezing and complaining of scratchy throat. Two days ago nose began to drip clear drainage, occasional dry, tickly cough; fever of 37.5°C. Today nose dripping continually and base becoming raw; continual wet, gurgly cough, nonproductive; no fever. Child no longer complaining of sore throat; no complaints of earache, stomachache, pain anywhere, diarrhea, constipation, or vomiting. Child's appetite less, but he is eating and asking for extra fluids. He was sleeping well until 2 nights ago when coughing woke him twice. Activity about the same except for taking an afternoon nap which he usually does not do. Continues to go to school.

Past History   None relevant

OBJECTIVE

Measurements   Temperature 37°C, height $43\frac{1}{2}$ in, weight 42 lb, BP 99/65

Physical Examination   (Showing extra attention to areas concerned with present illness would be recorded in this area)

ASSESSMENT   Normal 5-year-old with runny nose and cough

PLAN

Diagnostic Throat culture done

Treatment

1. Aspirin 5 grains every 4 hours during fever.

2. Robitussin cough medication 1 tsp every 4 hours for cough.

3. Cold mist vaporizer running in his room since last night.

4. Encourage fluids.

Educational May go to school if he feels like it. Safety around a vaporizer. Return to clinic if worse or for regularly scheduled well-child care.

The following history forms are used in the pediatric outpatient department at Colorado General Hospital. These forms are completed by the parents or the adolescent patient, and provide a starting point for the examiner, who reviews the material and uses it as a basis for building the remainder of the history.

Example 3 History Form for a Child from Birth through 5 Years

The pediatric clinic at Colorado General can provide either short-term emergency care or long-term continuous care. If your child is under the care of a private doctor or a convenient health clinic, we do not want to interfere with or duplicate the care you are receiving there.

My child usually gets his care at _____ and his last physical examination was _____ months or _____ years ago.

I am here for this visit only and my child receives care elsewhere. Yes _____   No _____

If your answer to the above question is Yes, there is no need to go any further with this questionnaire.

If you would like your child cared for in a private doctor's office or a public health facility more convenient to you, please ask to speak with one of the public health nurses.

If your child is not receiving care elsewhere and you want him to get his care here, you can help us take better care of him by answering the following questions:

If your child is over 3 years old, is he/she too sick today to have the eyes checked?   Yes _____   No _____

Is he/she too sick today or are you too rushed for us to test how he/she is developing? (approximately 15 minutes)   Yes _____   No _____

I.   *Pregnancy and Birth*   *Circle One (1)*

      1. Did you have any illnesses during your pregnancy?........................... Yes No
      2. Did you carry him/her for a full 9 months? Yes No
      3. Where was your baby born? _____
      4. How much did he/she weigh at birth? _____ lb _____ oz
      5. Did your baby have any trouble starting to breathe?........................... Yes No
      6. Did your baby have any trouble in the hospital? .... Yes No
      7. Did your baby go home with you when you left the hospital? .... Yes No
      8. How long did he/she stay in the hospital? _____ days

II.   *Feeding and Digestion*

      1. Did you baby have severe colic or any unusual feeding problems during the first 3 months of life?....................... Yes No
      2. If on vitamins, what kind and how much?

         _____

      3. If still on formula, which one do you use?

         _____

      4. Is your child's appetite usually good? Yes No
      5. Do any foods bother him/her? .... Yes No
      6. Does he/she often have diarrhea or runny bowels?............................... Yes No

III. *Baby Shots, Tests, and Development*

     Has your child had:

      1. A scar from smallpox vaccination? ...... Yes No Year _____
      2. All three of his/her DPT shots? .... Yes No Booster ____
      3. All three doses of polio vaccine by mouth? .... Yes No Booster ____
      4. Measles shot? .... Yes No
      5. Skin test for TB?....................... Yes No When _____
      6. Rubella (German measles) shot? .... Yes No
      7. Mumps shot? .... Yes No
      8. Did your child sit alone before 7 months of age? .... Yes No
      9. Did your child walk alone before 15 months of age?........................ Yes No
    10. Did your child say any words by $1\frac{1}{2}$ years of age? .... Yes No
    11. Is he/she as quick in learning as your other children? .... Yes No

IV. *Allergies*
Has your child had:
1. Eczema or hives?...................... Yes No
2. Wheezing or asthma?................... Yes No
3. Allergies or reactions to any medicines or injections such as penicillin? .... Yes No
4. Does he/she have a constant cold, hay fever, or sinus trouble?.................. Yes No

V. *Family-Social History*
1. Are both parents in good health? .... Yes No
2. Are there any other members of your child's immediate family (brothers, sisters, parents, grandparents, aunts, uncles) with a serious health problem (mental or physical)?.................... Yes No
List each problem and who has it.
_____
3. How many people live in your home? Children _____ Adults _____
4. With whom does the child live? (circle one) Both parents Mother Father Legal guardian Other_____
5. Does anyone help you take care of your child on a regular basis? .... Yes No

VI. *Infections, Illnesses, and Other Problems*
Has your child:
1. Had *more* than six (6) colds or throat infections each year?..................... Yes No
2. Had *more* than three (3) ear infections? .. Yes No
3. Had any trouble hearing? .... Yes No When _____
4. Had his/her hearing tested?............. Yes No When _____
5. Had any trouble seeing? .... Yes No
6. Had his/her eyes tested?................ Yes No When _____
7. Had any trouble with his/her teeth?...... Yes No
8. Seen a dentist recently? .... Yes No When _____
9. Had any trouble passing his/her urine? .. Yes No
10. Ever had a convulsion or fit or fainting spell?.................................. Yes No
11. Circle any of the following that your child has had: 3-day measles 10-day measles Chicken pox Mumps Whooping Cough Pneumonia
12. Had other diseases? _____ Had to stay in the hospital overnight?.... Yes No Age _____ Hospital _____ Reason_____

VII. *Accidents*
    1. Has your child had any serious accidents? .... Yes No
       Burns_____ Poisoning_____
       Cuts needing a doctor_____
       Broken bones_____
    2. Does your child use seat belts and/or a safety chair in your car? .... Yes No
    3. Do you know how to prevent infant smothering or choking?................. Yes No
    4. Do you have firearms (loaded or unloaded) in your home? .... Yes No

VIII. *Behavior and Discipline*
    1. Is he/she more difficult to raise than your other children? .... Yes No
    2. What is the most effective way of disciplining your child? (circle) Spanking
       Sending to room
       Taking privileges away
       Other _____
    3. Are you concerned about any of the following? (circle which ones) Bad temper
       Will not mind Holds his breath
       Jealous Sleep problems
       Thumb sucking Nail biting
       Speech problems
       Cannot toilet train
       Very shy
       Does not pay attention
       Overactive Slow to learn
       Eats dirt or paint

Reviewed by_____

Printed by permission of Dr. Burris Duncan, Colorado General Hospital.

Example 4 History Form for a Child from 6 through 12 Years

The pediatric clinic at Colorado General Hospital can provide either short-term emergency care or long-term continuous care. If your child is under the care of a private doctor or a convenient health clinic, we do not want to interfere with or duplicate the care you are receiving there.

My child usually gets his care at _____ and his last physical examination was _____ months or _____ years ago.

I am here for this visit only and my child receives his care elsewhere.
Yes _____ No _____

If your answer to the above question is Yes, there is no need to go any further with this questionnaire.

If you would like your child cared for in a private doctor's office or a public health facility more convenient to you, please ask to speak with one of the public health nurses.

If your child is not receiving care elsewhere and you want him to get his care here, you can help us take better care of him by answering the following questions:

I. *Pregnancy and Birth*   *Circle One (1)*
   1. Did you have any illnesses during your pregnancy?............................ Yes No
   2. Did you carry him/her for a full 9 months? Yes No
   3. Where was your baby born? _____
   4. How much did he/she weigh at birth? _____ lb _____ oz
   5. Did your baby have any trouble starting to breathe?............................ Yes No
   6. Did your baby have any trouble in the hospital? .... Yes No
   7. Did your baby go home with you when you left the hospital? .... Yes No
   8. How long did he/she stay in the hosptal? _____ days

II. *Baby Shots, Tests, and Development*
   Has your child had:
   1. A scar from smallpox vaccination? ...... Yes No Year _____
   2. All three of his/her DPT shots? .... Yes No Booster ____
   3. All three doses of polio vaccine by mouth? .... Yes No Booster ____
   4. Measles shot? .... Yes No
   5. Skin test for TB?....................... Yes No When _____
   6. Rubella (German measles) shot? .... Yes No
   7. Mumps shot? .... Yes No
   8. Did your child sit alone before 7 months of age? .... Yes No
   9. Did your child walk alone before 15 months of age?........................ Yes No
   10. Did your child say any words by $1\frac{1}{2}$ years of age? .... Yes No
   11. Is he/she as quick in learning as your other children?........................ Yes No

III. *Allergies*
Has your child had:
1. Eczema or hives?....................... Yes No
2. Wheezing or asthma?.................... Yes No
3. Allergies or reactions to any medicines or injections such as penicillin? .... Yes No
4. Does he/she have a constant cold, hay fever, or sinus trouble?................. Yes No

IV. *Accidents*
1. Has your child had any serious accidents?................................. Yes No
Burns_____   Poisoning_____
Cuts needing a doctor_____
Broken bones_____
2. Does your child use seat belts and/or a safety chair in your car? .... Yes No
3. Does your child know how to swim ...... Yes No
4. Do you have firearms (loaded or unloaded) in your home?................ Yes No

V. *Family-Social History*
1. Are both parents in good health? .... Yes No
2. Are there any other members of your child's immediate family (brothers, sisters, parents, grandparents, aunts, uncles) with a serious health problem (mental or physical)?.................... Yes No
List each problem and who has it.
_____
3. How many people live in your home? Children _____ Adults _____
4. With whom does the child live? (circle one) Both parents Mother
Father Legal guardian Other_____
5. Does anyone help you take care of your child on a regular basis? .... Yes No

VI. *Infections, Illnesses, and Other Problems*
Has your child:
1. Had *more* than six (6) colds or throat infections each year?..................... Yes No
2. Had *more* than three (3) ear infections? .. Yes No
3. Had any trouble hearing? .... Yes No
4. Had his/her hearing tested?............. Yes No When _____
5. Had any trouble seeing? .... Yes No
6. Had his/her eyes tested?................ Yes No When _____
7. Had any trouble with his/her teeth?...... Yes No
8. Seen a dentist recently? .... Yes No When _____

9. Had any trouble passing his/her urine? .. Yes No
10. Ever had a convulsion or fit or fainting spell?................................ Yes No
11. Circle any of the following that your child has had: 3-day measles 10-day measles Chicken pox Mumps Whooping Cough Pneumonia
12. Had other diseases? _____
    Had to stay in the hospital overnight?.... Yes No
    Age _____ Hospital _____
    Reason _____

VII. *Behavior and Discipline*
1. What school does your child attend? ____
   Grade _____
2. Does your child get along well in school? Yes No
3. Have you met with the teacher? .... Yes No
4. Is the teacher worried about any problems?................................ Yes No
5. What is the most effective way of disciplining your child? (circle) Spanking
   Sending to room
   Taking privileges away
   Other _____
7. Are you concerned about any of the following? (circle which ones) Bad temper
   Will not mind Holds his breath
   Jealous Sleep problems
   Thumb sucking Nail biting
   Speech problems
   Cannot toilet train
   Very shy
   Does not pay attention
   Overactive Slow to learn
   Eats dirt or paint

Reviewed by _____

Printed by permission of Dr. Burris Duncan, Colorado General Hospital.

Example 5 History Form for a Child from 13 through 18 Years

The pediatric clinic at Colorado General can provide either short-term emergency care or long-term continuous care. If you are under the care of a private doctor or a convenient health clinic, we do not want to interfere with or duplicate the care you are receiving there.

I usually get my care at _____ and my last physical examination was _____ months or _____ years ago.

I am here for this visit only and I receive my care elsewhere.
Yes _____   No _____

If your answer to the above question is Yes, there is no need to go any further with this questionnaire.

I am too sick today to have my vision and hearing checked.
Yes _____   No _____

If you would like to get your care in a private doctor's office or a public health facility more convenient to you, please ask to speak with one of the public health nurses. If you are not receiving your care elsewhere and you want to get your care here, you can help us with your care by answering the following questions.

I.   *Medical*   *Circle One (1)*

     A. *Immunizations?*

       Do you have your immunization records
       with you today? .... Yes No
       If not, please bring them on your next
       visit.

      1. Did you get your DPT immunizations as
         an infant?............................. Yes No
      2. Date of last tetanus booster _____
      3. Have you had the oral polio vaccine? .... Yes No
      4. Have you had a tuberculin skin test in the
         past year?............................. Yes No
      5. Do you have a smallpox scar? .... Yes No
      6. Have you had the German measles (rubella) vaccine? .... Yes No
      7. Have you had German measles?......... Yes No
      8. Have you had the measles (rubella) vaccine? .... Yes No
      9. Have you had measles (7-day)? .... Yes No
     10. Have you had the mumps vaccine? ...... Yes No
     11. Have you had mumps?.................. Yes No

     B. *Past History*
      1. Have you ever been hospitalized for illness or operations? .... Yes No
         Age_____ Hospital_____
         Reason_____
      2. Any other prolonged or serious illness?.. Yes No

3. Do you have any allergy (hives, wheezing, asthma, hay fever)? .... Yes No
4. Have you ever had a reaction (rash, hives, breathing difficulty) to any medications or injections such as penicillin? .... Yes No
5. Are you taking any medicines now? ...... Yes No
   If so, which ones? _____

C. *Family History*
1. Are both your parents in good health? ... Yes No
2. Are there any other members of your immediate family (brothers, sisters, parents, grandparents, aunts, uncles) with a serious health problem (mental or physical)? .... Yes No
   List each problem and who has it.

   _____

3. How may people live in your home? Children_____ Adults_____
4. With whom do you live? (circle one)
   Both parents   Mother   Father
   Legal guardian   Other_____
5. Do your parents get along well with each other? .... Yes No
6. Do you feel that your parents understand your problems? .... Yes No
7. Any long-term separations of the family? Yes No
8. Do you feel your parents (circle one)
   Are too strict   Are too old fashioned
   Do not care
   Favor your brothers and sisters over you
   Are fair
9. Could things be better at home? .... Yes No

D. *Accidents*
1. Have you ever had any serious accidents? .... Yes No
   Burns_____   Poisoning_____
   Cuts needing a doctor_____
   Broken bones_____
2. Do you use seat belts in your car? .... Yes No
3. Do you know how to swim? .... Yes No
4. Are firearms (loaded or unloaded) kept in your home? .... Yes No

E. *Review of Systems*
1. Do you have any of the following complaints? (circle which ones)
Headaches   Dizzy spells   Convulsions
Difficulty hearing   Blurred or double vision   Sinus trouble   Seizures
2. Do you wear glasses?_____ How long?_____
3. Last time you had your eyes checked_____
4. Do you have swollen glands of the neck or under the arms?...................... Yes No
5. Have you had pneumonia more than two times?.................................. Yes No
6. Do you get short of breath before other members of your class do?.............. Yes No
7. Do you smoke?_____ How many packs per day?_____
8. Do you have a chronic cough?........... Yes No
9. Do you have a heart murmur? .... Yes No
10. Do you have (circle)   Chest pain
Abdominal pain   Constipation
Diarrhea   Frequent vomiting
11. Have you ever had hepatitis (yellow eyes or skin)? .... Yes No
12. Have you had joint pain or swelling of joints?................................. Yes No
13. Have you ever had a kidney infection? ... Yes No
14. Does it burn when you pass your urine (water)................................. Yes No
15. Do you get up at night to urinate (pass water)? .... Yes No
16. Do you ever wet the bed?................ Yes No
17. Have you had venereal disease (VD)? .... Yes No
18. Do you have any questions about venereal disease? .... Yes No
19. Have you had recurrent fevers?.......... Yes No
20. Do you have problems with acne? .... Yes No
21. Do you have problems with your teeth? .. Yes No
22. Are you tired in the morning when you get up?.................................... Yes No

Individual Patterns
1. What grade are you in?_____ Are you satisfied with your grades? .... Yes No
2. Do you miss more than 3 days of school each month? .... Yes No
3. Is something slowing your progress at school?................................ Yes No

4. Do your teachers pick on you?........... Yes No
5. Is school (circle) A drag
   A means to an end Meaningless
   Worthwhile
6. What do you plan to do when you graduate? _____
7. Do you make friends easily?............. Yes No
8. Do you often feel left out?.............. Yes No
9. Do things get on your nerves easily?..... Yes No
10. Do you feel that you are a nervous person?................................. Yes No
11. Do drugs make you feel better?.......... Yes No
    Which ones? _____
12. Do you take drugs when you are alone?.. Yes No
13. Would you like to learn more about the prevention of pregnancy? .... Yes No

For Girls Only
1. Have you had your first period?_____ At what age?_____
2. Would you like to learn more about periods? .... Yes No
3. Do you have cramping with your periods? Yes No
4. Are your periods regular? .... Yes No
5. Are you taking the "pill?" .... Yes No
6. Would you like more information about the "pill?"............................ Yes No

Printed by permission of Dr. Burris Duncan, Colorado General Hospital.

BIBLIOGRAPHY

Batten, Joe D.: "Face-to-Face Communication," *Nursing Digest,* vol. 5, no. 1, pp. 89–90, Spring 1977.

Mansell, Ellen, and Shirlee Stokes: "Patient Assessment: Taking a Patient's History," *American Journal of Nursing,* vol. 74, no. 2, p. 293, February 1974.

Rosnoy, Melinda: "The Young Adult: Taking a Sexual History," *American Journal of Nursing,* vol. 76, no. 8, pp. 1279–1282, August 1976.

Weed, Lawrence L.: "Medical Records That Guide and Teach," *New England Journal of Medicine,* vol. 278, no. 3, pp. 593–600, 652–657, March 14 and 21, 1968.

Chapter 2

General Approach to the Physical Examination

The physical examination is an important tool in the evaluation of the child. It involves both the learning of a variety of specific skills and the organization of these skills into a system.

This system may vary with the age of the child. For example, the newborn infant does not protest when all clothing is removed or when laid down on the examining table. The examiner may coo at the infant or make "nonsense" talk in order to watch responses. The physical examination will usually begin with the feet and finish with the head; then the infant can be returned to the parent's arms for comfort. A 6 to 8 month old still may not object to having all clothing removed, but will probably protest when placed on the isolated examining table. The parent's lap usually works best for this age, and the examiner may want to begin the examination by listening to the child's chest while quiet and then start with the feet, systematically working towards the head. Again, the examiner should include time for play, for talking to the child, and for getting acquainted. Two year olds are usually difficult to examine; they do not like to have their clothing removed and usually do not want to be touched by the examiner. Many 2-year-olds are frightened and no one, including parents, seems able to comfort them. The examiner must decide what has to be accomplished, help the child get through the situation as best they can (kicking and biting are not allowed, but crying is), and finish the examination as quickly as possible. The 4 and 5 year olds are usually delightful to work with. They will gladly remove all their clothing (underpants are usually left on), stand before the examiner, or sit on the examining table or a parent's lap. Although the infant is examined while lying down, the older child is examined while standing or sitting, with little done when lying down. (Usually only inspection of the genitalia, palpation of the abdomen, and listening to the chest are done in the supine position.) Preschoolers like to help, to be talked to, and to listen to their own heart; they usually do not find any of the examination, including ears and mouth, objectionable. In examining the adolescent, it is probably best to begin with the head, leaving the genitalia examination until last. It is also important to assure the adolescent that all is well (if that is the case) during each part of the examination since bodily concerns are so common in the adolescent.

The physical examination should be used, not only to gather information about the child, but also to teach the child something about his or her body and health. The child who is interested in listening to his or her own heart may be the ideal candidate for some health teaching about keeping the heart healthy with exercise or proper diet.

Not only does the physical examination vary with the age of the child, but it varies with the type of physical examination to be performed. A complete physical examination includes using all basic skills and a review of every part of the body. The examiner must learn when this is appropriate and when modifications should be made. Most children coming for a well-child visit should have a complete, thorough physical examination. The child who is ill may need a complete physical or just an examination relevant to the complaint. However, the examiner must be careful not to miss important physical findings by abbreviating the physical too much. If the child is too ill for the complete examination when the nurse sees the child, it is important to make certain that either he/she has had one recently or will soon. The nurse must be thorough and methodical in doing the complete physical examination, but must also know how to adjust it to the situation and age of the child.

Physical examinations can be done under many conditions, but it is important to secure some privacy, the proper equipment, and some time for the nurse and the child and family to become comfortable in the setting. The atmosphere should be warm, friendly, and unhurried—this may take real effort when the nurse has a full waiting room. The physical examination begins the minute the child enters the room. The nurse should notice many things when first meeting the parent and child, make everyone in the room comfortable, and greet the child by name. If the child already appears frightened she should be encouraged to sit on the mother's lap or be given her own chair. The child should be allowed to play quietly with some toys while the nurse interviews the mother, thus letting the child adjust gradually to the situation. With increasing confidence, the nurse will become very proficient at completing the history and physical quite rapidly, even though giving the impression of having plenty of time for both the parent and child.

There are certain skills that are important in physical assessment, some of which will be new for many nurses, but the cornerstone of physical assessment is not a group of esoteric and complex skills; by far the most important part of the physical assessment is thoroughness. Every single part of the body must be examined with every applicable method of examination. By the end of the examination, there should be no accessible part of the body which has not been directly inspected and felt by the examiner. Nor should listening, or percussion, be omitted at any point of the examination where it would be helpful. Certainly, the best insurance for thoroughness is a system. Every examiner should adopt a systematic, logical approach to physical examinations. Once the nurse develops such a system, he or she should adhere to it as rigidly as possible. The examination always begins with an observation period concerned with the total child—appearance, behavior, and activity. Does the child appear to be happy, frightened, ill? Does the child seem small or large? Does the child have features or characteristics that are particularly striking? What is the general, overall impression the examiner gets from the child?

During the general observation period the nurse must decide where the examination will be done and if the child will have to be restrained. According to the age and condition of the child, and equipment available, the child may be examined on the examining table, the laps of the nurse and parent, or while standing up. An older child and a young infant can easily be examined on the examining table. The 8- to 15-month-old may be most comfortable on the parent's lap. This can easily be done if the nurse will move the chair in front of the parent's until their knees touch, then the child's buttocks can be supported on the nurse's lap and the head and shoulders on the parent's lap. This provides quite a satisfactory examining table. The nurse may decide during the initial observation that some help during the examination will be needed. Infants will frequently lie quietly if someone will hold a bottle or pacifier in their mouths. Older children may respond to a story or questions about their day, as the nurse begins the physical examination. Some children will hold a doll or stuffed toy or squeeze a toy during the examination. The apprehensive child may quiet down if the nurse does a physical examination on a doll while he or she watches and helps (see Fig.

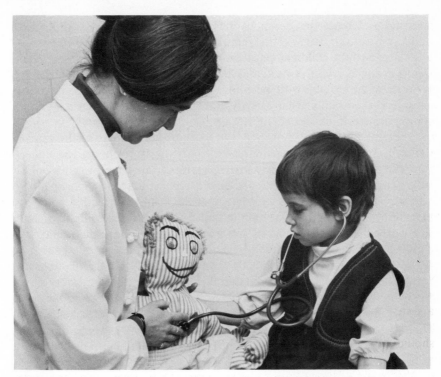

Figure 2-1 A child doing a physical examination on her doll.

2-1). If looking in the ears or mouth is particularly upsetting, the nurse may start by examining the parent's ears or mouth while the child watches.

A mirror over the examining table (so long as it is securely fastened) will often quiet the child under 1 year of age, as the child watches in the mirror. It is much nicer to have a cooperative child and avoid all restraints. But if this is impossible, the nurse must decide how to restrain the child and if he or she and the parent can manage or if a third person is needed. Specific ways of restraining will be discussed later.

When doing the physical examination, it is usually best to begin either with the head or the feet and proceed to examine methodically each adjacent part, gradually working up or down to the other end of the child. In this way, one is sure that absolutely nothing has been forgotten. There is an important exception to this rule when working with young children: it is best to do those parts of the examination that require a happy cooperative child at the first opportunity; so that if a young baby, for instance, is quiet at the beginning of the examination, the opportunity should be taken to listen to heart and lungs and to feel the abdomen. The examiner should then return to the usual routine and follow the rest of the system meticulously. A personal preference that seems to the authors to have some usefulness is that a system beginning with the feet and going to the head is most useful in infants and young children, since examination of the ears and throat often results in angry, crying protest, making the rest of the examination difficult. If the examination ends with these items, the parent can quickly comfort the child, and the examiner has already gathered all the important data from the physical examination.

For the older child, however, the more traumatic part of the examination is frequently getting undressed, particularly removing the underpants. In this case, it is often wise to begin with certain tests for neurological functions, since these resemble games and can be used as rapport-gaining devices. The examination is then begun at the head, since with a good explanation, the ear and throat examination is seldom threatening to a child of 3 years or older. If items of clothing are removed one at a time, the child's confidence will hopefully be gained, and by the time the pants are removed, her fears should be largely resolved. If this procedure is still traumatic, the child should be assured that the pants will be off for a very short time, and that the whole examination will then be finished. Another very helpful device in examining children of this age is to enlist their help in the examination whenever possible. It can make a 4-year-old feel very important if she is allowed to hold the stethoscope for you. She will also be interested in listening to her own heart through it (see Fig. 2-2). You can effectively use her own hand held over your's to palpate her abdomen (a procedure which greatly reduces the amount of voluntary guarding, as well as ticklishness encountered in children of this age). Showing her the "flashlight" (otoscope) that you will use and how it turns on and off will often fascinate her, as will a chance to thoroughly investigate the reflex hammer. If the child is exceptionally fearful, it will be wise to take more time in winning her confidence. When there are several children in the family to be examined on one day, it often pays to examine the least fearful child first, giving the others a chance to see just what will happen to them and that it will not be traumatic, while helping the first child feel important by being "first."

Traditionally, there are considered to be four basic methods of physical examination: inspection, palpation, auscultation, and percussion. Other methods of evaluation, such as using the sense of smell and taking specific types of measurement, are also important in certain parts of the examination. Inspection is certainly the most useful of the methods, although it is often the most difficult to learn. This is probably because we are so used to using inspection in everyday life in a rather haphazard manner. The nurse must be constantly on guard in a physical examination to observe not only for general inspection as we do in everyday life (although the gestalt we receive in this way is important), but also in a more detailed and meticulous fashion, seeing both the whole and each of the minute parts and their rela-

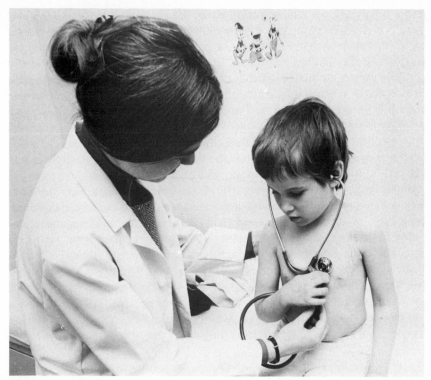

Figure 2-2 Child listening to her own heart.

tionships. Background knowledge of what is normal and what constitutes a normal condition is important to the nurse. The nurse must have sufficient knowledge to judge which things are significant and which are not. The vast majority of information will be gained from inspection with the naked eye. For certain parts of the body, however, special instruments, such as the otoscope or ophthalmoscope, will enhance vision.

Palpation generally follows inspection and is, perhaps, less familiar to the nurse. One usually thinks of palpation as meaning the act of touching and feeling, but it must not be forgotten that touch also includes the sense of temperature, vibration, position, and kinesthesia. Different parts of the hands are used for these different sensations. While the fingertips seem to be most discriminating in the area of fine tactile details, the back of the fingers are most sensitive to temperature, and the flat of the palm and fingers perceive vibrations such as cardiac thrills most accurately. All accessible parts of the body should be palpated thoroughly, using both light and deep palpation. Such different qualities as moisture, pulsatility, crepitus, and texture should all be appreciated wherever they are encountered. Information about bones, muscles, glands, masses, organs, vessels, hair, skin, and mucosa can be gained through palpation. Special types of palpation, such as ballottement, will be discussed under the appropriate parts of the examination.

The third method of physical examination is percussion. Basically, percussion is the method of determining the density of various parts of the body by the sound emitted by these parts when they are struck with the examiner's fingers. They can either be struck directly with the examiner's fingers (direct or immediate percussion), or the examiner may lay the middle finger of one hand flush against the body part to be percussed and then strike this finger with the index or middle finger of the other hand (bimanual, indirect, or mediate percussion). Different densities occur normally in different parts of the body. The terms usually used for these densities from least to most dense are tympany, hyperresonance, resonance, impaired resonance, dullness, and flatness. The sound emitted from gas-filled organs like the intestines or stomach is called *tympany,* while the sound produced by percussing a bone is said to be flat. Percussion is helpful in discovering unexpected densities, such as a solid mass where there should not be one. Mapping out the borders of certain organs like the heart can also be done by percussion. This is done by gradually comparing the differing densities of the organ one is mapping and the surrounding body tissues.

Auscultation theoretically refers only to sounds transmitted through the stethoscope. This is too narrow a meaning for its use in physical diagnosis, however, since listening with the unaided ear is often equally or even more important. The sound of the child's voice or the pitch of the infant's cry can be of critical importance. Although one first thinks of using the stethoscope to listen to breath and heart sounds, it must not be forgotten that it is equally useful in listening for bruits in the skull or thyroid, or for murmurs in the neck or abdomen.

Smelling, although not traditionally classed with the four methods of physical examination, can be, at times, of great help in evaluating a patient's physical status. Odors from the breath, sputum, vomitus, feces, pus, or urine can be extremely helpful.

Clinical measurements, such as height, weight, head circumference, temperature, pulse, respirations, etc., are quite familiar to the nurse, but their importance must not be overlooked. While the nurse actually may not have to perform the procedures, he or she is responsible for checking that they have been done and that they are accurate and must decide whether or not the results are within normal range. Clinical measurements have been universally incorporated into routines because they are extremely important in assessing physical health or illness.

All these techniques are incorporated into a complete, thorough, systematic physical examination. To avoid loss of interest, chilliness, and fatigue in the child, most examinations should be completed within 5 to 10 minutes. The nurse should make positive statements to the child and not allow a choice if there is no choice. The child can be told "Jane, now it is time to take off your clothes," rather than "Jane, will you take off your clothes?" Ideally, all clothing should be removed, but for the uncooperative child, one piece at a time may be removed. An older child may want to have a drape or hospital gown for modesty. The child should be positioned either on the examining table or the parent's lap, and the nurse must be comfortable, either standing beside the table or sitting in front of the parent and child.

Before beginning, the nurse must get all equipment ready for use. Depending on the age of the child, he or she may want to lay out the otoscope, stethoscope, reflex hammer, tongue blade, etc., within easy reach or introduce one instrument at a time, showing the child what it is and how it is going to be used. The examiner should begin the examination by moving slowly and avoiding sudden, jerky movements. The nurse should be gentle but firm in handling the child and should proceed as quickly as possible.

In using all the methods of physical diagnosis, the nurse will gradually become more and more proficient. The most important thing for the nurse learning physical assessment is to be familiar with the normal, and it is the normal which is stressed in this book. However, in order to appreciate the normal, it is frequently necessary to be familiar with the abnormals if only in order to compare. For this reason, some discussion of abnormalities is also included. Nurses must remember, however, that their basic responsibility is not usually one of differential diagnosis. Once the nurse is certain that a condition is abnormal and abnormal to a greater extent than what he or she can handle then the primary responsibility is to refer the patient to the physician. Although the nurse may find it interesting to diagnose the exact type of abnormality, this is not usually necessary. For purposes of clarity, the examination is broken down into sections of the body, and under each section where it is appropriate, there will be discussed six basic aspects of the examination: (1) why the child is examined; (2) what to examine: anatomy of area; (3) how to examine; (4) where to examine; (5) what to examine with; and (6) what to examine for.

BIBLIOGRAPHY

Alexander, M. M., and M. S. Brown: "Physical Examination: The Why and How of Examination," *Nursing '73*, vol. 3, no. 7, pp. 25–28, July 1973.

Greenhill, J. P.: "Physician Examination of Children and Adolescents for School," *Clinical Medicine*, vol. 80, no. 10, pp. 15–18, October 1973.

Luciano, Kathy, and Claire Shumsky: "Pediatric Procedures—The Explanation Should Always Come First," *Nursing '75*, vol. 5, no. 1, pp. 49–52, January 1975.

Chapter 3

The Skin

WHY THE CHILD IS EXAMINED

The skin comprises the greatest amount of body tissue that is directly accessible to the examiner. For this reason evaluation of the skin constitutes a major portion of the physical examination. It is important not only because its own health is essential to the proper functioning of the body, but also because it frequently mirrors the health of other systems in the body and can often be the only clue to disease elsewhere.

WHAT TO EXAMINE: ANATOMY OF THE AREA

The skin covers the entire body and has several functions: (1) It protects the deeper tissues from injury, drying, and foreign matter invasion. (2) It regulates the body temperature. (3) It helps in sensation, i.e., touch, heat, or cold. (4) It provides an avenue for excretion. (5) It participates in the production of vitamin D.

The skin varies greatly in different areas of the body. In thickness, for instance, it may vary from 0.5 to 1.5 mm, being thinnest over the earlobes and thick and horny on the palms and soles of the feet. It may be soft, smooth, and pliable as in babies or thick, wrinkled, and loose as in the elderly. It may contain few hair follicles, as on the palms of the hands, or many hair follicles, as on the scalp. Skin may also become extremely hard and form nails, or become elongated and form hair.

The skin is composed of two layers: epidermis and dermis. The epidermis is nonvascular stratified epithelium which varies in thickness. It contains five layers (see Fig. 3-1).

1 The stratum corneum (or horny layer) is the topmost surface and contains the remains of deeper cells. This layer continually desquamates, or sloughs off. It also contains keratin, an important fibrous protein.

2 Next is the stratum lucidum, a thin translucent layer.

3 The stratum granulosum underlies the stratum lucidum and contains several layers of flattened cells with large granules of keratohyalin, an early stage in the formation of keratin.

4 The stratum spinosum (or prickle-cell layer) contains polygonal cells that flatten as they move toward the surface.

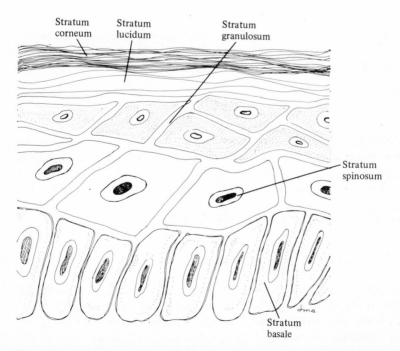

Figure 3-1 The layers of the epidermis.

5 The stratum basale (or basal layer) is the deepest layer which anchors the epidermis to the dermis. Within this layer lies melanin, the pigment that accounts for the black, brown, and tawny colors of the different races. Melanin consists of dark, very small closely packed granules. Most skin contains some melanin except in the case of albinos whose skin contains little or no melanin.

The dermis is tough, elastic, flexible, and highly vascular. It contains lymphatics and nerves and is composed of two layers: papillary and reticular. The papillary (or superficial) layer contains collagenous, elastic reticular fibers intertwined with superficial capillaries and covered by ground substances. The collagenous fibers are made up of a gluey white substance, forming the matrix for the elastic fibers which provide the flexibility and movement of the dermis. This layer causes the familiar ridges and furrows seen on the fingertips. Tracings of these patterns are called *dermatoglyphics.* The reticular fibers are important in wound healing and are interspersed irregularly throughout the ground substance, a nonvisible, semiliquid material which fills the spaces and bathes the cells.

The reticular layer is made up of fibroelastic connective tissue, including yellow elastic fibers. The deep layer of the reticular layer contains the sweat glands, sebaceous glands, hair follicles, and small fat cells and is attached to the adipose tissue of the subcutaneous fascia.

Discussion of the skin generally includes: (1) nails, (2) hair, (3)*sudoriferous* (sweat) *glands* and ducts, and (4) sebaceous (oil) glands and ducts.

Nails are flattened hard keratin cells (see Fig. 3-2). The outer surface is convex and contains:

1 An outer edge.
2 The nail plate, which is the exposed portion.
3 The lunula which is the white moon-shaped section near the proximal end of the exposed nail. The nail is not firmly attached to the deeper connective tissue at this point, thus giving the lunula its characteristic white color.
4 The eponychium which is a thin cuticular fold lying over the lunula.
5 The cuticle which is part of the stratum corneum (the first layer of the epidermis) of the finger.
6 The nail root (or fold).
7 The nail matrix from which the nail is produced.

Nails are formed on the dorsal surfaces of the fingers and toes by the fourteenth week of gestation. Fingernails are completely replaced every $5\frac{1}{2}$ months, while toenails take $1\frac{1}{2}$ years for total replacement.

Hair is found on every part of the body except the palms of the hands,

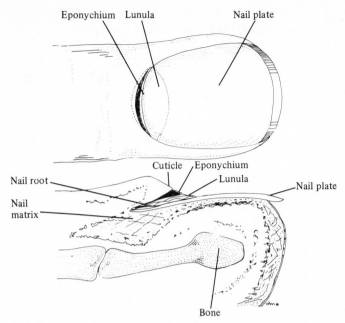

Figure 3-2 The nail.

soles of the feet, dorsal surfaces of the terminal phalanges, inner surfaces of the labia, and inner surfaces of the prepuce and the glans penis. Each hair consists of a root and a shaft. The root is implanted in the layers of skin and ends in the rounded hair bulb within the dermis. The hair bulb contains the papilla, a structure that produces the shaft of the hair follicle. The hair shaft is composed of an outer layer (the cuticle), a middle layer (the cortex), and the inner layer (the medulla); it may be round, oval, or flat and varies in thickness, length, and color. The hair lies in a deep cavity of dermal cells called the *hair follicle*. Each follicle contains a sebaceous gland and a bundle of smooth muscle fibers (arrectores pilorum muscles). When stimulated these muscles cause the sebaceous gland to secrete sebum and the hair shaft to stand erect.

There are several specialized types of hair. *Lanugo* is the first, fine hair to cover the body during fetal life; this hair generally disappears before or shortly after birth. Certain parts of the body are covered with fine, non-pigmented hair called *vellus*. *Terminal hair* covers all the ordinarily hairy parts of the body; it is more obvious, coarse, long, and pigmented.

Hair growth is cyclic. The active growth stage of the hair is called the *anagen stage*. The *catagen stage* is a transition from activity to nonactivity, and the *telogen stage* is the resting period. Rates of hair growth differ on different parts of the body. A normal scalp usually contains 80 to 85 percent of growing hairs, which grow at a rate of about 1 mm every 3 days or 2.5 mm a week. Adults lose between 20 to 100 hairs daily from their scalp. Body hair has a 3- to 4-month growing period, while facial hair (beard) has a 3- to 4-year growing period.

With the exception of the lips and certain parts of the genitalia, every part of the body has sweat or sudoriferous glands. An average body contains 2 to 5 million such glands, all of which are present at birth. These sudoriferous glands consist of a single duct, opening on the surface of the epidermis and are coiled and twisted deep in the dermis. The sweat glands open onto the surface of the skin on the palms, fingers, soles, and toes, they form pores (see Fig. 3-3).

Perspiration is the most important function of these glands. There are two types of perspiration: sensible perspiration is visible and produced by an emotional or thermal stimulus; insensible perspiration is microscopic and evaporates as it reaches the surface. Perspiration is composed of water, sodium, potassium, chloride, glucose, urea, and lactate. On an average day, a sedentary (inactive) individual will produce 1.5 liters of perspiration in 24 hours; but with dry, hot conditions this can rise to 6 liters in 24 hours.

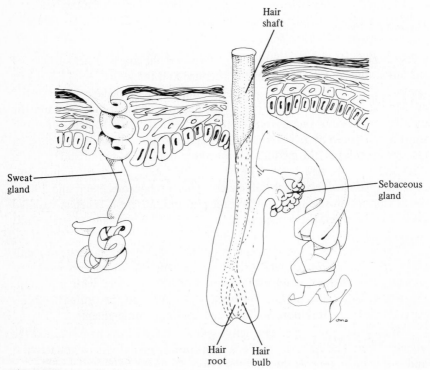

Figure 3-3 Structures piercing the epidermis.

Sebaceous glands are another type of excretory gland. They are combined with hair follicles and secrete sebum through the opening for these follicles. Sebaceous glands are found throughout the body, but are particularly abundant and active in the scalp and face. Their activity is controlled by hormones, testosterone increasing the activity and estrogen suppressing it.

HOW TO EXAMINE AND WHAT TO EXAMINE FOR

Skin is both inspected and palpated. It is first inspected for color. Normal skin is whitish pink, light brown, yellow-tinted, or deep black depending on race. Cyanosis may be seen in light-skinned people (skin with minimal melania) when unoxygenated hemoglobin reaches 5 mg/100 ml of blood. Dark-skinned persons may require additional unoxygenated hemoglobin to make the cyanosis visible. These changes can be caused by pulmonary disease, congenital heart disease, central nervous system disorders, or hypoglycemia. Normally, by 4 hours postnatally, an infant that was cyanotic at birth will show less cyanosis of the hands than of the feet. Infants with coarctation of the aorta, however, may show an even more striking difference, with the lower extremities distinctly more blue than the upper.

Jaundice is best seen in true sunlight by looking at the sclera, mucous membranes, or skin. Sometimes direct pressure to the skin blanches the blood and leaves only the yellow color. When the total serum bilirubin reaches 5 mg/100 ml in the newborn there is visible jaundice. Older children become visibly jaundiced at 2 mg/100 ml. A pale yellow-orange tint seen on the palms, soles, and nasolabial folds may be caused by carotenemia, or too much carotene in the blood. Children with this condition have white sclera rather than yellow. Certain drugs may cause this, as may excessive dietary intake of carrots or other yellow vegetables. Often physiologic jaundice appears about 24 hours after birth and disappears by the second week. This is usually normal, but may also be due to an abnormal condition such as erythroblastosis, ABO incompatibility, sepsis, viral hepatitis, or bile duct obstruction. Even if it is physiological, it requires treatment if serum bilirubin levels become excessively high. Erythroblastosis fetalis, on the other hand, causes jaundice at birth or within the first 12 hours.

Paleness of the face, conjunctiva, mucous membranes, and nail beds may be indicative of anemia; however, this is a subjective sign and should always be validated by laboratory studies. Pallor in the newborn may indicate shock or circulatory failure.

The infant with a beefy-red color over his entire body may be suffering from hypoglycemia. Sometimes one-half of a newborn's body is red and the other half pale (harlequin sign). This usually is transitory, and not a pathologic condition. The examiner should also inspect the skin for pigmentation. Pigmentation over exposed areas may be from sun and wind. This may cover large areas of skin or may present as many small pigmented areas called *freckles*. Small, light brown patches are called *café-au-lait spots* and may be indicative of fibromas or neurofibromatosis. Usually a small number of patches are considered to be a normal variation; seven or more should make the examiner suspicious of possible underlying pathology. *Vitiligo* (absence of pigment) may appear as irregular splotches of white in an otherwise melanotic skin.

The skin is also tested for *turgor*. This is best done by taking a large pinch of skin on the lower abdomen. Normal, hydrated skin rises with the pinch but quickly falls when released. Dry, dehydrated skin will remain in the elevated position much longer and return only very slowly to its normal position. Turgor is also tested by feeling the calf of the leg. It should feel firm. Newborns, premature infants, and dehydrated infants have loose, extra skin at the calf. Localized edema may be pitting or nonpitting. If a finger is pressed firmly against the skin and the impression remains, the child has pitting edema. This is due to an increased, abnormal amount of extracellular fluid. Pitting edema is frequently seen first over the ankles and sacral region. Children with long-term heart disease, malnutrition, kidney disorders, and certain parasitic diseases, will display pitting edema. Some children have a puffy appearance but finger pressure leaves no mark. This is referred to as *nonpitting edema* and is seen in children who are cretins as well as in some with other conditions. Localized edema may also be caused by allergies, hives, insect bites, or contact dermatitis. Children with certain contagious childhood diseases may also display puffy faces and eyelids.

Texture of the skin is very important. It should be smooth, soft, and flexible. Skin that is rough and dry may be caused by frequent bathing, cold weather, vitamin A deficiency, or hypothyroidism. Scaliness may occur on several parts of the body. Scaliness between the toes and fingers may be due to ringworm. Profuse scaling of the soles and palms is usually caused by *scarlet fever*. Infants with scaliness of the diaper area may be recovering from a diaper rash. Eczema also causes scaliness over the cheeks, behind the ears, behind the knees, and at the elbows. This usually begins when the infant is about 2 months old and may last until he is 2 years old.

Scaliness over the scalp (especially the anterior fontanel) associated with a red macular rash over the forehead, cheeks, neck, and chest may be due to *seborrhea,* which usually clears with firm shampooing.

Scaliness and desquamation is seen in many normal newborns. It can be quite pronounced over the feet and ankle creases and usually clears with no special attention. Babies with a lot of desquamation are thought to be postmature.

A crackling sensation when the skin is pressed may be due to subcutaneous emphysema associated with some bone fractures and lung disorders.

Some newborns have an abundant amount of *vernix caseosa,* a cheesy white material covering the entire body. Formerly this was vigorously scrubbed off, but the present trend is to leave it on in order to protect the skin.

Very obese children or children who have lost a great deal of weight may have *striae* over the abdomen and thighs. These are pale white or pink stripes. They may fade with age, but generally they will not disappear.

Observation of the skin may also include a look at the dermatoglyphics of the palms and fingers (see Fig. 3-4). A good light and magnifying glass (such as the otoscope) are essential. A more detailed description of this patterning is given in other books, but generally, a normal person's ridges fall into arches, loops, and whorls on the fingers; the palm displays a triradius (three palmar lines meeting) at the wrist area. These patterns will vary in children with such specific diseases as *Down's syndrome, Trisomy 18 syndrome,* and *XO syndrome.* Children with Down's syndrome frequently display the prominent simian line straight across the palm; however, this can also be seen in some normal children (see Fig. 3-4).

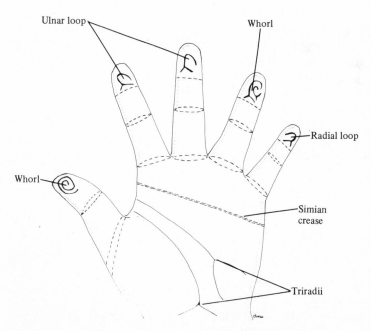

Figure 3-4 Dermatoglyphics of the palm with a simian line.

It is difficult to evaluate skin sensitivity. A child who reacts to skin touch may be just irritable or may be suffering from systemic disease, central nervous system disease, or skin problems. Further investigation is usually needed.

Inspection and palpation may reveal a variety of skin lesions, some being just a variation of normal, but some indicating pathology. *Milia* are small yellow plaques appearing on the nose and cheeks which usually dissolve in a few weeks. *Miliaria* is prickly heat, characterized by tiny red, irritated lesions. Keeping the baby cool, with less restrictive bedding and clothing, will generally clear up this condition. *Mongolian spots* are bluish discoloration of the skin, usually seen over the coccygeal area most often in black and Mexican-American babies. These spots sometimes disappear with time. *Erythema toxicum neonatorum* (erythema means reddened area) is a condition in which a rash of pinpoint, red-based *macules* may appear on the cheeks or trunk during the first 3 days of life. They sometimes appear and disappear within an 8-hour period and should not be a matter of concern.

Hemangiomas are vascular lesions present at birth. They should be noted for size, color, and shape. Authorities differ on the exact classification of hemangiomas. *Superficial infantile hemangiomas* are frequently seen as irregular blotchy pink patches over the eyelid or bridge of the nose of the newborn. They gradually fade and are usually gone by 2 years of age. *Port wine stain* (nevus flammeus) is present at birth as a flat, reddish capillary lesion. It is more common around the scalp and face and may be superficially or deeply involved in the dermis. It may be associated with convulsions as part of the Sturge-Weber syndrome. *Strawberry mark* (hemangioma simplex) is a soft, red, raised lesion present at birth. It may occur anywhere on the skin and sometimes enlarges during the first 6 to 10 months of life before spontaneously shrinking and disappearing. Treatment is not generally suggested, since it often leaves a scar. *Cavernous hemangioma* is a reddish, soft, rounded lesion found on any portion of the skin; it may disappear spontaneously.

Other abnormalities of the skin may also be noted. A nontender, fluid-filled mass felt in the superficial layers of the skin may be a *cyst.* Cysts found on the hand or wrist may be ganglions; cysts found in other parts of the body may be tumors. Both types of cyst need further investigation.

Trauma to the skin produces *ecchymoses* (bruises), a collection of blood beneath the skin causing the top layers to turn bluish purple and become firm and tender to the touch. Active, normal children can have many ecchymoses, usually below the knees and elbows. Children with such diseases as hemophilia, the purpuras, or leukemia display many bruises all over their bodies and have a history of decreased play and activity. Children who are battered or abused often display bruises, but in peculiar places, and have a history of odd and unusual falls or accidents.

Erythema nodosum appears as painful, red tender nodules 2 to 4 cm across, along the shaft of the leg. These often occur in connection with some systemic disease, such as streptoccocal infections, rheumatoid arthritis, or a reaction to a drug. *Erythema marginatum* is seen in children with rheumatic fever. This lesion is a flat 1- to 2-cm circular reddened area with a definite border. These areas may change from hour to hour. Erysipelas produces erythema that is localized, tender, and firm, with raised borders. Early diaper rash also produces erythematous eruptions.

In describing lesions of the skin it is necessary to know certain terms. The term "primary lesion" refers to a lesion as it originally appears before scratching or other things occur to change it. The nurse-practitioner should be familiar with the seven basic types of primary lesions:

1 A *macule* is a flat, small (no larger than 1 cm) lesion different in color from the surrounding skin. Macules are seen in rubeola, rubella, scarlet fever, and roseola infantum.

2 A *papule* is elevated, sharply circumscribed, small (1 cm or less), and colored. Papules are seen in ringworm, pityriasis rosea, and psoriasis.

3 A *vesicle* (or blister) is a small (under 1 cm) sharply defined lesion filled with clean, free fluid. Vesicles are seen in herpes simplex, varicella, poison ivy contact dermatitis, and herpes zoster.

4 *Bullae* are large vesicles—any vesicle over 1 cm—often seen on the soles and palms in scarlet fever and in connection with sunburn.

5 A *pustule* is an elevated, sharply circumscribed lesion filled with pus—measuring less than 1 cm—seen in impetigo, acne, and staphylococcal infections.

6 A *wheal* is an elevated, white-to-pink, edematous lesion that is unstable and associated with *pruritis*. Wheals are evanescent, that is, they appear and disappear quickly. The borders of a wheal are less well defined than those of a vesicle. Wheals are seen in mosquito bites, hives, urticaria.

7 *Petechiae* are tiny, reddish purple, sharply circumscribed lesions in the superficial layers of epidermis. They can be a sign of severe systemic disease, such as meningococcemia, bacterial endocarditis, and nonthrombocytopenic purpura, and should be referred immediately if there is any possibility of such illnesses.

Secondary lesions result from some alteration—usually traumatic—to the primary lesion.

1 *Scales* are the dried fragments of the sloughed dead epidermis, seen in diseases like seborrhea and tinea capitis.

2 *Crusts* are accumulations of dried blood, scales, pus, and serum such as those seen in infectious dermatitis.

3 *Excoriation* is the mechanical removal (for instance, a scratch or scrape) of the epidermis that leaves the dermis exposed.

4 *Erosion* is the loss of the superficial portions of the epidermis.

5 *Ulcers* are sores resulting from destruction and loss of epidermis, dermis, and possibly the subcutaneous layers.

6 *Fissures* are vertical linear cracks through the epidermis and dermis.

7 *Scars* are formations of dense connective tissue resulting from destruction and healing of skin.

8 *Lichenification* is a thickening of the epidermis and dermis due to chronic irritation.

Sweating is an important function of the skin. It is necessary both for excretory purposes and for heat regulation. The sweat mechanism of a newborn is immature and visible sweat may not be seen during the first month of life. It may be seen sooner if the infant has brain irritation, a sympathetic nervous system disorder, or a mother who is a chronic morphine user. Sweating may normally be produced by exercise, crying, excessively hot environment, or eating, but excessive sweating may be an indication of fear, fever, hypoglycemia, hyperthyroidism, or heart disease.

While checking the skin, it is important to observe the nails. Normally the nail beds should be pink and convex. Nail color should be noted. Cyanosis is easily seen in nail beds. Postmature infants may have yellow nail beds, while children with porphyria may have darkened nail beds. A hemorrhage under the nail (from trauma) causes darkening of the nail. Fungal infections may also be evident, and may cause the nails to become pitted. Paronychia, which is an infection around the nail, is frequently seen in children.

Another important aspect of evaluating the skin is the examination of the hair. Normal head hair should be clean and shiny, cover the entire head, and be of generally the same color. Hair distribution is important to note. Hair covers the entire body, but is normally most easily detected on the head, eyebrows, and eyelashes. Newborns may have lanugo over the shoulders, back, and sacral area. Long eyelashes may be familial or a sign of a possible chronic disease. Hairiness over the arms, legs, and other parts of the body may be familial or a sign of excessive vitamin A, hypothyroidism, or Cushing's syndrome. Tufts of hair over the spine and sacral area may mark spina bifida or spina bifida occulta. Hair on other parts of the body begins to develop with puberty. Pubic hair appears between ages 8 and 12 years, followed by axillary hair about 6 months later. Boys usually develop facial hair 6 months after the appearance of pubic and axillary hair. Curling of the pubic hair is thought to signify the onset of sperm formation.

Hairiness should be noted. Normally the scalp hair begins high over the forehead and extends midway down the back of the neck; infants of Spanish-Mexican descent, however, may have hairlines that normally begin at the middle of the forehead. Infants with some types of chronic debilitating syndromes have hair very low on the back of the neck.

Hair texture should also be evaluated. Normally, hair may be thick and coarse, thin and fine, straight, or curly. Very brittle dry, coarse hair is often associated with hypothyroidism. Some nutritional disturbances also effect hair texture.

Hair may be yellow, brown, black, red or various shades of these colors. Infants or children with a single patch of white hair (called a "white forelock") may have a disease known as *Waardenburg's syndrome.* Of these children 20 percent may be deaf bilaterally. Children with reddish rust color hair may have severe nutritional deprivation, usually a lack of protein.

WHERE TO EXAMINE

It is of utmost importance, that at some time during the examination, the nurse carefully inspect and palpate every square inch of skin, hair, mucous membranes, and nails. It will be necessary to smooth out creases carefully and to open folds wherever appropriate. Although each section of skin is usually inspected and palpated while the examiner is evaluating the relevant area of the body, it is also important to inspect the skin as a whole either at the beginning or the end of the examination. In this way, the examiner will be more likely to pick up changes, such as color or texture, between areas of skin.

WHAT TO EXAMINE WITH

For the most part, the skin is examined without specialized equipment. The nurse must rely heavily on her techniques of inspection and palpation. Good lighting, preferably natural lighting, is by far the most essential equipment. Other minor equipment is sometimes also used. A microscope slide, for instance, is often pressed flush against the skin to better evaluate jaundice; a Wood's lamp is sometimes used for inspection of fungus. Other specialized tests, such as smears, cultures, and patch and intradermal tests, might also be considered here.

GLOSSARY

bullae vesicles over 1 cm in diameter
café-au-lait spots small light-brown patches on the skin
cavernous hemangiomas soft, reddish rounded lesions present at birth
crust a collection of dried blood, scales, pus, and serum

cyst   a nontender fluid-filled mass felt in the superficial layers of the epidermis and dermis

dermatoglyphics   tracings of patterns seen as ridges and furrows on fingertips

ecchymoses   a collection of blood beneath the skin, causing the top layers to turn bluish purple and become firm and tender to the touch; a bruise

erosion   the loss of the superficial portions of the epidermis

erythema toxicum neonatorum   a pinpoint red-based macule on cheeks and trunks of newborns

excoriation   the mechanical removal of the epidermis, leaving the dermis exposed; a scratch or scrape

fissure   a vertical linear crack through the epidermis and dermis

hemangioma   a collection of blood vessels, forming a benign tumor

lanugo   the first, fine hairs to cover the body during fetal life

lichenification   thickening of epidermis and dermis due to chronic irritation.

macule   a colored, flat skin lesion

miliaria   prickly heat

papule   an elevated sharply circumscribed small (less than 1 cm in diameter) lesion which may be a variety of colors

petechia   a tiny reddish purple, sharply circumscribed lesion in the superficial layers of epidermis

port wine stain (nevus flammeus)   a flat reddish hemangioma present at birth, usually found around the scalp and face, with the dermis superficially or deeply involved

pruritis   an itching condition

pustule   an elevated, sharply circumscribed (less than 1 cm) lesion filled with pus

scales   dried fragments of the sloughed dead epidermis

scar   a formation of dense connective tissue as a result of destruction of skin

seborrhea (or cradle cap)   an overproduction of sebum from the sebaceous glands producing whitish yellow, greasy scales over scalp

strawberry mark (or hemangioma simplex)   a soft red, raised lesion present at birth

striae   pale white or pink stripes frequently seen in obese children

sudoriferous glands   sweat glands

superficial infantile hemangiomas   irregular blotchy pink patches covering the eyelid or bridge of the nose of a newborn

turgor   the normal fullness and resistance seen in healthy skin

ulcer   destruction and loss of epidermis, dermis and subcutaneous layers

vernix caseosa   a cheesy, white material covering the entire body of some newborns

vesicle (or blister)   a small (under 1 cm) sharply defined lesion filled with clean, free fluid

vitiligo   absence of pigment in the skin

wheal   an elevated, white to pink, edematous lesion which is unstable and associated with pruritis

Chapter 4

The Lymphatic System

WHY THE CHILD IS EXAMINED

Because the lymphatic system acts as a drainage system for wastes from the entire body, it is often a very sensitive indicator of health or illness. It is most frequently useful as an indicator of either localized or generalized infection, but it can also give the examiner clues concerning certain hypersensitivities and metabolic and lymphoid diseases.

WHAT TO EXAMINE: ANATOMY OF THE AREA

The lymphatic system is almost as extensive as the vascular system and consists of:

    1 A network of capillaries which collect lymph from the organs and tissues

55

2 A system of collecting vessels which carry the lymph from the lymphatic capillaries to the bloodstream via openings in the neck
3 A series of lymph nodes which are filters for the collecting vessels
4 Certain lymphatic organs such as the tonsils, spleen, and thymus

Lymph is a clear, watery fluid which flows within its own system of vessels, and mixes with blood only at the jugular and subclavian veins within the neck, the point at which the lymph is emptied into the bloodstream.

Although the lymph nodes are scattered throughout the lymphatic system, the examiner is interested in those lymph nodes found in four main areas: the head and neck, the axillae, the arms, and the groin (inguinal region).

The greatest number of palpable nodes are concentrated in the area of the head. The nodes to be palpated in this area are: *posterior auricular* (postauricular), *occipital* (preoccipital), *superficial cervical, submental, submandibular, mandibular, parotid* (preauricular), and *inferior deep cervical.* Nodes up to 3 mm in diameter are normal in all areas, but nodes in the cervical and inguinal areas may normally be as large as 1 cm. Normal nodes can be easily moved under the fingers during palpation. The examiner should be concerned about nodes which feel as though they are attached to underlying tissue. This type of node is said to be "fixed" or "immobile." Normal nodes are nontender and cool. In acute infections, nodes will frequently present as tender, warm, and large.

Knowledge of the drainage system will often be helpful in locating the source of infection. Foot and leg infections cause the inguinal nodes to enlarge, as does the common diaper rash. Finger and arm infections cause the *epitrochlear* and *axillary* nodes to enlarge; scalp infections, rubella, pediculosis, and tick bites can cause occipital nodes to swell; and mouth and throat infections usually cause cervical gland swelling. Generalized glandular disease (adenopathy) is often a symptom of systemic disease. See Table 4-1 for a more complete listing of the drainage system.

The upper limbs contain the axillary and epitrochlear nodes. Five to six small groups of nodes lying at the lateral edge of the pectoralis major muscle are called the axillary nodes; they drain the arm, thoracic wall, and breast. The epitrochlear nodes are on the medial aspect of the arm, slightly above humerus and ulnar junction at the elbow. They drain the lymph vessels of the fingers and forearm.

The inguinal nodes lie along the inguinal ligament and the saphenous vein and are easily palpated along the crease separating the thigh from the abdomen. These inguinal nodes drain the entire lower limb, gluteal area, perineal area, and all the skin from the lower abdominal wall.

Table 4-1 Lymphatic Drainage System*

Chain	Location	Areas drained
1. Occipital (or suboccipital)	At nape of neck; lower occipital bone	Scalp (diseases: pediculosis, seborrhea, rubella, tick bites, chicken pox, head scratching, external otitis)
2. Posterior auricular (or postauricular)	Behind ear	External acoustic meatus; scalp behind ear (rubella, facial skin, anterior pinna)
3. Preauricular	Directly in front of ear; temporal	Conjunctivitis, styes, chalazions
4. Superficial cervical (or poststernocleido-mastoid)	Chain lying over the sternocleido-mastoid muscle at the upper half of the neck	Tongue, tonsils, pinna, parotid, scalp, neck, thorax
5. Deep cervical (or jugular)	Begins with tonsilar node at angle of jaw and proceeds under sternocleidomastoid muscle, ending posterior to this muscle in the supraclavicular chain	Most of the tongue, tonsil, pinna, and parotid
6. Submaxillary (submandibular or mandibular)	Under the jaw bone halfway between the chin and ear	Tongue, submaxillary gland, medial conjunctiva, lips and mouth, central lower lip, floor of mouth
7. Submental (sublingual)	Directly below chin	Tip of tongue, skin of cheek
8. Tonsillar	The first of the deep cervical chain at angle between ear and jaw	Mouth, throat, superficial facial tissues
9. Supraclavicular	Directly over medial area of clavicle	Head, abdomen, breast, thorax, and arm
10. Posterior cervical	Along anterior border of trapezius muscle	Scalp and neck
11. Infraclavicular	Below the clavicle	Breast, anterior thoracic wall
12. Lateral axillary	Along head of humerus	From all of arm except what goes to epitrochlear
13. Central axillary	High in medial axilla	Arm, breast, anterior and posterior thoracic wall
14. Subscapular (posterior axillary)	Lateral edge of scapulae, deep in posterior axillary fold	Posterior thoracic wall and part of the arm
15. Pectoral (anterior axillary)	Lower border of pectoralis major, inside the anterior axillary line	Anterior thoracic wall, most of the breasts
16. Epitrochlear	Medial, inner aspect of elbow	Ulnar surface of forearm, little, middle and ring finger
17. Horizontal inguinal	Parallels the inguinal ligament, running diagonally toward crotch	Skin of lower abdominal wall, external genitalia (except testes), anus
18. Vertical inguinal	Runs vertically at upper, inner aspect of thigh	Drains most of the leg (same drainage system as the greater saphenous vein) and gluteal

*From the Workbook/Video Series: *A Programmed Approach to Pediatric Assessment* by Marie Scott Brown, Blue Hill Educational System, 1976. Used with permission.

HOW TO EXAMINE

The lymphatic system is examined by both inspection and palpation. Auscultation and percussion are not used for this examination. It is best to examine that part of the lymphatic system in each body area as you examine that body area. Thus, the nurse should incorporate the four main areas of lymph nodes into the general system of examination. It is important, however, not to forget to evaluate the general status of the entire lymphatic system when the examination is finished, since a generalized *lymphadenopathy* has implications which may be different from localized lymphadenopathy.

WHERE TO EXAMINE

Although the lymphatic system permeates the entire body in both a deep and superficial level, not all areas of it are accessible to the examiner. That part of the system which is accessible, and should be examined during every physical, consists primarily of four groups of nodes: those located around the head and neck areas (see Fig. 4-1), the axillary nodes, the arm nodes, and the inguinal nodes.

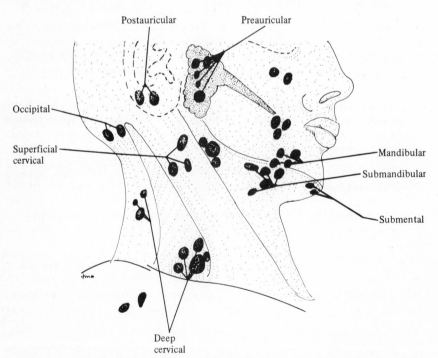

Figure 4-1 Lymph nodes of the face and neck.

WHAT TO EXAMINE WITH

For this part of the examination, no specialized instruments are necessary. The nurse's observational skills are crucial and he or she must depend on them entirely.

WHAT TO EXAMINE FOR

When examining the lymphatic system, the nurse is primarily concerned with evaluating any lymphadenopathy. Lymph nodes are often palpable in normal infants and children, but they should always be evaluated carefully. Small firm nodes are called *shotty,* and are generally normal in moderate amounts. These are signs of past infections that are often found in the inguinal area from past diaper infections and in the cervical area from past respiratory infections. If lymph nodes are enlarged, warm, tender or perhaps even red, it is a sign of current infection and the source of the infection should be found. Lymphadenopathy may be caused by an infection of any type: bacterial, viral, or fungal. If the examination reveals localized lymphadenopathy, the anatomy of the drainage system must be reviewed to locate the infection. Tonsillitis and pharyngitis, for instance, usually cause cervical adenitis, but stomatitis may result in submaxillary adenopathy. Swelling of the occipital and postauricular nodes may indicate some infection of the scalp, usually seborrheic dermatitis or pediculosis. Infections occurring along the arms will result in swelling of the epitrochlear and axillary lymph nodes, while those along the legs will result in lymphadenopathy of the inguinal and femoral areas.

Certain infectious diseases have characteristic distributions of lymphadenopathy. Rubella, for instance, is accompanied by inflamed nodes in the occipital, posterior cervical, and posterior auricular chains. Scarlet fever is characterized by cervical adenitis. Generalized lymphadenopathy is typical of mononucleosis; in this disease, the nodes are felt to be discrete and firm. Usually they are not tender and may be anywhere from $\frac{1}{2}$ to 3 in in diameter. Mumps, chickenpox, measles, Salmonella infections, eczema, histoplasmosis, sarcoidosis, or bacteremia may also result in generalized superficial inflammation of lymph node chains, but the nodes are usually smaller in these diseases.

Vaccinations may also cause lymphadenopathy. Smallpox and other vaccinations injected into the arm may cause axillary node enlargement, while generalized adenopathy may be found after a typhoid inoculation. Vaccination given in any area may cause palpable nodes in nearby localized areas.

Conditions other than infections may also result in lymphadenopathy. Drugs such as Dilantin or diseases such as systemic lupus erythematosus, rheumatic fever, and juvenile rheumatoid arthritis may also result in enlarged lymph nodes. Cancerous illnesses, such as leukemia, Hodgkin's disease, several types of sarcoma, neuroblastoma, and cancer of the thyroid may be accompanied by lymphadenopathy. Sickle cell anemia, Cooley's anemia, hemolytic anemia, and certain metabolic diseases such as cystinosis and Gaucher's disease may also be typified by this symptom.

BIBLIOGRAPHY

Roach, Lora B.: "Assessing Skin Changes: The Subtle and the Obvious," *Nursing '74,* vol. 4, no. 3, pp. 64–67, March 1974.

Roberts, Sharon L.: "Skin Assessment for Color and Temperature," *American Journal of Nursing,* vol. 75, no. 4, pp. 610–613, April 1975.

GLOSSARY

axillary lymph nodes the five to six small groups of lymph nodes lying at the lateral edge of the pectoralis major muscle

epitrochlear nodes lymph nodes on the medial aspect of the arm, slightly above the humerus and the ulnar junction at the elbow

lymph a clear, watery fluid flowing through the lymphatic system

lymphadenopathy an enlargement of the lymph nodes

occipital lymph nodes lymph nodes located over the occipital bone

posterior auricular (postauricular) lymph nodes several small lymph nodes lying behind the ear

"shotty" lymph nodes small, firm lymph nodes usually indicating a past infection

submandibular lymph nodes small lymph nodes felt below the jaw

submental lymph nodes small lymph nodes felt along the posterior border of the jaw

superficial cervical lymph nodes shallow lymph nodes felt in the cervical regions of the neck

Chapter 5

The Head, Face, and Neck

WHY TO EXAMINE

The head, face, and neck are vital areas of the physical examination. The brain and the organs of vision, hearing, and speaking are all located here; it is obvious how important their adequate functioning is to the future happiness of the child. Parents also are very concerned with these areas, especially in regard to cosmetic questions. Particularly in the newborn period, some of the most important parts of the physical examination, such as taking careful serial head circumferences, are a part of this examination.

WHAT TO EXAMINE

The skull and face comprise a vault designed to protect the brain and certain other vital centers of the central nervous system. The skull is divided into two sections: (1) the cranium and (2) the facial skeleton. The first of these, the cranium, is composed of 7 bones, joined together by immovable sutures; these are 2 frontal bones, 2 parietal bones, 1 occipital bone, and 2 temporal bones. These bones are soft and separated at birth; the *fontanels,* unossified membranous spaces, are found at the junctions between the frontal and parietal bones and the parietal and occipital bones (see Fig. 5-1).

Most infants are born with 6 fontanels, but the most prominent are the anterior and the posterior. However, some infants have an additional opening (sometimes referred to as a third fontanel) along the *sagittal suture* between the anterior and the posterior. This is present in some children with Down's syndrome, but can also be present in normal infants. The spaces between the skull bones are called *sutures* and are frequently palpable at birth. The *coronal suture* goes from ear to ear across the top of the skull, while the sagittal suture divides the parietal bone, thus running at a right angle to the coronal suture. The *lambdoidal suture* separates the parietal bones from the occipital bones. The facial bones number 14 and are immovable except for the *mandible.* These include the mandible, the *maxilla,* 2 *nasal bones,* 2 *zygomatic bones,* 2 *sphenoid bones,* 2 *ethmoid bones,* 2 *lacrimal bones,* and 2 *vomer bones.* All these bones are present at birth, but

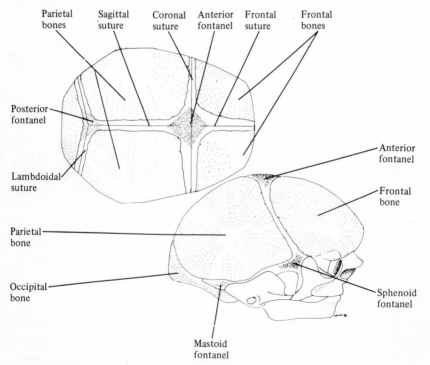

Figure 5-1 The infant skull bones showing fontanels and sutures.

the mandible and maxilla are very small, giving the head a flat, squashed shape (see Fig. 5-2).

The vertebral column is considered as a whole elsewhere, but the bones of the neck will be considered separately here; these are the first 2 vertebrae. The cranium rests directly on the atlas, or first cervical vertebra, a small vertebra with no body. The *atlas,* in turn, rests on the second vertebra called the *axis.* The two form a pivot for rotation of the head.

Vertebrae 3 through 6 are not easily palpable, but the seventh vertebra has a long spinous process and is used for identification when palpating the spinal column.

The muscles considered in this area are skull muscles, facial muscles and neck muscles.

The cranium is covered with tough and thick, subcutaneous fascia, and it is below this fascia that the broad, muscular layer called *epicranius* is found. Contraction and relaxation of these muscles control wrinkling of the forehead, raising of the eyebrows, and some facial expressions.

The muscles of the face are many and varied. They are generally described in connection with certain orifices, that is, the muscles of the ear, of the eye, of the mouth, and of the nose.

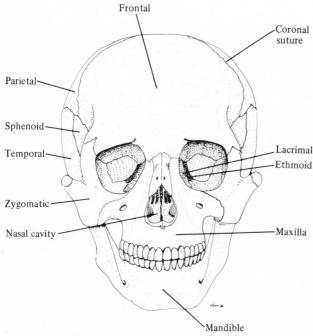

Figure 5-2   The facial bones.

The muscles of the neck may be divided into six categories, beginning with the superficial and going deeper and in several directions (see Fig. 5-3). The subcutaneous fascia varies from thin on the anterior neck to thick and tough on the posterior areas. The superficial cervical muscle is the *platysma* which attaches below the clavicle and runs upward to the edge of the mandible. It assists in opening of jaws. The lateral cervical muscles are the trapezius and sternocleidomastoid. The trapezius is a neck and back muscle which originates near the protuberance of the occipital bone and spreads downward along the cervical and thoracic vertebrae and the clavicle and scapula. This gives the muscle a slightly triangular shape. It acts to turn the head and raise the shoulders. The sternocleidomastoid is a thick, tough muscle running from the mastoid area behind the ear to the sternum and clavicle regions. It is instrumental in turning the head to either side. The *suprahyoid, infrahoid, anterior vertebral,* and *lateral vertebral* muscles are the deep muscles of the neck and contribute to the sideways movement.

The skin covering the subcutaneous fascia and muscle on the skull is thicker than on any other part of the body. It contains abundant, tightly spaced hair follicles, sebaceous glands, and subcutaneous fat. Thus the scalp has five tightly packed layers: the skin, subcutaneous tissue, ep-

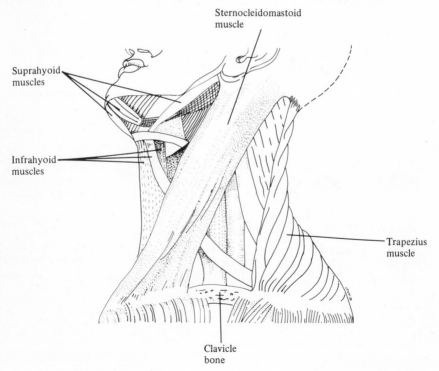

Figure 5-3 The neck muscles.

icranius, connective tissue, and *pericranium.* The face and neck are covered with a layer of skin containing hair follicles and sebaceous and sweat glands.

Circulation for the entire head and neck is supplied through the two common carotid arteries: the external and the internal. The external carotid artery carries blood to the head, face, and neck, while the internal supplies the structures within the cranium. Blood is drained from the head, neck, and face through two deep and superficial veins of the face, four veins from the cranium, and three large veins in the neck. The neck contains the external and internal jugular veins.

The face and head form a highly sensitive, highly coordinated area with many nerve innervations. The most important nerves in this area are the cranial nerves. There are 12 pairs, which are discussed in the chapter on the nervous system.

There are also some additonal structures within the neck to be considered (see Fig. 5-4). The trachea (windpipe) is a cartilaginous, membranous tube extending from the larynx to the bronchi. Posteriorly it lies against the esophagus and anteriorly the isthmus of the thyroid gland covers it. Males have larger tracheas than females; in children the trachea is deeply buried in the neck and is more movable than in adults.

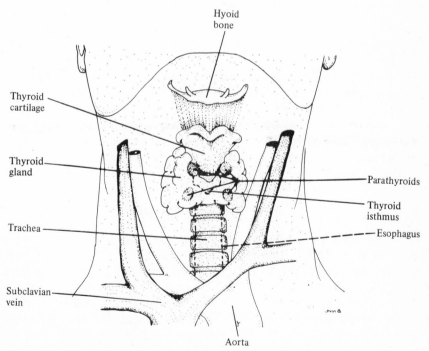

Figure 5-4 The neck structures.

The thyroid gland is an extremely vascular endocrine gland located at the fifth or sixth tracheal ring. Like all endocrine glands, the thyroid has no ducts and secretes hormones directly into the bloodstream. It contains a right and left lobe connected by a neck called the *isthmus* and secretes thyroxine which is essential for normal body growth. The diet must contain adequate amounts of iodine for thyroxine to be produced. The *parathyroid glands* are flat, oval disks, averaging 6 by 4 mm located on the thyroid gland along the dorsal borders of the lateral lobes. These are endocrine glands which secrete *parathyroid*, a hormone needed for calcium metabolism.

HOW TO EXAMINE

Examination of the head, face, and neck, including the ears, nose, mouth, and eyes may be uncomfortable; therefore, it might be best to do this part of the examination last on the young child and then return the child to the parent for comforting. Much of the observation of the head, face, and neck can be done while watching the child on the parent's lap. Palpation is also important; the examiner should feel every part of the head, face, and neck. Remember to begin by assessing the whole (shape, size, symmetry) and proceeding to a more specific examination of the fontanels and other details. (See charts at the end of this chapter.)

WHERE TO EXAMINE

All parts of the head, face, and neck must be included in this part of the examination. Most of these areas will be accessible to direct inspection and palpation, but in certain areas, some manipulation of parts may be necessary. Movable parts should be inspected and palpated in both the quiet, resting state and in motion. For instance the head and neck should be rotated either passively or actively so that the examiner can adequately check all positions.

WHAT TO EXAMINE WITH

Few specialized instruments are needed for the examination of the head, face, and neck. This area does, of course, include the eyes, ears, and other special features, but the instruments for their examination will be discussed separately. A stethoscope will sometimes be used for auscultating *bruits;* a Wood's lamp may be needed for evaluating the scalp; a flashlight with a rubber cuff attachment will be used at times for transillumination; and a tape measure will be important for measuring head circumference.

WHAT TO EXAMINE FOR

The examiner will want to first observe the head and face for symmetry, paralysis, weaknesses, head shape, and movement. Often this can be done when the child cries, laughs, or wrinkles the forehead. Symmetry is usually regained in the newborn period by the end of the first week. Small, rounded depressions in the frontal and parietal bones are a normal result of the birth process and should disappear soon after birth. Any prominent bulges or swelling should be observed and felt for size, location, and density. Frontal bulges are known as *bossing* in infants. This may be the first indication of rickets or syphilis. *Cephalohematoma* (bleeding below the periosteum of the skull bones) is normally restricted to one bone, unless it is associated with a skull fracture. *Caput succedaneum* (edema of the scalp) generally crosses the suture lines. Prominent foreheads sometimes seen in children may be a sign of Hurler's syndrome or rickets. The shape of the head may be long or broad, or may assume a squashed appearance. Some races are noted for specific head shapes. For example, members of the Nordic race are characterized by long heads. The head shape must be observed from all angles. The examiner must look at it from the front, the sides, and the top; otherwise, a flat occiput may be missed. Prematurity will sometimes be the cause of long, narrow heads in children. Premature closing of the suture lines may cause many abnormal shapes, depending on which sutures close. The child may present with *oxycephaly, scaphocephaly, plagiocephaly* or *trigonocephaly.* Any indication of premature closure of the sutures must be thoroughly investigated, since the first 2 years of a child's life are vital for brain growth. The size of the head is extremely important in infancy and childhood and should be a routine part of every examination. Head size changes proportionally throughout life (see Fig. 5-5). The normal head size is between 32 and 38 cm at birth, the average being around 34 cm.[1] In the infant the head is generally 2 cm larger than the chest. However, during childhood the head is generally 5 to 7 cm smaller than the chest. The head is measured with a metal or paper tape measure (cloth has a tendency to stretch and give an inaccurate reading). The measurement is taken around the greatest circumference, with the tape placed over the occipital protuberance and midforehead (see Fig. 5-6). As can be seen from Figure 5-5, a single measurement can be meaningless. It is important to obtain a series of measurements to ascertain that growth is occurring at the proper rate.

Heads are generally measured at every visit until the child is 2 years old. Any sudden increase or failure to increase at the rate predicted by the graph should be explored immediately. Some terms in describing head size are:

[1] Gerhard Nellhaus, "Head Circumference from Birth to Eighteen Years," *Pediatrics,* vol. 41, no. 1, pt. 1, pp. 106–133, 1968.

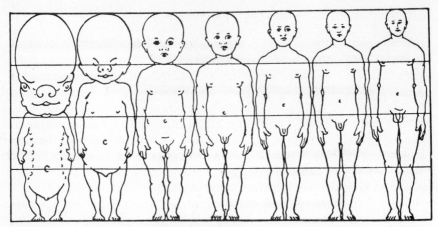

Figure 5-5 The Stratz chart of proportional size. (*From Stratz, modified by Robbins et al, Growth, Yale University Press, 1928. Original source, C.M. Jackson in Morris, Human Anatomy, 5th ed., P. Blakiston's Son and Co., Philadelphia, 1914*).

normocephalic (normal-size head), *microcephalic* (small-size head for body size and age), *macrocephalic* (large-size head for body size and age), and *hydrocephalic* (indicating excessive fluid in the cranial cavity). The examiner must observe and feel the fontanels in infants. Infants are born with six fontanels, but generally only two are easily palpated: the anterior and the posterior. A third fontanel may be normal but should be further investigated; it may occur along the sagittal suture betwen the anterior and posterior fontanels. The anterior fontanel may be small or absent at birth and then enlarges to an average of 2.5 by 2.5 cm. Ninety-seven percent will close between 9 and 19 months of age. Early closure is not a reason for concern so long as head growth is proceeding normally. Late closure may be due to cretinism, rickets, syphilis, Down's syndrome, osteogenesis imperfecta, or hydrocephalus, and these possibilities must be investigated. The posterior fontanel, which is often not palpable at birth, averages 1 by 1 cm. It will close by 1 to 2 months of life. Fontanels are observed for their number and position and for their bulging, flattened, or sunken appearance. They are palpated for size, pulsations, and tenseness. The size should be recorded by both dimensions, not just "anterior fontanel 2 cm," but "anterior fontanel 2 by 3 cm." Pictures may be helpful. Slight pulsation of the fontanels is within normal range, but definite, great pulsations may be an indication of intracranial pressure and should be investigated thoroughly.

The scalp is observed and palpated for sutures, scaliness, infections, and hair. Sutures may appear as prominent ridges at birth because of the overriding of the edges during the delivery. These usually flatten by 6 months. Some infants have wide spaces along the suture lines, giving the impression of very large fontanels. Cranial margins adjacent to these

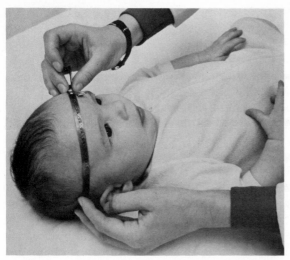

Figure 5-6 Placement of measuring tape when measuring the head circumference.

sutures can be appreciably depressed by palpation in many normal infants. An osseous ridge may be palpable along the sagittal and metopic suture lines. Although they do not actually close until adult life, suture lines should not be palpable after 5 or 6 months of age. The coronal, sagittal, and lambdoidal sutures are normal breaks in the skull, any other ridges or breaks may indicate fractures. In American Indian children however, there may be one additional horizontal suture in the occipital bone.

The scalp should not be dry or flaky. In an infant this is usually an indication of cradle cap. As the examiner's fingers palpate each area of scalp, they should feel for the occipital lymph nodes. These usually are present only with infections of the scalp, roseola infantum, or rubella. The hair is observed for color, texture, distribution, amount, and presence of nits or pediculi. Hair can be any one of a number of colors, but the color should be faily even throughout the hair strand. Children with a white streak of hair running from their forehead towards the crown of their head may have Waardenburg's syndrome and should be carefully evaluated for deafness. Children with kwashiorkor (protein deficiency disease) may display patches of reddish, coarse hair throughout their regular hair color. Generalized malnutrition may result in dry, gray hair. There is little or no hair pigment in children with albinism. Hair should have a smooth, fine texture. If it is brittle and chopped looking, hypothyroidism or ringworm may be present. It should be evenly distributed over the entire scalp, beginning with a hairline at the forehead and going to the nape of the neck. Normal children of certain racial backgrounds and some with such syndromes as Hurler's syndrome or cretinism have hairlines beginning midforehead and excessive hair. *Alopecia* (bald spots) may be familial or due to ringworm. It may also be a sign of hair pulling, an indication of serious emotional problems. All of an infant's hair is often replaced by 3 months of age; the new hair is usually of a darker color. Bald spots over the occiput may appear if an infant has been lying in the crib, face up, for extended periods of time.

The head is observed for control, position, and movement. Control comes with age; most infants have some head lag as they are pulled to a sitting position until about 3 months. Control is attained gradually, but should be almost complete by 3 months. If much head lag remains at this age, the nurse should be suspicious of an abnormality. This may be the first sign of cerebral palsy or other neuromuscular deficit. Children should be observed for the position they hold their head in while in a resting position. If it is constantly held at an angle, *torticollis* or hearing or vision difficulties should be suspected. Movement is also important. Passive range of motion must be done for the infant, but the older child can follow a toy or bright light so that the examiner can evaluate the full movement. The head should move easily and smoothly from left to right and towards the ceiling and floor. Any jerking, tremors, or inability to move in one direction must be investigated.

The face is observed for the spacing of the features, symmetry, paralysis, skin color, and skin texture. Looking at the child, face to face, the examiner should be able to note eyes set at the same level, nostrils of the same size, lips equal on both sides of the midline, and ears set at the same level on both sides of the head. There will normally be slight differences in each side, but any major differences are important to note. Eyes that are at the same level but very wide set are called *hypertelorism. Hypotelorism* is the condition in which the eyes are set unusually close together. Any clefts or dimples are also noted at this time.

The skin should be a good color and smooth over the entire face; there should be no pallor, cyanosis, or jaundice. The examiner must also turn the child's head to each side to evaluate symmetry and spacing of features. Normally the top of the pinna of the ears crosses an imaginary line drawn from the lateral corner of the eye to the most prominent protuberance of the occiput; referred to as the eye-occiput line. Ears that do not cross the line are said to be low set and must be investigated since this is often associated with mental retardation or kidney abnormalities. From the side, the child's chin can also be checked. Infants normally have very little chin; however, a marked decrease in chin, called *micrognathia,* is abnormal and must be investigated promptly, since the child may have breathing difficulties if the tongue falls backward and blocks the nasopharynx area. The cheeks should be palpated for tone and muscle strength. Infants normally have very fat, well-developed cheeks for sucking. If hyperirritability, tetany, or hyperventilation are suspected, *Chvostek's sign* can be elicited by tapping the cheek just below the zygomatic bone. The sign is positive if that side of the face shows a grimace. It is present in children normally under 1 month of age.

As the examiner finishes the head and face, he or she should move on to the neck. The neck is also observed for symmetry, size, shape, control of movement, and pulsation; it is palpated for pulsations, strength, and position of the trachea and thyroid. The neck should be symmetrical from all angles. It is normally short in infants and difficult to see, but if the shoulders are supported, the head may be tilted back and forth for a look at its symmetry and size. Posteriorly the neck should be checked for *webbing*—the presence of loose, extra folds of skin. These are often associated with certain syndromes and should be investigated further.

Movement and control may be checked by rotating the head in all directions. As the head turns to the right, it is important to palpate along the left sternocleidomastoid muscle for strength, tone, and presence of any hematomas. By turning the head to the left, the procedure is repeated along the right sternocleidomastoid. Strength in the neck can be tested in older children by having the child look over the right shoulder while the examiner attempts to force the face to rotate forward. This is repeated with the child looking over the left shoulder.

Excessive pulsations observed and palpated in the neck may be signs of cardiac problems. The neck is also palpated for the location of the trachea, which should be felt as a series of cartilaginous rings. It should be midline, descending towards the sternum. In the infant this can be done only by supporting the shoulders and head and tilting the head back to expose the short neck area. The thyroid can be palpated as a firm, smooth mass which moves upward with swallowing. It is difficult to palpate in infants and is often not felt in normal adults. It may be palpated with the examiner in front of or behind the child. From the front the examiner has the child flex the head forward slightly while using one hand to palpate along both sides of the trachea. From behind, the examiner places two or three fingers of both hands on either side of the trachea below the thyroid cartilage. In either case, the trachea is first palpated from the top to the bottom noting the hyoid, circoid, and thyroid cartilages. The thyroid isthmus is then located slightly below the thyroid cartilage. Using it as a landmark, the examiner's fingers are then moved to one side and downward. The examiner's hand then palpates behind the sternocleidomastoid and pushes inward and toward the trachea holding the thyroid lobe on that side steady; the other hand is then inserted behind the other sternocleidomastoid and palpates that thyroid lobe against the first hand which supplies a steadying effect. The procedure is then repeated on the opposite side. In rare instances the thyroid can be auscultated for bruit.

The above are procedures normally done in examining the head, face, and neck. There are several procedures that can also be done if the examiner suspects certain conditions. They are not normally done at each examination. *Craniotabes* is the softening of the outer layer of the skull. Premature infants or children with rickets, syphilis, hypervitaminosis A, and hydrocephaly will display craniotabes, that is, a ping-pong snapping sensation of the scalp when the examiner's fingers are firmly pressed behind and above the ears in the temporoparietal region along the suture lines. This can also be present in normal children up to 3 months of age.

Children with increased intracranial pressure will domonstrate Macewen's sign, a resonant, cracked-pot sound heard when the finger is used to percuss the skull. In an infant with an open fontanel, this sound is normal, but once the fontanels are closed the sound is indicative of a pathologic condition.

Children suspected of having intracranial lesions, hydrocephalus, or decreased brain tissue should have their skulls transilluminated. A special rubber ring is fitted to a flashlight for the procedure. The room must be completely darkened as the rubber ring of the flashlight is pressed firmly against the skull. A small ring of light extending beyond the rubber edge is normal, but any increased area of light around the edges denotes abnormality. Normal transillumination is 1 cm in the occipital area to 2 cm in the frontoparietal area. Infants with anencephaly will transmit the light placed at the occiput through the eyes. The flashlight must be moved over the skull covering both sides, front and back.

BIBLIOGRAPHY

Alexander, M., and M. Brown: "Physical Examination: The Head, Face and Neck," *Nursing '74,* vol. 4, no. 1, pp. 47–50, January 1974.
Mechner, Francis: "Patient Assessment—Examination of the Head and Neck," *American Journal of Nursing,* vol. 75, no. 5, pp. 1–24, May 1975.

GLOSSARY

alopecia   lack of hair in spots that normally have hair
anterior vertebral muscle   a deep muscle of the neck that aids in sidewise movement
atlas   the first cervical vertebra supporting the cranium
axis   the second cervical vertebra forming a pivot for the atlas and cranium
bossing   the rounded bulges, as of the frontal bones of the cranium
bruits   abnormal sounds heard during auscultation of certain parts of the body, for example, the thyroid or cranium
caput succedaneum   the clear fluid trapped under the scalp, but on top of the pericranium and not confined to one bone
cephalhematoma   a soft, fluctuating mass of blood trapped beneath the pericranium and confined to one bone
Chvostek's sign   a facial grimace elicited when the zygomatic bone is tapped
coronal suture   the space separating the frontal from the parietal bones of the skull and interrupted by the anterior fontanel

craniotabes a softening of the outer layer of the skull

epicranium the skin, muscles, and fasciae of the scalp

ethmoid bone one of the 14 facial bones

fontanels unossified membranous intervals of the infant skull

hydrocephalic excessive fluid in the cranial cavity

hypertelorism wide-set eyes, with a broad flat nasal bridge

hypotelorism close-set eyes, with a small nasal bridge

infrahyoid muscle one of the deep muscles of the neck controlling sideway movements

lacrimal bone one of the 14 facial bones

lambdoidal suture the suture separating the parietal bones from the occipital bones and interrupted by the posterior fontanel

lateral vertebral muscle one of the deep muscles of the neck aiding in sideway movements

Macewen's sign a resonant,cracked-pot sound heard when the finger is used to percuss the skull of a child with increased intracranial pressure

macrocephalic designating a large-sized head for body size and age

mandible the one movable facial bone which forms the lower portion of the oral cavity

maxilla the bone forming the upper portion of the oral cavity

microcephalic designating a small-sized head for body size and age

micrognathia an abnormally tiny mandibular bone

normocephalic designating a normal-sized head

oxycephaly a dome-shaped head caused by the coronal sutures closing prematurely

parathyroid glands flat, oval endocrine glands located on the dorsal borders of the thyroid gland

parathyroid hormone a hormone secreted by the parathyroid glands and needed for calcium metabolism

pericranium the periosteum covering the cranium

plagiocephaly a deformity of the skull due to irregular sutures which cause the cranium to assume a twisted, asymmetrical shape

platysma muscle the superficial cervical muscle attaching below the clavicle and running towards the mandible, necessary for opening the jaws

sagittal suture the suture dividing the right from the left parietal bone with the anterior fontanel on the anterior end and the posterior fontanel at the posterior end

scaphocephaly a narrow, long cranium due to early closure of the sagittal suture

sphenoid bone one of the 14 facial bones

suprahyoid muscle one of the deep muscles of the neck aiding in sideway movement

suture a closure or juncture between bones, as of the head or skull

torticollis asymmetry of the neck muscles causing the head to be tilted to one side

trigonocephaly a flattened frontal skull bone giving the head a flat anterior shape

vomer bone one of the 14 facial bones

webbing the loose, extra folds of skin seen in the posterior neck area

zygomatic bone one of the 14 facial bones forming the upper cheek area

Inspection of the Head, Face, and Neck*

Head	Yes	No	Not appli-cable	Describe (where appropriate)	Significance
A. Size					
1. Large (macrocephaly)					May be normal variant; may indicate hydrocephaly; needs consecutive head measurements graphed against normal.
2. Small (microcephaly)					May be normal variant or microcephaly; again needs to be graphed against normal variant; microcephaly often associated with mental retardation; may indicate cranial stenosis.
3. Normal					
B. Shape					
1. Normal					
2. Long					May be racial variant of Nordic races; also common in prematures; may indicate cranial stenosis.
3. Broad					May indicate cranial stenosis.
4. Symmetrical					Symmetry usually attained by the end of the first week; before that molding is prominent in a normal infant of vaginal delivery.
5. Prominent bulges					Small, rounded depressions in frontal and parietal bones result from vaginal deliveries and disappear in about a week; cephalohematoma, caput succedaneum also common in newborns.
6. Prominent forehead					May be present in syndromes such as Hurler's; "bossing" may be the first indication of rickets or syphilis.
C. Hair					
1. Distribution normal					
2. Low hairline in back					Often present in children with cretinism or Hurler's syndrome; also common in certain races such as Mexican-American.

3. Low hairline in front		
4. Amount		
a. thin		May be present in malnutrition or hypothyroidism; may be normal variant.
b. thick		Usually a normal variant.
c. alopecia		May be due to hair pulling, ringworm, or familial traits.
d. normal		
5. Color		
a. even		Normal.
b. white streak		Sometimes a normal variant, but can be a sign of Waardenburg's syndrome.
c. reddish tips		May indicate malnutrition.
D. Scalp		
1. Nits		Require treatment and education.
2. Pediculi		Same as above.
3. Flaky		May indicate beginning seborrhea or dandruff.
4. Dry		May need change of shampoo or less frequent washing.
5. Oily		Same as above.
6. Dandruff		Same as above.
7. Other		

*These charts are meant to be used by beginning students as they perform their first physical assessments. Each item should be examined on the child and then checked off on the checklist. The significance of the items follows in the right-hand column.

75

Inspection of the Head, Face, and Neck (*Continued*)

Face	Yes	No	Not appli- cable	Describe (where appropriate)	Significance
A. General shape					
1. Symmetrical					Symmetricality expected by about 1 week.
2. Moonface					May indicate adrenal problems.
3. Paralysis					May indicate neurological or muscular problems.
B. Bones and muscles					
1. Muscle atrophy or absence					May indicate neurological or muscular pathology.
2. Muscle hypertrophy					Same as above.
3. Enlarged bones (acromegaly)					May indicate acromegaly.
4. Receding chin					May be familiar; common in newborns, but excessive degree may indi- cate Pierre-Robin syndrome.
5. Other					
C. Skin					
1. Color					
a. cyanosis					Same significance as elsewhere; area around lips is a common place to see cyanosis.
b. ruddiness					Same significance as elsewhere.
c. pallor					Same significance as elsewhere.
d. jaundice					Same significance as elsewhere.
e. hyperpigmentation					Same significance as elsewhere; port wine stain likely in this area.
f. vitiligo					Same significance as elsewhere.
g. other					

2. Lesions			
a. birthmarks			Strawberry marks, port wine stain, stork bites all common here.
b. milia			Common and normal particularly during first month.
c. scars			Necessitates history taking for etiology.
d. acne			Indicates need for treatment, education, and possibly referral.
e. other			
3. Edema			Same significance as elsewhere.
a. general			Fluid retention.
b. periorbital			In infants, edema commonly begins here.
4. Dry			May indicate need for lotion, cream, or less bathing; may be variant of normal; can indicate hyperthyroidism.
5. Oily			May need more frequent cleansing.
6. Texture smooth			Irregularities should be noted.
7. Other			
D. Facial features: general placement			
1. Symmetrical			Features are generally not completely symmetrical but if striking differences are noted, then investigate possible paralysis.
2. Wide set eyes			May indicate cranial deformities; often associated with mental retardation syndrome; may be a variant of normal.
3. Narrow set eyes			May be a variant of normal or associated with cranial bone deformity.
4. Ear pinna crosses eye occiput line			Pinnas falling completely below this line usually indicate renal problems or mental retardation.
5. Ear attachment less than 10°			Same as above.
6. Other			

Inspection of the Head, Face, and Neck (*Continued*)

Face	Yes	No	Not appli-cable	Describe (where appropriate)	Significance
E. Specific facial features					
1. Lips full and symmetrical					Usually normal.
2. Bushy eyebrows					Can be familial or racial variant (such as Mexican-American); also associated with syndromes such as Hurler's.
3. Scant eyelashes					Common in prematures; absent outer two-thirds found in Treacher-Collins syndrome.
4. Brows meet in middle					Same as 2.
5. Epicanthic folds					Common in Orientals; 5 percent of Caucasians have this which is generally outgrown by age 10; is also associated with Down's syndrome.
6. Mongolian folds (epiblepharon)					Normal racial variant in Orientals.
7. Other					
Neck					
A. General					
1. Size					
a. long					Neck is generally quite short in infants, gradually increasing in length.
b. short					
2. Shape					
a. webbing					Webbing may occur in a number of mental retardation syndromes.
b. visible bulging thyroid					Visible thyroid is almost always enlarged.

c. visible bulging on muscles			Bulging especially on the sternocleidomastoids often indicates a hematoma although other tumors or masses are possible.
d. visible tilting of head			Children often tilt their heads if vision in one eye is bad or if one sternocleidomastoid muscle is abnormally short.
3. Symmetrical from all angles			Major asymmetry requires further investigation.
B. Skin			
1. Color normal			Same significance as elsewhere.
2. Markings			Same significance as elsewhere.
3. Other			
C. Underlying Muscles, Bones, and Other Structures			
1. Masses or cysts			Can be benign or cancerous, need further investigations.
2. Excessive pulsations			May indicate cardiac problems.
3. Trachea midline			Asymmetricality indicates abnormal underlying pressure or adhesions.
4. Visible cricoid cartilage			Normal variant, particularly in adolescent boys.
5. Visible thyroid cartilage			Same as above.
6. Visible thyroid gland			Visible thyroid gland is almost always enlarged.
7. Visible lymph gland			Indicates enlargement.
8. Visible sternocleidomastoid muscle			Normal, particularly when turning head.
9. Other			

79

Palpation of the Head, Face, and Neck

Face	Yes	No	Not applicable	Describe (where appropriate)	Significance
A. Hair					
1. Coarse					May indicate hypothyroidism.
2. Brittle					Same as above.
3. Other					
B. Scalp					May be a normal variant.
1. Oily					Usually a normal variant; indicates need for more frequent or different kind of shampoo.
2. Dry					Usually a normal variant; indicates need for less frequent or different kind of shampoo; also occurs with hypothyroidism.
3. Other					
C. Palpable lymph nodes					
1. Occipital					Usually indicates present or past infection of the scalp, roseola, or rubella.
2. Postauricular					Usually indicates infection of the ear, mastoid, or scalp.
D. Fontanels					
1. Anterior–opened					Expected to close between 9 and 19 months of age; early closure is a concern only if head growth stops. Late closure may indicate cretinism, syphilis, rickets, hydrocephalus, Down's syndrome, or other problems.
closed					
size					Size and shape vary considerably in the normal child.
shape					

2. Posterior—opened		Expected to close by 1–2 months of age; significance of early or late closure is same as above.
closed		
size		
shape		
3. Third fontanel—size		Located along saggital suture between anterior and posterior fontanels; may be a normal variant but is also commonly present in Down's syndrome.
shape		
E. Sutures		
1. Coronal		
a. overriding		Should not be palpable after 5–6 months; may be overriding at birth or may have a marked gap between them.
b. wide		
c. closed		
2. Saggital		
a. overriding		Same as above.
b. wide		
c. closed		
d. other		
3. Lamboidal		
a. overriding		Same as 1.
b. wide		
c. closed		
d. other		

81

Palpation of the Head, Face, and Neck (*Continued*)

Face	Yes	No	Not appli-cable	Describe (where appropriate)	Significance
A. Skin					
1. Normal texture					Same significance as elsewhere.
2. Nodules, cysts, etc.					
3. Other					
B. Normal bone and muscle contours					Same significance as under inspection.
C. Sinus tenderness					
1. Frontal					May indicate sinusitis.
2. Maxillary					Same as 1.
D. Lymph nodes					
1. Preauricular					May indicate present or past infection of ear or scalp.
2. Tonsillar					May indicate present or past infection of mouth or teeth or ear or scalp.
Neck					
A. Skin					
1. Normal texture					Same significance as elsewhere.
2. Palpable masses					
B. Neck structure					
1. Cricoid cartilage palpable					Normal.
2. Thyroid cartilage palpable					Normal; much larger in adolescent males.

3. Hyoid bone palpable				Normal.
4. Thyroid isthmus palpable				Can be normal but may indicate enlargement.
5. Thyroid lobes palpable				May be normally palpable but can indicate enlargement.
6. Thyroid lobes enlarged				Enlargement can be from hypo- or hyperthyroidism.
7. Sternocleidomastoid a. symmetrical				Torticollis may cause asymmetricality.
b. equal length bilaterally				Same as above.
c. masses				May be any tumor or mass, but in an infant, it is commonly a hematoma from the birth process.
8. Lymph nodes a. submandibular				May indicate infection from mouth, throat, face.
b. submental (or submaxillary)				Same as above.
c. superficial cervical chain				Same, may indicate infection from ear, scalp, face, mouth or throat.
d. deep cervical chain				Same as above.
e. supraclavicular				May indicate infection including cancer from breasts.

83

Percussion of the Head, Face, and Neck

Head, Face, and Neck	Yes	No	Not applicable	Describe (where appropriate)	Significance
1. Macewen's sign ("cracked pot" sign)					Normal if child still has open fontanels; otherwise, may indicate fracture.
2. Sinus tenderness					Sinusitis.

Auscultation of the Head, Face, and Neck

Head, Face, and Neck	Yes	No	Not applicable	Describe (where appropriate)	Significance
1. Bruits in the skull					Sometimes a normal variant, but can indicate underlying vascular problems.
2. Bruits in the neck					May indicate underlying vascular problems.

Source: These checklists are printed with permission from Blue Hill Videotape Incorporated and are part of a more complete programmed learning approach to the physical examination, which includes a workbook and series of videotapes. The materials can be purchased from Blue Hill Educational Systems, Inc., 52 South Main Street, Spring Valley, New York 10977.

Chapter 6

The Eyes

WHY THE CHILD IS EXAMINED

A careful eye examination is an important part of every physical. The eye is obviously a vital part of the human body and the practitioner will discover that every parent shows particular concern over the health of their child's eyes. Many parental questions will focus on this area for both cosmetic and health reasons. Will my baby's eyes stay this shade of blue? Will these folds over my baby's eyes go away? Can my child see well? Are my child's eyes healthy? All are common questions which the nurse will encounter frequently. The eye examination is also important because the eyes will frequently give the nurse clues as to the general and systemic health of the child. The color of the sclera may be the clue that makes the nurse further investigate the possibility of liver disease, osteogenesis imperfecta, or certain other diseases. The shininess of the child's eyes can also be important to a general assessment of his or her health. A very careful and thorough ocular examination, then, is a necessary part of the health evaluation of every child the nurse sees.

WHAT TO EXAMINE: ANATOMY OF THE AREA

For purposes of study, the eye can be divided into the eye proper and its surrounding structures: the ocular orbit, muscles controlling movement, eyebrows, eyelids, eyelashes, tarsal glands, conjunctiva, and lacrimal apparatus (see Fig. 6-1).

The eye is situated in the orbit which is a bony cavity formed by the bones of the upper face (palatine, lacrimal, zygomatic, sphenoid, ethmoid, maxillary, and frontal bones); it is cushioned with fat for extra protection. There are 7 ocular muscles to control the movement of the eye. The levator palpebrae superior is a thick, long muscle which attaches behind the eyeball and stretches anteriorly to the eyelid; it raises the upper eyelid. The rectus superior, rectus inferior, rectus medialis, and rectus lateralis surround the eyeball on all four sides joining at the posterior portion of the eye. They act singly to move the corneal surface in different directions. The obliquus superior runs parallel to the levator palpebrae and acts as a pulley as it attaches to the bulb of the eye. The obliquus inferior is small and thin, attaches near the sclera, and runs across the other muscles. Both the obliquus superior and obliquus inferior work in refining the movements of the recti muscles.

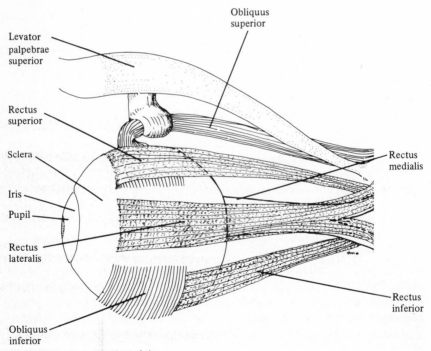

Figure 6-1 The muscles of the eye.

The eyebrows are arched prominences above the eye orbit, which consist of thickened skin and many thick short hairs. It is moved in various directions by the orbicularis oculi, corrugator, and frontalis muscles.

The eye is also protected by the two eyelids which are narrow, moveable layers of skin, areolar tissue, glandular fibers, conjunctiva, and muscle. The lower lid is smaller, contains no muscle layer, and is less mobile than the upper lid; the upper lid is large and contains the levator palpebrae superioris muscle for upward movement. The elliptical space left by the open eyelids is called the *palpebral fissure.*

Eyelashes are thick, curved hairs connected to the moveable edges of the eyelids, which add further protection for the surface of the eye. The hairs may be long or short and arranged in double or triple rows; they are surrounded by modified sudoriferous glands called *ciliary glands.*

Embedded in the connective tissue of the lids on the posterior surface are *meibomian glands* (modified sebaceous glands).

The conjunctiva is a mucous membrane lining the eyelids and portions of the sclera. It is composed of two parts: the palpebral portion and the bulbar portion. The palpebral portion lines the eyelids and is thick, opaque, vascular, and covered by many papillae; the bulbar portion lies loosely over the sclera and is thin and clear, containing no papillae and very few blood vessels.

The lacrimal apparatus consists of the lacrimal glands, lacrimal ducts, lacrimal sac, and *nasolacrimal duct.* The *lacrimal gland* is the size of a large peanut and similar in structure to the serous salivary glands; it is lodged in the lacrimal fossa of the frontal bone where its function is to secrete tears. Each eyelid also contains one lacrimal sac, and one nasolacrimal duct (see Fig. 6-2).

The eye proper sometimes called the *eye bulb,* is composed of three layers: (1) the outer, fibrous layer containing the anterior cornea and the posterior sclera; (2) the vascular, pigmented tunic containing the choroid, ciliary body, and *iris*; and (3) the inner nervous tunic containing the *retina.* The outer layer makes up a large part of the eye proper. Its cornea is thin, transparent, and convex; it forms the anterior one-sixth of the covering, and is a five-layered membrane. The thick, tough, opaque, nonelastic membrane covering the remaining five-sixths of the eye is the sclera. Muscles are inserted into the scleral surface. The vascular layer is composed of choroid, ciliary body, and iris. The choroid lies in the posterior five-sixths of the eye with the optic nerve penetrating it. It is a deep chocolate color, thin, and highly vascular. The ciliary body is a thick, vascular surface extending from the posterior optic nerve opening to the sclerocorneal junction. The ciliaris muscle attaches to the ciliary body and is the major muscle in accommodation. The iris is the colored, round, contractile disk suspended in the aqueous humor between the cornea and the *lens.* It contains four layers and

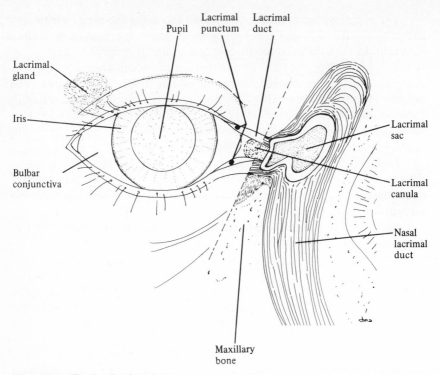

Figure 6-2 The lacrimal system

the center is perforated to form the pupil. The color of the iris is determined by the amount of pigment present and its distribution within the layered membrane (see Fig. 6-3).

The inner layer of the eye is divided into a posterior portion containing many nerves and an anterior portion containing no nerves. The retina proper is the most important structure of the posterior inner layer. It forms the *optic nerve* which receives the images from external objects. It is soft, semitransparent, made up of ten layers and contains *rhodopsin* (or visual purple) which gives it a lavendar color. The *macula* is an oval yellowish area at the exact center of the posterior retina. The *fovea centralis* is the central depression in the macula, the area where vision is most perfect. The optic nerve exits through the optic disk, which is located 3 mm to the medial side of the macula; the blind spot of the retina is the depressed center of this optic disk (see Fig. 6-4).

The anterior, nonnervous portions are called the *pars ciliaris retinae* and the *pars iridica retinae.*

There are five structures for refraction within the eye proper: the *cornea, aqueous humor, vitreous body, zonula ciliaris,* and *crystalline lens.* [The cornea has already been discussed.] The aqueous humor is an alkaline watery fluid secreted by the ciliary process which fills the anterior and

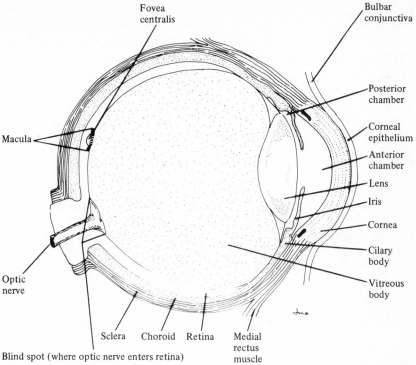

Figure 6-3 A cross section of the eye.

Labels: Fovea centralis, Bulbar conjunctiva, Posterior chamber, Corneal epithelium, Anterior chamber, Lens, Iris, Cornea, Cilary body, Vitreous body, Macula, Optic nerve, Blind spot (where optic nerve enters retina), Sclera, Choroid, Retina, Medial rectus muscle

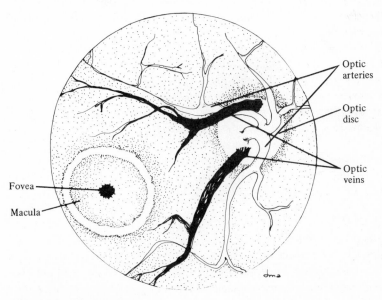

Figure 6-4 The retina.

Labels: Optic arteries, Optic disc, Optic veins, Fovea, Macula

posterior chambers of the eyeball. The vitreous body is a transparent semi-gelatinous substance filling the main cavity of the eye; the retina and ciliary processes maintain its nutritional balance. The zonula ciliaris (or suspensory ligament of the lens) attaches the ciliary body to the lens by several fibers, which helps to position the lens and change its shape. The crystalline lens is a transparent, soft cortical body, biconvex in shape, which is suspended between the suspensory ligaments; it is contained within a thick, transparent elastic membrane called the capsule.

HOW TO EXAMINE AND WHAT TO EXAMINE FOR

The primary method of examination used in evaluating the eye is inspection. In both the external and internal parts of the eye, the nurse's observational skills are the single most valuable tool. Palpation of the eye is also important and may reveal certain conditions of the eye more readily than will inspection. Auscultation is not used frequently, but may be important for detecting bruits. Percussion is not generally used in examining the eye. Some specific methods of examination, such as the cover test and ophthalmoscopic examination, will be described in more detail later in this chapter.

There should be a definite system in examining the eye. The nurse may begin with the lids. The eyelids are carefully inspected and palpated (see Fig. 6-5). They are examined for *ptosis* or drooping of the lid. Ptosis may be congenital and acquired. Congenital ptosis is often inherited, and a family history should be taken. Some babies are born with ptosis; frequently this type of ptosis disappears with maturation, but any infant with ptosis should

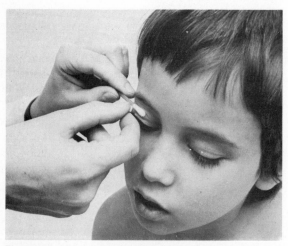

Figure 6-5   The lid being everted for inspection.

be examined for the jaw-winking reflex or *Marcus Gunn phenomenon*. In this reflex, moving the jaw to one side results in the child raising the opposite eyelid. In infants, sucking may cause this same response. This type of ptosis may be due to paralysis of the superior rectus muscle or to oculomotor nerve damage.

Acquired ptosis may occur in several conditions, such as polio, encephalitis, meningitis, pineal tumors, Horner's syndrome, or myasthenia gravis. Whatever the cause, it is important for the nurse to make certain that the ptosis does not obstruct the child's vision in one eye (it should not cover the pupil), since this can cause *amblyopia* (loss of vision in the covered eye) in the same way that strabismus does. *Pseudoptosis* is a type of ptosis caused by the weight of the upper lid, ususally due to edema.

The upper lid should also be examined for *retraction*. If the nurse finds that the upper lid does not cover the usual area of the globe (or eyeball), she must discover why. It may be that the globe is protruding, as in exopthalmus or advanced hydrocephalus, where the sclera is exposed above the iris and there is a downward displacement of the iris and pupil. Hyperthyroidism may also be accompanied by a widened palpebral fissure due to retraction of the lids. This results in a wide-eyed staring expression. The examiner must also ascertain that the lids are long enough to cover the eye. *Lagophthalmos* (lids which do not close entirely) may result from facial nerve paralysis or from a congenitally shortened muscle. Whatever the cause, if the cornea or bulbar conjunctiva remains exposed, a consultation should be sought, since this may result in damage to the exposed portion of the eye due to dust or other environmental irritants.

Blepharospasm (excessive blinking) is another situation which may be encountered in the examination of the eye. This may be due to a tic or habit or may be a sign of eyestrain or irritation.

Strabismus (squinting) should be noted, and where it occurs, a thorough visual examination is imperative.

Upward slanting of the eyes may be indicative of Down's syndrome, while the opposite (downward) kind of slanting may be indicative of Treacher Collins syndrome (see Fig. 6-6). (This may also be accompanied by a notched lower lid called a *coloboma*).

The *setting sun expression* in which sclera is exposed above the iris may be elicited by rapidly lowering the infant from a sitting to a supine position. This sign may be present in some normal full-term infants and in many premature infants. Children with hydrocephalus and brainstem lesions may also exhibit this sign.

Many types of infections may be discovered while examining the eyelids. *Styes,* or *hordeola,* are inflammations of the sebaceous glands near the lashes. They can be painful, red, tender, and swollen. The immediate cause is almost always staphylococcal infection; however, when they recur

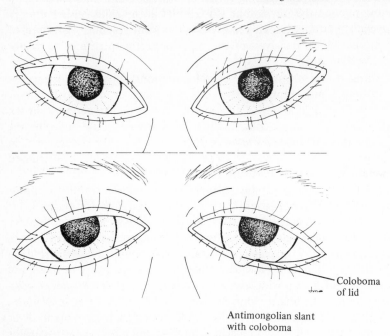

Mongolian slant

Coloboma of lid

Antimongolian slant with coloboma

Figure 6-6 Mongolian and antimongolian slants.

frequently, the clinician should look for an underlying reason, such as poor general health or poor vision which causes the child to irritate the lids by rubbing the eyes constantly.

Internal hordeolum is an acute inflammation of the Meilbomian glands, which causes pain in the upper lid. It is also usually caused by infection with staphylococci. If chronic it can result in a sensation of sandiness under the lid, and if the upper lid is everted, a vertical yellow line across the tarsus can be seen.

Chalazions are another frequent finding of the lids. They are granulomas of the internal sebaceous glands and tarsus. They consist of localized, nontender, firm, discrete swellings. These small, hard, slow-growing nodules are covered with freely moveable skin and are usually located on the bulbar part of the lid next to the tarsal plate. They produce no subjecttive symptoms, but they can often be palpated through the lid and can be seen as enlarged erythematous glands if the lid is everted.

Furuncles, or boils, are staphylococcal infections of the hair follicles while *carbuncles* are large loculated furuncles. Both are relatively common findings in this area of eyelids, eyelashes, and eyebrows.

Marginal blepharitis is another fairly common finding on the eyelids. It consists of red, scaly crusted lid edges. If this is caused by staphylococci, the scales will cling and leave open lesions if removed; pustules may form around the base of the lashes and the Meibomian glands may contain pus. If the blepharitis is part of a seborrheic dermatitis, the scars are waxy, greasy, and come off easily.

Eyelids must also be inspected for nits or lice. This condition, called *phthiriasis,* is usually caused by head lice, although pubic lice may occasionally be involved.

The lids must be examined for positional faults. There are two possible malpositions of the eyelids: (1) *ectropion,* or a rolling out of the lids, and (2) *entropion,* or a rolling in of the lids. Ectropion may be a result of scar tissue formation or of spastic or paralytic muscles. Whatever the cause, it usually requires surgical correction. The everted part of the lid develops a velvety red appearance and is accompanied by an *epiphora* (excess tearing) which frequently causes an eczematous reaction of the lower lid. Entropion, or turning in of the lid, can also be caused by scars or muscle spasticity (usually from inflammation). It is present normally in many Oriental children. It is harmless unless the lids scrape the cornea and cause abrasion (see Fig. 6-7).

Epicanthal folds are vertical folds of skin covering the inner canthus. They may be present in Oriental infants, and 20 percent of Caucasian newborns have them also. In 97 percent of Caucasian children the folds will disappear by 10 years of age. If they fail to disappear, surgery may be performed for cosmetic reasons. Epicanthal folds can also be a sign of Down's

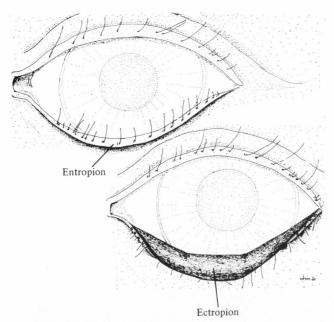

Entropion

Ectropion

Figure 6-7 The eye with ectropion and entropion.

syndrome, hypercalcemia, glycogen storage disease, or renal agenesis. This type of fold is quite different from a Mongolian fold, or *epiblepharon,* which is a horizontal fold in the upper lid, overhanging the superior tarsus. This fold is normal in Asiatic and is found occasionally in Caucasian children. It will generally disappear by the end of the first year. The nurse must be sure, however, that it does not rub the cornea.

Edema of the lids must also be noted; it may indicate hyperthyroidism, ethmoid sinusitis, measles, infectious mononucleosis, nephritis, nephrosis, chronic upper respiratory infections, sinusitis, or allergies.

The eyelashes of the child must be examined. A lack of pigment may indicate *albinism.* Lashes which are absent on the inner two-thirds of the lid may be seen in children with Treacher Collins syndrome. They may be particularly bushy in Hurler's syndrome or absent in premature infants.

The lacrimal apparatus, including glands and ducts, must also be assessed. Enough lacrimal fluid for tearing is not usually present until the third month of life or later, but if the lacrimal duct is not patent, the minimal lacrimal fluid present in the young infant may overflow into tears. For this reason, excess tearing before the age of 3 months must be further investigated. Such a blockage can be caused by an accumulation of debris or by a thin congenital membrane covering the punctum. The parent of such an infant should be taught to massage the infant with each feeding, exerting pressure with her index finger directly under the punctum and then sweeping the finger down and out of the general area of the gland. If no results are obtained by 6 months, the punctum is probably covered by a thin membrane and will need to be probed. If the blockage was caused by an accumulation of debris, the massage will usually unplug the duct. The clinician must be very careful in this situation, however, since a clogged lacrimal duct predisposes a child to infection of the lacrimal sac (*dacryocystitis*). This will be manifested by swelling and redness below the inner canthus; by local conjunctivitis; by a turbid, yellow secretion; and at times by a palpable mass. In this situation, massage is contraindicated since it may spread the infection.

Other conditions that may be encountered in the lacrimal apparatus are disorders of tearing. *Dysautonomia* is a condition in which tears are produced in inadequate amounts. Epiphora, or excessive tearing, may result from an allergy or inflammation, a foreign body, a plugged lacrimal duct, or *exophthalmos.*

Dacryoadenitis, or inflammation of the lacrimal gland, may also be found. Usually, this is accompanied by pain within the temporal edge of the orbit, although it may be painless if it is chronic.

Next, the conjunctiva is examined. Both the palpebral and bulbar parts must be evaluated carefully. *Chemosis,* or edema of the conjunctiva, is encountered at times and is usually an indication of infection. Infections of the conjunctiva can be of many types, and a more thorough description of them will be found in a book on ophthalmology. Suffice it to say here that there are many different types of physical findings that may indicate *conjunctivitis*. The so-called cobblestone or ground glass appearance consists of enlarged follicles in the palpebral conjunctiva, which impart a bumpy appearance to the membrane. This can indicate allergic conjunctivitis. Conjunctivitis may also be suspected with highly erythematous palpebral and bulbar conjunctiva. Mucoid secretions or plaques on the bulbar conjunctiva may indicate similar problems.

The pallor of anemia can be reflected in the palpebral conjunctiva; and vitamin A deficiency may result in dryness and hyperemia of this area, sometimes accompanied by *Bitot's spots* (irregular yellows patches).

The *pinguecula,* if irritated from wind, sand, or other causes, may darken and begin to encroach on the iris and even into the pupil (see Fig. 6-8). This is called *pterygium.*

Next, the orbit of the eye must be assessed. Sunken, blank eyes are a matter of concern. They may be an indication of a malnourished or dehydrated baby or a baby severely ill for any reason. *Microphthalmia,* or very small orbits, are another condition the nurse must be alert for. They may be a sign of encephaloophthalmic dysplasia, toxoplasmosis, or retrolental fibroplasia.

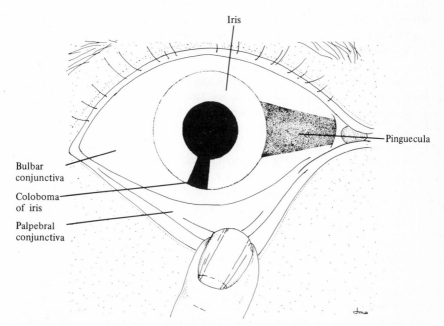

Figure 6-8 The front of the eye displaying a coloboma of the iris and a pinguecula.

There are also rare occasions when a careful examination of the orbit will reveal a small meningocele.

Spacing of the orbits should also be evaluated. Hypertelorism, or abnormally widely spaced eyes, may be present in normal children, but is frequently associated with various syndromes of mental retardation or Waardenburg's syndrome. Hypotelorism, or eyes that are abnormally closely spaced may indicate an absence of the nasal bridge or trigonocephaly.

Prominent supraorbital ridges should also alert the nurse to the possibility of ectodermal dysplasia, gargoylism, or Marfan's syndrome.

Assessing the condition of the ocular muscles is a very important part of the eye examination. Full range of motion must always be checked; it is particularly important to remember to include the movement of the eyes in diagonal directions. *Noncomitant,* or *paralytic strabismus,* occurs as a result of a paralyzed extraocular muscle; this type will frequently not be evident when a child stares straight ahead, but will become apparent only at some point in a complete range of motion. Usually this type of strabismus is posttraumatic and will probably not disappear at all if it is not gone by 1 or 2 months after the trauma. The other type of strabismus is called *concomitant strabismus* and will appear no matter in which direction the eyes are gazing. However, the examiner must frequently be quite astute to discern mild degrees of this type of strabismus. It is very important that this be picked up as early as possible, since amblyopia or loss of vision can occur if it persists for any length of time; this loss may not be reversible. Many infants exhibit concomitant strabismus in early life. This can be a normal condition in a very young infant. However, any child who is still exhibiting this type of strabismus by 6 months of age (some ophthalmologists say by 3 months of age) should be referred for specialized evaluation. Any infant younger than this should be followed closely and referred only if the strabismus is constant rather than intermittent, if it is getting worse or showing no improvement, or if there is any sign of vertical rather than horizontal strabismus. These conditions should be referred very early. Some children will exhibit not a *tropia* (overt strabismus), but only a *phoria* (tendency toward strabismus), particularly when tired to sick. Mothers must be questioned regarding this situation since it will frequently not be present when the child is being examined (see Fig. 6-9).

There are two very important screening tests which should be performed on every child over 6 months of age to rule out subtle strabismus. The first is *Hirschberg's test* in which the room is darkened and a penlight is shone into the child's eyes. The reflection of the light should be in exactly the same position on each pupil. If there is even a slight difference, strabismus may be present. This test is particularly useful in children with pseudostrabismus. Often pseudostrabismus occurs when an epicanthal fold makes the eyes appear crossed even when they are not. In this situation, two types

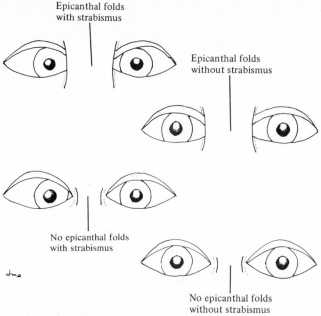

Epicanthal folds with strabismus

Epicanthal folds without strabismus

No epicanthal folds with strabismus

No epicanthal folds without strabismus

Figure. 6-9 Strabismus.

of mistakes can occur. The nurse may be unaware that this will make the child appear cross-eyed and will refer him with no further evaluation. This will result in overreferral. The other possible mistake is that a nurse who is familiar with the fact that epicanthal folds will result in this appearance may dismiss the child without further study. This mistake is far worse. It must be remembered that even though a child has epicanthal folds, it is also possible for him to show true strabismus. Here is where Hirschberg's test is so useful.

The second screening test that should be done on all children over 6 months of age is a cover test. In this test, the child is asked to focus on an object within 12 inches of the eyes. The child must be encouraged to hold the eyes perfectly still or the test cannot be performed. The examiner then holds his or her hand or a small card in such a way that it occludes the vision of one eye but does not touch it. Both eyes must remain open, however. The card is held there several seconds and then quickly removed. The covered eye is observed closely as the card is withdrawn. There should be no movement of this eye. A slight jerking movement of the previously covered eye indicates that some amount of strabismus is present. The same procedure should then be followed with the opposite eye. Finally, the test should be repeated with the child focusing on a distant object. Again, both eyes must be tested.

Finally, the eye proper is examined. This consists of the cornea, sclera, iris, pupil, and lens. The cornea is examined for any enlargement or clouding. These signs, along with dilatation of the pupil, epiphora, and a thin, bluish white sclera, may indicate infantile glaucoma. Clouding or opacities may also indicate Hurler's syndrome or cystinosis.

The cornea should further be inspected for any ulceration. Most often such ulcers are a result of a herpes infection and may begin with a gray or yellowish cornea, accompanied usually be a reddened conjunctiva, intense pain, photophobia, and lacrimation. Ciliary flush is usually a good indication that an infection of the deeper structures exists, and it appears as congested, hyperemic vessels forming a partial or complete reddened circle around the limbic area of the eye. The cornea should further be examined for any dermoids or any evidence of abrasion or irritation.

The sclera may also provide important information. It should be inspected for any irregularities or local manifestations such as *staphyloma* (a small area of outpouching where parts of the sclera seem to be pushed forward and may take on an slightly bluish tinge). The color is important. Jaundice may be best detected in the sclera, particularly in the fornices where the yellow may appear darker. Some sclera may appear slightly brownish. This can be normal in all races although it is more frequent in blacks, as is the occurance of darker brown irregular blotches scattered throughout the sclera. In *alkaptonuria,* large pie-shaped patches of brown pigment pointing toward the limbus may be found. The sclera of newborns will usually be slightly bluish, but a darker blue may indicate osteogenesis imperfecta or glaucoma.

The iris and pupil are examined as a unit. An irregular iris may be due to adjacent adhesions from previous inflammation and should be carefully investigated. Dulling of the color of the iris, ciliary flush, a small pupil, and an eye soft and tender to palpation, particularly when accompanied by pain and throbbing in the ocular area, may indicate iritis.

Anisocoria (difference in pupil size) can be normal, and 5 percent of the normal population mainfests this condition. However, it should make the nurse highly suspicious concerning the possibility of central nervous damage, and a complete and thorough neurological examination should be performed on any child with anisocoria who has not had this condition noted on previous examinations.

Pupil size is quite important. Dilatation of the pupil may be a clue to retinoblastoma, intracranial damage, glaucoma, or poisoning from atropine or barbiturates. A constricted pupil, on the other hand, may indicate morphine poisoning or intracranial damage. Pupils should always be checked for their equality in size and reaction to light. The reaction to light should be checked both directly and consensually. A pupil reacts to light directly if the pupil into which the light is shone constricts; it reacts consensually if it constricts when the light is shone in the opposite eye. Accommodative constriction is also important. To test this, the nurse should have the child look far off into the distance (the authors have found that, to be effective, this must be a distance of some miles through a window); then the child is asked to focus quickly on something within 12 or 14 inches of the eyes. The pupils should dilate when looking into the distance and constrict when focusing on a nearby object. Obviously this test cannot be done on an infant or very young child.

The color of the iris should also be evaluated. The permanent color of the iris will be manifested in 50 percent of children by 6 months of age and in all children by 12 months. A pinkish or blue iris color may appear in albinism.

Brushfield' spots (a light or white speckling of the iris) may occur in normal children, but, particularly in its more striking appearance, may be an indication of Down's syndrome or other syndromes associated with mental retardation.

Heterochromia, or irises of different colors bilaterally, can be normal or can be associated with Waardenburg's syndrome or with chronic low-grade infection of the iris. Even in normal children, heterochromia is associated with a higher incidence of cataracts as they grow into adulthood.

Coloboma can occur on many structures. Earlier in this chapter, coloboma of the eyelid was discussed. A coloboma of the iris is also sometimes found. The notch may include only the iris or may extend through the choroid and retina. If it involves only the iris, there is usually no problem, but vision may be impaired if the retina is involved.

A *Kayser-Fleisher ring* is another possible finding in this area. It consists of a brown or grayish green circle at the limbus and can be a sign of Wilson's disease. It may be unilateral or bilateral and can be partial or complete.

Nystagmus, (the involuntary, rapid, jerky movements of the eye) is another important condition of the eye; it can be horizontal, vertical, or rotary, and can be a result of vestibular, neurological, or ocular causes. The ocular causes include cataracts, astigmatism, muscle weakness, poor vision, albinism, and retrolental fibroplasia. Short periods of nystagmus in an infant who is not yet focusing can be normal, but any continuous nystagmus, even in infants, should be referred. Children of all ages may demonstrate slight nystagmus when gazing from the far corners of their eyes; this should be considered normal.

Finally, in the external examination of the eye proper, the lens should be considered. The primary defects that may be revealed on physical examination in this area are *cataracts* and *dislocated lenses.* Cataracts are opacities of the lens. Some can be seen by flashing a light into the eye; this is particularly useful if done at an angle. Some, however, need an opthalmoscopic examination, at times even with a *slit lamp* and with dilatation for peripheral opacities. When a flashlight or *otoscope* light is shone directly into the pupil, it should produce a red reflex in much the same way that when the headlights of a car shine directly into a cat's eyes, the eyes will appear bright red or orange. If, rather than a circular red reflex, an opaque density surrounded by the red reflex appears, this may be an indication of a cataract. For the most part, however, if there is any reason to suspect a cataract, the child should be seen by an ophthalmologist. Causes of cataracts include maternal rubella or toxoplasmosis, galactosemia, hypoparathyroidism, Lowe's syndrome, or trauma.

A dislocated lens may be seen on ophthalmoscopic examination, but should be suspected with a trembling iris that moves in quick horizontal movements. Trauma, Marfan's syndrome, or homocystinuria can all cause dislocated lenses.

The final part of the ocular examination to be discussed in this chapter is the use of the *ophthalmoscope*. Only a very brief description of it will be given here. It should be stressed again that the authors do not feel this should be the nurse's responsibility, except as a part of a neonatal physical examination where the nurse is merely looking for the red reflex, or in unusual situations where there is occasion to use this skill extensively and constantly. Even then, it will probably take the nurse a long time to feel very confident in the findings.

When using an ophthalmoscope, the examiner must be sure that the child will hold her eyes still (see Fig. 6-10). She should be asked to focus on a specific object in the room and told to try to keep her eyes on that object during the entire examination. It should be explained that the examiner may step in front of the child's eyes, and in that case, the child should pretend that she can still see the object and continue to hold her eyes still. The room should be darkened, admitting perhaps a small amount of light from a door left slightly ajar. The examiner holds the ophthalmoscope in the right hand and looks through his or her own right eye into the child's right eye. The reverse is true for the examination of the left eye. The ophthalmoscope should be held firmly against the examiner's own forehead and the dial should be turned to the black plus numbers, beginning at about $+8$ to $+10$. With the ophthalmoscope at this setting, the examiner begins the evaluation at a distance of about 12 in from the patient. At this point, the red reflex should be visible and opacities in it should be noted. The nurse must then approach to within about 3 in of the patient and turn the ophthalmoscope dial to successively smaller plus numbers and then through the red minus numbers to about -5 for an optimal look at the retina. The exact number at which the view is optimal depends on the refractory ability of both the examiner's eyes and the child's eyes. When dialing to smaller and smaller numbers, the nurse should also be approaching closer to the patient's

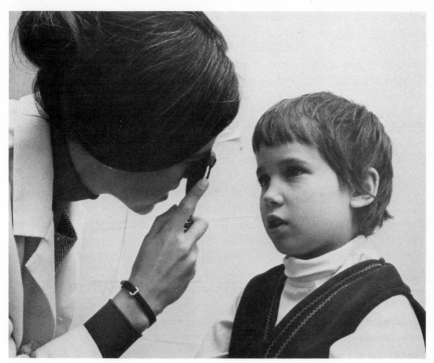

Figure 6-10 Proper usage of the opthalmoscope.

forehead, and by the time the optimal view of the retina is found, the nurse should be almost touching foreheads with the child.

Five parts of the internal examination will be discussed: the red reflex, the optic disc, the macula, the fundus and vessels, and the vitreous and aqueous humors.

The red reflex has been discussed previously in this chapter, and it should be obtained on all newborn examinations by looking directly into the eye with a flashlight or the ophthalmoscope. It should be orange-red and the color should be fairly uniform; no dark or opaque spots should be seen.

The optic disc should be evaluated as to size, shape, color, margins, and physiologic depression. The practitioner must learn the normal size by experience. The important thing to remember is that everything else found on the fundus is measured in "disc diameters," abbreviated "DD's." The size indicated by one disc diameter is the size of the optic disc in that eye. The optic disc is usually round but sometimes vertically oval. Any irregularities may indicate adjacent disease. The color should be creamy pink and lighter than the surrounding fundus. In the center of the optic disc should be an indented area called the physiologic depression. This depression should be grayish in color and slightly temporal of center. It should never extend all the way to the disc margin. The disc margins should be smooth and may be slightly darker in color than the rest of the disc. They may be surrounded by a white, clearly demarcated ring called the *scleral ring* which sometimes has a pigmented crescent adjacent to it on the temporal side. These are normal findings, although they are also frequently absent in normal eyes.

Some conditions that may be encountered in evaluating the optic disc should be mentioned. A small optic disc associated with a pallid color may indicate atrophy, while blurred margins accompanied by an obliterated depression and a reddened disc covered with large tortuous vessels may indicate *papilledema.*

The macula is a small circular landmark, 1-disc diameter in size with a tiny gleaming light near its center, the fovea centralis. It is located 2-disc diameters temporal to the disc; if it is not seen the examiner can ask the child to look directly into the light; this will center it. However, this is a light-sensitive area and the child will not be able to gaze directly into a light for any length of time.

The fundus is usually an orange-red color, although it is lighter in albinos and darker in blacks and some other individuals. There is a wide range of individual variation even within a race. Whatever color is present, however, should be fairly uniform throughout the fundus although the outside periphery may be slightly lighter. White blotches scattered throughout the area may indicate scarring.

There are both arteries and veins in the area. The arteries are one-fourth narrower than the veins and reflect a light reflex from their center. The veins are slightly wider, have no light reflex and manifest slight pulsations.

Abnormalities should be suspected if these vessels are notched at the crossing, if they are abnormally tortuous, if they manifest hemorrhages or exudates, or if the veins show no pulse.

When the examiner finishes inspecting the most posterior surfaces, the dial on the ophthalmoscope should be turned gradually to the black, or plus numbers, going from zero to each higher number in turn. The examiner will then be able to see in succession the posterior vitreous, the anterior vitreous, the lens, and finally, at about the $+15$ or $+20$, the examiner will be focusing on the iris and cornea. No opacities or irregularities shold be seen in any of these structures.

WHERE TO EXAMINE

The entire external eye, orbit, and surrounding tissue must be thoroughly evaluated. The internal eye may also be evaluated ophthalmoscopically, but this examination is quite difficult and requires a great deal of practice. The nurse working primarily with young children will not usually have occasion enough to keep up skill in this area. For this reason, this chapter has discussed only the basic elements of the ophthalmoscopic examination.

WHAT TO EXAMINE WITH

The external eye, for the most part, is examined by gross inspection. A penlight or some other good source of light such as an otoscope head is needed to test the strabismus. A cover card may be used for the cover test although many clinicians use their hand in place of such a card. An ophthalmoscope is necessary only if an internal examination is to be done. This is not generally part of a routine physical examination of the child.

BIBLIOGRAPHY

Campbell, Milton, et al.: "Office Diagnostics: Fundoscopy for the Office Clinician," *Journal of Practical Family Medicine: Patient Care,* vol. 10, no. 21, pp. 86–98, December 1976.

Mechner, Francis: "Patient Assessment: Examination of the Eye, Part I," *American Journal of Nursing,* vol. 74, no. 11, pp. 1–24, November 1974.

_____: "Patient Assessment: Examination of the Eye, Part II," *American Journal of Nursing,* vol. 75, no. 1, pp. 1–24, January 1975.

O'Neill, John: "Strabismus in Childhood," *Pediatric Annals,* vol. 6, no. 2, pp. 74–90, February 1977.

Robb, Richard: "Children's Ophthalmologic Problems," *Hospital Practice,* vol. 12, no. 4, pp. 107–115, April 1977.

Rogers, Gary L.: "Strabismus," *Pediatric Nursing,* vol. 1, no. 6, pp. 11–13, November–December 1975.

Stager, David: "Amblyopia and the Pediatrician," *Pediatric Annals,* vol. 6, no. 2, pp. 91–108, February 1977.

Staton, Y.: "Responsibility of the Pediatrician and the Family Physician for Prevention of Blindness in the Preschool Child," *Journal of the Florida Medical Association,* pp. 926–928, October 1968.

Von Nooden, G. K.: "Diagnosis and Management of Eye Muscle Problems in Childhood," *Surgical Clinics of North America,* pp. 885–894, August 1970.

Watson, P. G.: "Diseases of the Cornea," *Practitioner,* pp. 759–768, June 1969.

Weinstein, G. W.: "Signs and Symptoms of Ocular Disease," *Occupational Health Nurse* (Auckland), pp. 7–12, May 1971.

Wirtschafter, J. D., and I. P. Stapp: "Strabismus Cover Test Demonstrator," *American Journal of Ophthalmology,* pp. 760–762, March 1971.

GLOSSARY

amblyopia   loss of vision caused from constant disuse of the eye
anisocoria   the condition in which one pupil is larger than the other

aqueous humor a clear watery secretion that fills the anterior and posterior chambers of the eye

Bitot's spots irregular yellow patches on the palpebral conjunctiva, caused by vitamin A deficiency

blepharospasm excessive blinking

cataract a clouding of the lens

chalazion (Meibomianitis) a cyst of the Meibomian glands

chemosis edema of the conjunctiva

ciliary glands the modified sweat glands found throughout the eyelashes

coloboma a notch; especially a notch of the lid or the iris of the eye

conjunctiva a thin layer of mucous membrane lining the inner portion of the eyelids and part of the sclera

conjunctivitis inflammation of the conjunctiva

cornea the transparent, anterior portion of the fibrous layer of the eye which is contiguous with the sclera

dacryoadenitis inflammation of the lacrimal gland

dacryocystitis infection of the lacrimal sac

dysautonomia production of an inadequate amount of tears

ectropion a condition in which the borders of the eyelids turn out

entropion a condition in which the borders of the eyelids turn in

epiblepharon (Mongolian fold) a horizontal fold in the upper lid, overhanging the superior tarsus

epicanthal folds vertical folds of skin covering the inner canthus of the eye

epiphora excessive tearing

exopthalmos the condition in which the globe of the eye protrudes from the socket

eye bulb the eye proper, consisting of the outer layer with its cornea and sclera, the middle layer with its choroid, ciliary body and iris, and its inner layer with its retina

fovea centralis the central depression of the macula

heterochromia the condition in which an individual has irises of different color

hordeola (styes) inflammations of the sebaceous glands near the lashes

internal hordeola (styes) inflammation of the Meibomian glands

iris the colored, round, contractile disc surrounding the pupil

Kayser-Fleisher ring a brown or grayish green circle at the limbus, may be a sign of Wilson's disease

lacrimal gland gland lodged in lacrimal fossa to secrete tears

lacrimal sac small pouch in eyelid

lagophthalmos a condition in which the upper and lower eyelids do not completely meet, causing incomplete closure

lens the transparent biconvex structure immediately behind the pupil whose function is to focus light rays on the retina

macula an oval yellowish area at the exact center of the posterior retina where vision is most perfect

Marcus Gunn phenomenon (jaw-winking reflex) the phenomenon in which movement of the jaw to one side causes the child to raise the opposite eyelid

marginal blepharitis red, scaling, crusted lid edges often caused by *Staphylococcus* infection

Meibomian glands a sebaceous gland between the tarsal plate and the conjunctiva

microphthalmia small orbits

nasolacrimal duct lower continuation of the lacrimal sac

noncomitant (paralytic) strabismus strabismus that occurs as a result of a paralyzed extraocular muscle

nystagmus involuntary, rapid, jerky movements of the eye

palpebral fissure elliptical space left by the open eyelids

papilledema swelling of the optic nerve where it enters the retina

phoria a latent tendency toward strabismus

pinguecula a yellowish triangular thickening of the bulbar conjunctiva, extending from the outer canthus to the limbic area

pseudoptosis ptosis caused by the weight of the upper lid, usually due to edema

pterygium an increase in growth of the pinguecula due to irritation, usually from wind

ptosis drooping of the upper eyelid

retina the inner layer of the eye whose function is to receive images focused upon it by the lens

retinoblastoma a malignant glioma of the retina

rhodopsin (visual purple) a lavendar pigment found in the retinal rods

strabismus (squint) a disorder of the eye in which both eyes are unable to fixate on the same object at the same time due to lack of coordination of the optic axes

tarsal glands modified sebaceous (fat-producing) glands located between the skin and the conjunctiva of the eyelid in the area of the tarsal plate

tarsal plate the supporting plate of the upper and lower eyelids

tropia overt strabismus

vitreous body a clear semigelatinous mass which fills the cavity of the eyeball

zonula ciliaris the suspensory ligament that attaches the ciliary body to the lens and helps to position the lens and change its shape

Inspection of the Eye *

Eyebrows	Yes	No	Not applicable	Describe (where appropriate)	Significance
1. Scant					Common in the premature.
2. Bushy					May be a racial variant, particularly in Mexican-American infants; may also indicate a syndrome such as Hurler's.
3. Meet in midline					Same as above.
4. Missing					Same as 1.
5. Other					
Eyelids					
1. Ptosis					Can be congenital or acquired; congenital may be familial; acquired may be due to polio, encephalitis, Horner's syndrome, a pineal tumor, or a number of other diseases; it requires further investigation as to cause. If either type covers the pupil, correction is necessary to prevent amblyopia in the young child.
2. Squinting					May indicate refraction error.
3. Mongolian slant					Can be a sign of Down's syndrome.
4. Antimongolian slant					Can be a sign of Treacher-Collin's syndrome.
5. Excessive blinking					May indicate a tic, eyestrain, photophobia, or irritation.
6. Retraction of the upper lid					May indicate hyperthyroidism or hydrocephalus.
7. Lagophthalmos					May need correction if much of the eye is continually exposed; can result from facial nerve paralysis or proptosis of the globe or can be congenital.
8. Setting sun expression					Can indicate hydrocephalus.

9. Lashes a. missing			Common in prematures; may indicate self-destructive hair and lash pulling; absent on inner two-thirds of lid.
b. ectropian			May be spastic, paralytic, or mechanical; result of scar tissue; usually requires surgery since it can expose the conjunctiva to irritation.
c. entropian			May be a racial variant as with Oriental children; may also result from scars, spasticity, or inflammation; can cause considerable abrasion of the cornea if severe.
10. Edema			In an infant edema may become manifest in the eyelids before anyplace else; can indicate local trauma or any systemic problem which causes edema such as hyperthyroidism, ethmoid sinusitis, pertussis, measles, infectious mononucleosis, nephritis, nephrosis, chronic allergies.
11. Hemangioma			Common birthmark which will usually fade in a few months if mild, in a few years if severe, rarely it will be lifelong.
12. Epicanthal fold			May indicate hypercalcemia, glycogen storage disease, renal agenesis or Down's syndrome; can also be a normal variant—particularly in the Oriental child; 20 percent of white children have them and 97 percent of these disappear spontaneously by 10 years.
13. Coloboma			May indicate underlying coloboma of the retina.
14. Epiblepharon			Normal variant; usually disappears by 1 year of age.
15. Blink reflex			Absent in certain neurological problems.
16. Infections a. marginal blepharitis			If waxy, greasy and easily removed, probably part of seborrhea; if crusty, scaley and hard to remove, maybe a staphylococcal infection.
b. chalazion			Will probably not recede spontaneously but needs surgery.
c. hordeolums (styes)			Almost always a staphylococcal infection; look for a secondary cause such as children with poor vision who constantly rub their eyes or systemic staphylococcal infection.

*These charts are meant to be used by beginning students as they perform their first physical assessments. Each item should be examined on the child and then checked off on the checklist. The significance of the items follows in the right-hand column.

107

Inspection of the Eye (*Continued*)

Eyelids	Yes	No	Not applicable	Describe (where appropriate)	Significance
17. Hematoma					The "black eye" of local trauma; can also be caused by extravasation of blood from elsewhere in the skull.
18. Other					
a. exophthalmos					Hyperthyroidism.
b. enophthalmos					Congenital.
c. other					
Lacrimal System					
1. Absence of tears					Tears normally appear at about 3 months. Later than this, absence of tears may indicate ectodermal dysplasia or eye desease.
2. Epiphoria					Usually from a plugged lacrimal duct; can also be from infection or photophobia, allergy, foreign body.
3. Cystic mass directly under temporal side of eyebrow (dacroadenitis)					May indicate infection of lacrimal gland.
4. Exudate					Possible infection.
5. Erythema, swelling below inner canthus					May indicate dacrocystitis.
6. Other					
Pupil					
1. Nystagmus					Can result from vestibular, ocular, or neurological pathologies.

2.	Anisicoria		Five percent of the normal population manifests this, but when a new occurrence, may indicate central nervous system damage.
3.	Direct constriction to light (right)		Lack of constriction may indicate serious neurological problems.
4.	Direct constriction to light (left)		Same as above.
5.	Hippus		A normal variant.
6.	Consensual constriction to light (right)		Same as 3.
7.	Consensual constriction to light (left)		Same as 3.
8.	Accommodative constriction to light (right).		Same as 3.
9.	Accommodative constriction to light (left)		Same as 3.
10.	Accommodative convergence		Same as 3.
11.	Dilation		May indicate retinoblastoma, intracranial damage, glaucoma, or atropine/barbiturate poisoning.
12.	Constriction		May indicate morphine poisoning, use of street drugs, or intracranial damage.

Lens

1.	Cataracts		Only superficial ones will be visible without an ophthalmoscope.
2.	Dislocated lens		Not usually visible without an ophthalmoscope; needs immediate referral; may cause a trembling in the iris with horizontal movement.

109

Inspection of the Eye (*Continued*)

Muscles	Yes	No	Not applicable	Describe (where appropriate)	Significance
1. Full range of motion (right)					Limited range of motion in any direction may indicate neurological or muscular problem.
2. Full range of motion (left)					Same as 1.
3. Strabismus					Strabismus (as seen in the Hirshberg's or cover test) at any point in the range of motion should be referred since suppression of vision can occur, particularly with the young child.
Orbit					
1. Sunken orbit					May indicate dehydration, malnourishment, micropthalmia (present in such diseases as toxoplasmosis, retrolental fibroplasia, and encephalo-opthalmic dysplasia).
2. Meningocele visible					This is rare but important if seen.
3. Prominent supraorbital ridges					May accompany ectodermal dysplasia, gargoylism, or Marfan's syndrome; may also be a variant of normal.
4. Bluish tinge					A slight amount is normal; excessive discoloration may indicate osteogenesis imperfecta or glaucoma.
5. Pie-shaped patches of brown pointed toward the limbus					Alkaptonuria.

Cornea

1. Dermoids		Warrants referral; usually indicative of irritation.
2. Ulcerations		Warrants immediate referral.
3. Enlargement		Possible glaucoma.
4. Clouding		Possible glaucoma; may accompany Hurler's syndrome or cystinosis.
5. Cataracts		Only superficial ones will be visible.
6. Other		

Iris

1. Coloboma		May indicate an underlying coloboma of the retina.
2. Brushfield's spots		May be a normal variant; is also associated with Down's syndrome.
3. Injection		"Ciliary flush"—usually indicates a serious underlying infection.
4. Heterochromia		May be normal variant but is also associated with Waardenburg's syndrome or low grade chronic infection of the iris; even when a normal variant, is associated with a higher incidence of cataract as the child grows older.
5. Pink or blue		May indicate albinism.

Conjunctiva

1. Palpebral		
a. cobblestone appearance		Chronic allergy—often local reaction to mascara in adolescent girls.
b. injection		Irritation from rubbing, foreign body, or infection.

111

Inspection of the Eye (*Continued*)

Conjunctiva	Yes	No	Not appli-cable	Describe (where appropriate)	Significance
2. Bulbar					
a. peripheral injection					Irritation from rubbing, foreign body, or peripheral infection.
b. central injection					Usually due to chronic irritation, e.g., from environments with many sand- or windstorms; note whether it encroaches into the iris.
c. visible pinguecula					A normal variant.
d. pterygium					Usually due to chronic irritation, e.g., from environments with many sand- or windstorms; note whether it encroaches into the iris.
e. dry, hyperemic					May indicate irritation or vitamin A deficiency.
f. Bitot's spots					Vitamin A deficiency.
Sclera					
1. Abrasions					May or may not be visible to naked eye; usually accompanied by severe pain and require immediate referral.
2. Local outpouchings					Staphyloma.
3. Jaundice					May be best visible in the sclera, particularly in a dark-skinned child; if skin is yellow but sclera is not, this is an important clue to carotinemia.

Palpation of the Eye

Eye	Yes	No	Not appli-cable	Describe (where appropriate)	Significance
1. Skin texture normal					May detect signs of dehydration.
2. Palpable masses					May indicate lacrimal system infection or other masses or nodules.
3. Eyebulb firmness					A soft eyebulb may indicate extreme dehydration.

Auscultation of the Eye

Eye	Yes	No	Not appli-cable	Describe (where appropriate)	Significance
1. Bruits present (not routinely done)					May indicate vascular system abnormalities.

Source: These checklists are printed with permission from Blue Hill Videotape Incorporated and are part of a more complete programmed learning approach to the physical examination, which includes a workbook and series of videotapes. The materials can be purchased from Blue Hill Educational Systems, Inc., 52 South Main Street, Spring Valley, New York 10977.

113

Chapter 7

The Ears

WHY THE CHILD IS EXAMINED

A thorough examination of the ears is an important part of every physical examination. Certainly ear infections are one of the most common of the early childhood infectious diseases. Ear disease can present with classic textbook symptoms: painful ears, fever, upper respiratory infection, etc., but it can also present, particularly in young children, with symptoms that seem totally unrelated, such as nausea and vomiting or generalized symptoms like lethargy. For this reason, the ears of every sick child, no matter what the presenting complaint, must be carefully examined. Likewise, the ears of every well child must be examined, since ear infections, particularly in infants, are frequently found with no symptoms at all.

WHAT TO EXAMINE: ANATOMY OF THE AREA

The ear is divided into three parts: external, middle, and internal ear. The portion of the ear protruding from the head is called the *auricle*, or pinna,

114

and is composed of a thin sheet of cartilage covered with skin. It is sometimes useful to know the specific names of the areas of the auricle in order to be able to describe the findings of the examination more accurately. The prominent, outer rim of the auricle is called the *helix,* while the *antihelix* is the area parallel and anterior to it. *Concha* is the term given to the deep cavity at the middle of the pinna, the entrance to the meatus. Lying anteriorly is the protuberance called the *tragus* and opposite it is the *antitragus.* The bottom, elastic portion of the pinna is called the *lobe.*

The position of the pinna is important. The tip of it should cross the *eye-occiput line* (an imaginary line drawn from the lateral aspect of the eye to the most prominent protuberance of the occiput). The angle formed by this line and the long axis of the ear should be almost vertical; if it is more than 10° from vertical, the examiner should make specific notation of it and look closely for further abnormalities (see Fig. 7-1).

The external meatus is a canal approximately 2.5 cm long, leading from the concha to the tympanic membrane. This canal follows an S-shaped curve; first inward, then forward and downward. This is important to remember when attempting to straighten the canal for vision. The curvature is slightly different in infants and young children, and this must be remembered when examining each age group. The canal is formed by cartilage at the outer opening and by bone toward the inner end. This skin lining is very thin and easily broken (see Fig. 7-2).

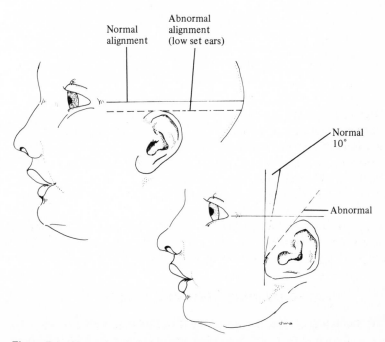

Figure 7-1 Normal and abnormal ear alignment.

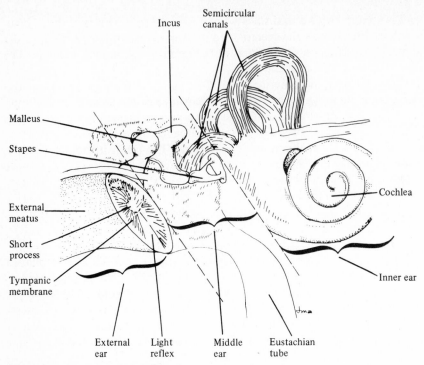

Figure 7-2   Ear canal and ossicles.

The middle ear is an air-filled space within the *temporal bone,* consisting of the *tympanic membrane,* the *malleus, incus,* and *stapes.* The tympanic membrane, or eardrum, is a thin, almost transparent membrane, angled inferiorly and medially so as to join the floor of the meatus at an angle of about 55 ° (see Fig. 7-3). This vertical and horizontal inclination is greatly exaggerated in the infant and young child. This is an important fact for the examiner to bear in mind, since the inexperienced examiner will often interpret this normal angle as a bulging of the pars flaccida. The posterosuperior quadrant is closest to the examiner when looking down the canal; the anteroinferior quadrant is the farthest. The tympanic membrane may be divided into four portions for easy reference: anterointerior quadrant, anterosuperior quadrant, posteroinferior quadrant, posterosuperior quadrant. Due to looseness of the top quadrants, this area is designated the *pars flaccida,* while the lower, more taut area is called the *pars tensa.* The white dense fibrous ring surrounding the tympanic membrane is called the tympanic ring or *annulus.* It completely surrounds the tympanic membrane with the exception of the superior portion between the anterior and posterior malleolar folds.

Directly behind the tympanic membrane lie three moveable ossicles: the malleus, incus, and stapes. The malleus is a small, inverted T-shaped bone

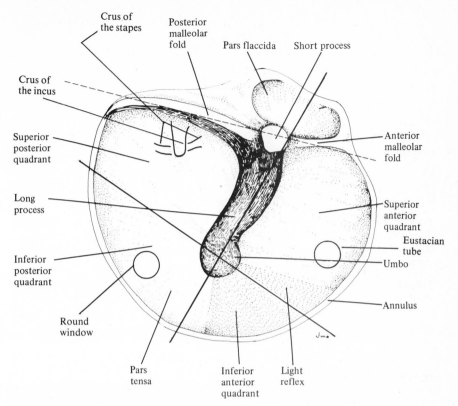

Figure 7-3 Tympanic membrane and landmarks.

often compared to a hammer. The long end of the malleus is attached to the inner surface of the tympanic membrane. This attachment causes the tympanic membrane to be drawn inward, creating a concavity called the *umbo.* Part of this bone, the manubrium, protrudes visibly through the membrane as an important landmark—the long process. The incus is the middle bone and serves to connect the other two ossicles. In certain tympanic membranes, particularly retracted ones, part of the incus called the crus can be seen. The short end is attached to the malleus and the long end to the stapes.

The innermost of the three bones is called the stapes and resembles a stirrup in shape. The head of the stapes is connected to the incus and the flat base attaches to the fenestra vestibuli (oval window) which leads to the vestible of the inner ear. Again, part of the stapes (the crus) may be seen through the tympanic membrane in certain normal or retracted eardrums.

The inner ear contains some of the essential organs of hearing which receive the sound waves entering the canal. The main parts of the inner ear are the vestibule, semicircular canals, and cochlea. The detailed description of these organs is not the subject of this book, and the reader is referred to a good anatomy book.

Throughout the external ear canal the blood vessels and nerves can be very near the surface. This means the nurse must be very careful, since the examination of these parts can often be painful or draw blood very easily.

HOW TO EXAMINE

The examination of the ears can be virtually painless if the child will cooperate or can be helped to cooperate. It is most important that he remain absolutely still during the examination. The older, cooperative child may be willing to stand in front of the examiner or to sit on the examining table or the parent's lap. The younger child (1 to 3 years old) may do better held on the parent's lap or on the examining table. If the lap is chosen, turn the child to the parent's side. Have the parent hold the child's head firmly against the chest with one hand and use the other hand to restrain the child's arm and chest (see Fig. 7-4). The child's legs can be secured between the

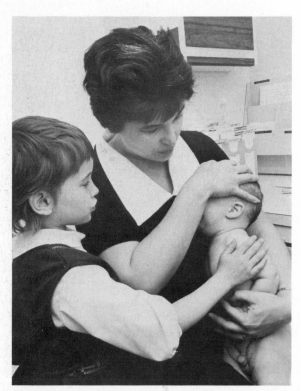

Figure 7-4   Child being restrained in the upright position.

parent's knees. If using the table, the child should be placed on his back with his head turned to one side and his arms held straight over his head. The parent may stand at the head of the table and firmly hold the child's arms at his elbows. The examiner leans on the child's chest and can then use both arms for examining the ear. The infant from birth to 1 year of age is best examined on the table in this fashion (see Fig. 7-5).

The child should be told she is going to have her ears looked at and should be given a chance to become accustomed to the *otoscope*. The nurse may show the child that it is a funny-looking flashlight and let her watch the light hit her palm. Once the initial introduction is made, the child is positioned. Place the speculum of the otoscope at the edge of the meatus, turning the child's head back and forth so she may become accustomed to the feel of something at her ear. If the child is sitting, remember that the tympanic membrane is at a 55 ° angle and that the child's head should be tilted away from the examiner in order to bring the membrane into an upright position. Because the canal is curved, the auricle must be firmly gripped and pulled to straighten the canal for a view. Since the canal curves upward in infants, the ear is pulled down; in the older child, the canal has a downward and forward position, and the ear must be pulled up and back. As the child becomes accustomed to the feel, tell her you are going to take a longer look in this ear; and slowly insert the speculum and take a look. Then repeat this procedure with the other ear. Even though there is no pain connected with the examination, most children dislike the feeling of being restrained and will cry. Often babies will cry until the speculum is inserted and then stop while the actual visualization is taking place. With young chil-

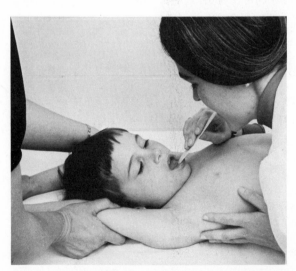

Figure 7-5 Child being restrained on the examining table.

dren, it is probably best to examine the ears last and then let the child recover from the ordeal in the parent's arms.

As with other parts of the body, the most important part of the examination is observation. With the exception of palpation of the outer auricle and the mastoid, the entire ear examination is done by observation—first with no instrument and then with the otoscope. Observation of the outer ear should include several points. Location of the ears on the head is important. Ar they low set? Are both ears at the same level? Are they flat against the head or protruding? Size of the ears should also be evaluated. Are they bigger or smaller than normal? Do they have large hanging ear lobes? The nurse must inspect the shape of the ears as well. The helix should be checked for the normal amount of curvature and the presence of the tragus. Color must be considered as must any discharges. Observation of the canal includes looking at the amount and texture of the cerumen and checking for any furuncles. Inspection of the canal requires the use of the otoscope. The otoscope consists of (see Fig. 7-6):

1 A handle, often containing the batteries.
2 The neck.
3 The head, containing the lens, the rim for attaching the speculum, a bulb, and often a small spigot for a pneumonic device.
4 Speculums are sized 2,3,4, and 5 mm and 9 mm for the nose. For the ears, most examiners do not use the 2-mm ones, because they are too small and could easily go too far into the canal.

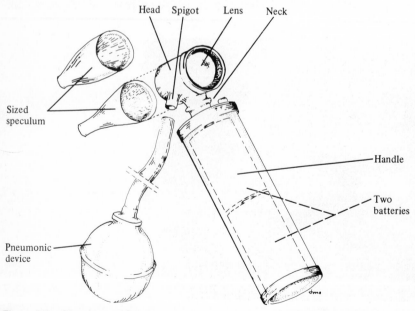

Figure 7-6 Otoscope parts.

Two batteries fit into the handle of the otoscope. It is extremely important to check the batteries to make certain they are still fresh. Regular batteries may last between 1 and 2 weeks, depending on the amount of use. Long-life batteries will last considerably longer and may be worth the added expense. The batteries should not be used when they give off a yellow light rather than a white. If the otoscope is going to be unused for several weeks, remove the batteries so they do not corrode the inside of the handle. To extend the life of the batteries, the otoscope should be turned on just as the speculum enters the ear and should always be turned off immediately after withdrawal. An extra bulb should always be available in case one burns out during an examination. Bulbs do not burn out gradually and there is generally no warning of when a replacement will be needed. The newer fiberoptic halogen otoscopes do not use either batteries or bulbs but must be recharged in a wall socket.

The speculum should be cleaned with an alcohol sponge after each use. The largest possible speculum which fits the child's ear should be used. It should be securely fastened to the otoscope handle.

When first learning to use an otoscope, it is important to hold it correctly (see Fig. 7-7). Hold it like a pencil with the head down and the heavy handle resting between your thumb and forefinger. This may seem awkward in the beginning. The examiner's hand should be firmly placed on the child's head. This is especially important with younger children who may move away suddenly. This method of bracing allows the speculum to move with the child's head and prevents the examiner from perforating the tym-

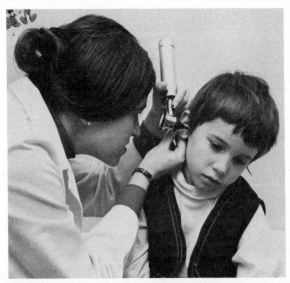

Figure 7-7 The correct way to hold the otoscope for the examination of the ear.

panic membrane with the speculum. The free hand can be used to pull the ear to straighten the canal. It should be pulled in a direction appropriate to the age of the child. Slowly insert the speculum $\frac{1}{4}$ to $\frac{1}{2}$ in into the canal, looking at the canal as the speculum passes.

When examining the tympanic membrane, the nurse is looking for six main characteristics: color of the membrane, the *light reflex,* the umbo, the *long process,* the *short process,* and membrane mobility.

The color of the tympanic membrane is normally a light, pearly gray, translucent color. The light reflex is a small cone of light reflected from the otoscope light. It should be a rather sharply demarcated triangular shape pointing posteriorly (away from the nose). A diffuse or spotty light reflex is not usually normal and requires further investigation. At the top of the light reflex is the umbo. This is the end of the malleus and is so firmly attached that it causes a protuberance of the tympanic membrane. It is seen as a small, round, white opaque spot. Looking anteriorly and superiorly to the umbo the examiner can see the long process of the malleus. This often appears as a whitish line extending from the umbo to the end of the tympanic membrane. At the upper end of the long process is the short process of the malleus. This presents as a small downward projection through the tympanic. The annulus is another important landmark; it is the fibrous ring surrounding the periphery of the tympanic membrane. It must be inspected carefully, since this is a common spot to find perforations. The examiner should locate this landmark and follow it completely around the periphery of the drum; it will appear whiter and denser than the rest of the membrane. The annulus should form a circle which is complete except for a small missing portion between the anterior and posterior malleolar folds.

Six other landmarks are the anterior malleolar folds, the posterior malleolar folds, the crus of the incus, the crus of the stapes, the round window, and the chorda tympani nerve. These landmarks are not so constant as the previously discussed ones, but the nurse should know their locations. They are included in the diagram for that reason. Frequently the view in the speculum shows only a portion of the tympanic membrance and the otoscope must be adjusted to see the remainder. With practice, the head of the otoscope can be slightly and gently maneuvered to see the entire membrane without causing discomfort to the child.

It is extremely important that the tympanic membrane always be tested for mobility (see Fig. 7-8). A normal tympanic membrane should move smoothly when air pressure is exerted against it. If the middle ear contains fluid, the tympanic membrane will not move or will move in a stickly or jerky fashion when air pressure is applied. This air pressure is exerted through the *pneumatic tube* either by squeezing the attached bulb or by removing this bulb and alternately blowing out and sucking in with the end of the tube in the examiner's mouth. The speculum must fit the canal snugly for this procedure to be effective. If air can be heard rushing out of the

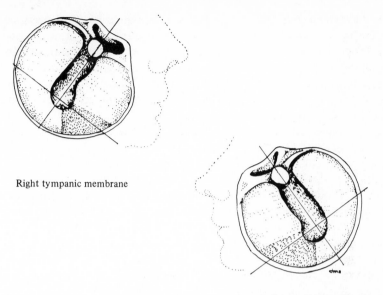

Right tympanic membrane

Left tympanic membrane

Figure 7-8 The right and left tympanic membranes with landmarks.

canal when the examiner blows, it usually indicates that the speculum is not large enough to produce the air-tight seal that is necessary. A larger speculum should be tried.

No examination of the ear is complete without examining the child for hearing. Tests for hearing are discussed later in this book.

WHERE TO EXAMINE

The entire ear, both inside and outside, must be examined carefully. The mastoid process directly behind the pinna must also be included. This is particularly important when ear infection exists, since mastoiditis is sometimes associated with this condition. An edematous tender area is usually the presenting symptom. If this condition does exist it must be thoroughly investigated, since, not only should it be treated for its own sake, but the infection can spread directly from the mastoid area to the brain.

WHAT TO EXAMINE WITH

An otoscope is the usual instrument utilized in the examination of the ear. This can be either the type that plugs into an electrical outlet in the wall or the battery type. The fiberoptic light is now used most commonly with both types as is a halogen light source (an extremely bright type of light). The speculum end is generally one of three types. The first has a space between the magnifying glass and the speculum. This type is best for curetting ears. However, it is impossible to use a pneumonic tube with it, an indispensable device in pediatrics. The second type of speculum attachment has the magnifying glass directly attached to the speculum and an attachment for a pneumonic tube. This is somewhat more difficult to handle when curetting, but it is possible. The third and newer type of otoscope combines the advantages of both of the first two by having a sliding magnifying glass which when in place creates an airtight sea for pneumonetry, but which can also slide to one side to allow the examiner to curette.

Specialists in ear, nose, and throat almost always use and strongly recommend a head mirror. The light source with a head mirror is far superior to that of an otoscope; however, few clinics are set up to utilize this type of equipment since it requires a gooseneck lamp. Also, the examiner does not have the aid of magnification. If the nurse is practicing where a gooseneck lamp is available, it is certainly recommended that he or she learn to use the head mirror. The nurse will find it excellent equipment for examination not only of the ear, but of the nose and throat as well.

WHAT TO EXAMINE FOR

The following are some minor conditions nurses need to be aware of when examining ears. For a discussion of more serious ear conditions the reader is referred to *Ambulatory Pediatrics for Nurses* (Brown and Murphy, 1975).

The external ear should be examined for malformation, nodules, cysts, or any type of lesions. The canal should be examined for any abnormalities, such as furuncles, foreign bodies including insects (a common problem in the young child), *polyps,* and swelling of the walls of the canal.

An important aspect of the ear canal which deserves careful evaluation is *cerumen.* Cerumen (ear wax) is a mixture of sebum from sebaceous glands and the excretion of apocrine sweat from the glands in the ear canal. The cerumen may be of several consistencies. Yellow cerumen tends to be soft and wet, while black and brown cerumen is often drier and harder. No one has been able to report the purpose of cerumen. The best hypothesis is that it is produced to carry foreign matter away from the tympanic membrane and avoid damage to that area.

A small amount of cerumen is harmless, and the examiner can look past it when examining the tympanic membrane. Parents should be taught how to clean the ears and should be told not to worry about the cerumen. Ears are best cleaned with a wash cloth during the regular bath. If wax has been a problem before, the parent may use a medicine dropper to put a few drops of liquid soap into the canal at the beginning of the bath; this should be thoroughly rinsed out at the end. The nurse must be sure an intact tympanic membrane exists before advising this procedure. The use of cotton-tipped applicators for cleaning out wax should be discouraged. It only pushes the wax further toward the tympanic and makes it very difficult to remove. It can also be potentially dangerous. The use of bobby pins or other pointed objects should be discouraged. If there is excessive wax in the ears and the tympanic membrane cannot be visualized, the wax must be removed. There are two methods available and they depend on the type of wax present (dry, scaly, wet, sticky, etc.) and the condition of tympanic membrane. If the wet sticky type is present, it is best to dig it out with a curette (No. 0-1 with blunt ends). This can be a painful and often bloody procedure. No matter what the age of the child, he must be restrained. It may take the examiner, the parent, and an additional person. The child should lie on the table with the head to one side. Some clinicians hold the otoscope in one hand, the lens slid to the halfway point, and the curette inserted through the head rim into the ear. Others hold the otoscope to one side of the ear so that the light falls into the canal but the curette is not put through the speculum but directly into the ear. The closeness of the blood vessels and nerves to the surface make it very easy to draw blood and cause pain. With practice, the nurse will learn to avoid pain and blood, in most cases. Curettes come in several sizes; usually Nos. 0 and 00 are used on children.

If the wax is dry, hard, and scaly, irrigation may be the only way to remove it. However, the examiner first must be certain that the tympanic membrane is intact, otherwise water is forced straight into the middle ear. This is a messy procedure and cannot be done on a child who will not cooperate. The equipment needed will be a large water syringe, a large basin of warm water (not hot), a small ear or kidney basin, and four to six towels. The child sits and is draped with towels. The syringe is filled with warm water and squirted with force at the superoposterior canal wall. If the water is not warm enough, the child will become dizzy. It will take several pans of water and about 20 minutes to remove the wax from each ear. As pieces of wax float out, the procedure can be stopped for a look through the otoscope to see if the tympanic membrane is in view. The child who comes in complaining of ear pain and who has an ear full of dry scaly wax, should have his ears curetted rather than irrigated. The examiner cannot take the chance that the tympanic membrane is broken.

The tympanic membrane is, of course, of utmost importance in an evaluation of the ear. As previously mentioned, the examiner must search meticulously, both centrally and peripherally, for perforations. Further disorders of the eardrum will not be considered in this book. The reader is referred to a book on otolaryngology.

The inner ear is not immediately accessible for physical examination and the tests used to determine its functioning are rather complex and not routinely done. The nurse need not concern herself with these tests. If she is worried about the functioning of the inner ear, the child should be referred to a physician.

BIBLIOGRAPHY

Brown, Marie S., and Mary A. Murphy: *Ambulatory Pediatrics for Nurses,* McGraw-Hill, New York, 1975.

Mechner, Francis: "Patient Assessment: Examination of the Ear," *American Journal of Nursing,* vol. 75, no. 3, pp. 1–24, March 1975.

Stool, Sylvan E., and Joseph Anticaglia: "Electric Otoscopy—A Basic Pediatric Skill," *Clinical Pediatrics,* vol. 12, no. 7, pp. 420–425, July 1973.

GLOSSARY

annulus the white dense, fibrous ring surrounding the tympanic membrane

antihelix the area parallel and anterior to the helix of the auricle

antitragus the protuberance lying anterior to the concha

auricle (pinna) portion of the ear protruding from the head

cerumen (ear wax) a combination of sebum and apocrine sweat produced within the ear canal

concha the deep cavity lying at the midauricle

eye-occiput line the imaginary line drawn from the outer corner of the eye to the most protuberant part of the occiput

helix the prominent, outer rim of the auricle

incus the middle bone connecting the malleus and stapes within the middle ear

light reflex a small cone of light reflected from the otoscope light

long process the whitish line extending from the umbo to the end of the tympanic membrane when looking in the ear. It is the long end of the malleus.

malleus a small, inverted T-shaped bone attached to the inner surface of the tympanic membrane in the middle ear

pars flaccida the flaccid portion of the tympanic membrane superior to the anterior and posterior malleolar folds

pars tensa the lower, tightly stretched area of the tympanic membrane inferior to the anterior and posterior malleolar folds

pneumonic tube the rubber tubing and bulb that can be attached to many otoscope heads when testing mobility of the tympanic membrane

polyps growths arising from mucous membrane tissue

short process a sharp protuberance seen through the tympanic membrane extending downward from the long process

stapes the innermost of the three ossicle bones. It is attached to the incus and fenestra vestibuli (oval window) of the inner ear

temporal bone the cranial bone that contains the middle ear

tragus the anterior protuberance of the concha

tympanic membrane the thin, transparent membrane covering the ossicles and dividing the outer and middle ear

umbo an indentation of the tympanic seen at the top point of the light reflex. It is the long end of the malleus firmly attached to the inner surface of the tympanic membrane

Inspection and Palpation of the Ear*

Mastoid process	Yes	No	Not applicable	Describe (where appropriate)	Significance
1. Tenderness					Indication of mastoiditis or local superficial irritation (e.g., furuncle, etc.).
2. Erythema					Same as above.
3. Swelling					Same as above.
4. Other					
Auricle (Pinna)					
1. Concha					
2. Helix					
3. Antihelix					All normal landmarks; note any irregularity, signs of infection, etc.
4. Tragus					
5. Antitragus					
6. Lobe					
7. Darwinian tubercle					A variant of normal.

*These charts are meant to be used by beginning students as they perform their first physical assessments. Each item should be examined on the child and then checked off on the checklist. The significance of the items follows in the right-hand column.

127

Inspection and Palpation of the Ear (*Continued*)

Auricle (Pinna)	Yes	No	Not appli-cable	Describe (where appropriate)	Significance
8. Placement a. does it touch eye–occiput line					An ear completely below the eye-occiput line is associated with renal problems and mental retardation syndromes.
b. does it deviate more than $10°$ from a line perpendicular to the eye-occiput line					Same as above.
External canal					
1. Scaling					May indicate otitis externa.
2. Redness					May indicate otitis externa or other irritation such as furuncles or child picking at ears.
3. Swelling					Same as above.
4. Polyps					May need removal.
5. Tenderness					Same as 3.
Tympanic membrane					
1. Annulus					Normal landmark.
2. Pars flaccida					Normal landmark; may show first signs of otitis media.
3. Pars tensa					Normal landmark.
4. Long process					Same as above.
5. Short process					Same as above.

128

6. Umbo			Same as above.
7. Anterior folds			Same as above.
8. Posterior fold			
9. Light reflex			Same as above.
10. Chordae tympanii			
11. Crus of the incus			Same as above; cannot usually be seen; visibility is more likely with retraction.
12. Round window			Same as 10.
13. Entrance to Eustachian tube			Same as 10.
14. Holes			Perforation; needs referral.
15. Bubbles			Indicates fluid, usually serous otitis.
16. Fluid level			Indicates fluid, usually serous otitis.
17. Retraction			May indicate beginning serous otitis.
18. Mobility good			Normal.
19. Bulging			Indicates otitis media.
20. Redness			May indicate beginning or advanced otitis media.

Source: These checklists are printed with permission from Blue Hill Videotape Incorporated and are part of a more complete programmed learning approach to the physical examination, which includes a workbook and series of videotapes. The materials can be purchased from Blue Hill Educational Systems, Inc., 52 South Main Street, Spring Valley, New York 10977.

129

Chapter 8

The Nose

WHY THE CHILD IS EXAMINED

As the beginning of the respiratory system the nose may give several clues as to how the rest of the system is functioning. It is also important in its own right since it can be the site of several disease processes, particularly those of an allergic nature.

WHAT TO EXAMINE: ANATOMY OF THE AREA

The respiratory system is composed of the nose, nasal passages, nasopharynx, larynx, trachea, bronchi, and lungs. This chapter shall be concerned with those structures accessible to physical examination, that is the nose, nasal passages, and paranasal sinuses.

The nose is divided into the external nose and internal nose, or nasal cavity. The base of the nose contains orifices called *nares* (*nostrils*) and is separated by a cartilaginous membrane called the *median septum*. The

130

upper third of the nose is bone—nasal bones and the frontal processes of the maxilla; the remainder of the nose is cartilage and fibroadipose tissue.

There are three muscles connected with the nose: the *procerus, nasalis,* and *depressor septi.* The procerus inserts between the eyebrows and runs toward the apex of the nose; it is the muscle used to wrinkle the nose. The nasalis runs along the side of the nose and helps keep the nares open during normal breathing. The depressor septi runs from the maxillary area toward the upper portion of the nose. It is the antagonist to the other two muscles.

The blood supply of the external nose comes from the external and internal carotid arteries; the nasal lymphatic system drains into the submandibular nodes in the area directly below the angle of the mandible. Nasal nerve supply originates from the fifth and seventh cranial nerves.

The internal nose is divided into two symmetrical, equal chambers separated by the nasal septum; the front portion of the nasal septum is cartilaginous, and the posterior section is bony. At birth, the septum is straight, but becomes deviated by adulthood causing the two cavities to be unequal in size. The cavities have two openings: (1) the anterior cavity is the vestibule where the nares are located, and it is thickly lined with small hairs; and (2) the posterior cavity or *choana* leads to the throat. The lateral walls of the cavities are divided into the superior, middle, and inferior nasal conchae (sometimes referred to as *turbinate bones*) and the superior, middle, and inferior meatuses. The superior turbinate is part of the ethmoid bone, and the smallest and most difficult to visualize. The middle turbinate is also part of the ethmoid bone and is intermediate in size. The inferior turbinate is a separate bone with a mucous membrane very rich in blood vessels. It is most easily visualized and most strongly affected by vasoconstrictors. Occasionally people have a fourth turbinate named the *supreme turbinate,* located high above the superior (see Fig. 8-1).

The *meatuses* are drainage tubes with openings that correspond to the turbinates lying directly above them. The superior meatus is short and drains from the sphenoethmoid recess, or pocket, above the superior turbinate. The middle meatus lies under the middle turbinate and drains the maxillary, frontal, and anterior ethmoid sinuses. The inferior meatus lies below the inferior turbinate and may change from large to small, depending on the amount of drainage. The nasolacrimal duct empties here. If there is a supreme turbinate there is a supreme meatus to drain from that area.

The olfactory region of the nose is located high on the superior turbinate and may be disturbed or absent if nasal obstruction becomes so great that air currents cannot reach the olfactory mucosa.

The nasal cavity is lined with a mucous membrane which is thick and vascular over the turbinates and septum, and is thin over the meatuses, the floor of the cavity, and the sinuses. The blood supply for the internal nose is similar to that for the external nose; it comes from the external and internal

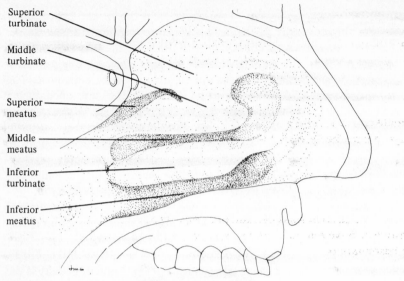

Superior turbinate
Middle turbinate
Superior meatus
Middle meatus
Inferior turbinate
Inferior meatus

Figure 8-1 A side view of the internal nasal cavity.

carotid arteries. The arterial blood flows into the anterior ethmoid artery and the sphenopalatine artery which form a fine network of small vessels towards the tip of the nose. These are called *Kisselbach's triangle* and frequently are the site of bleeding in *epistaxis*.

The lymphatic system of the internal nose drains into three areas: the submandibular nodes, the retropharyngeal nodes (deep in the neck), and the superior deep cervical nodes.

The nerve supply for the internal nose is more complex than that of the external. The main source is the fifth cranial nerve, but the nasal mucosa has a distribution of parasympathic and sympathic fibers as well.

The *paranasal sinuses* are air-filled spaces lined with mucous membrane. There are eight all together—four on each side. These sinuses are the *ethmoid*, the *maxillary*, the *frontal*, and the *sphenoid*. The ethmoid sinus is made up of many small cavities and lies behind the frontal sinus and near the superior part of the nasal cavities. It is composed of the frontal, lacrimal, sphenoid, and palatine bones and the maxilla. The maxillary sinus is the largest of the sinuses (sometimes called the *antrum of Highmore*) and lies along the lateral wall of the nasal cavity. Most of it is carved out of the maxilla. The average adult maxillary sinus will hold 9 to 20 ml of fluid. The frontal sinuses are located behind the superciliary arches of the frontal bone. They are separated by a septum and usually the two cavities are not symmetrical. The sphenoid sinus lies deep within the skull behind the ethmoid sinus. It lies within the sphenoid bone and is divided by a septum into two unequal parts. The ethmoid and maxillary sinuses are present at birth, while the sphenoid is a minute cavity at birth and is fully developed after puberty; the frontal sinus is absent at birth and develops at around 7 to 8 years of age. All sinuses are lined with ciliated mucous membrane which is continuous from the nasal cavity; they drain into the nasal cavity and out through the various nasal meatuses (see Fig. 8-2).

The nose must be able to perform a varity of functions. Since it provides the entry of air into the respiratory system, it must temper the air, humidify, and filter it. By the time the air hits the trachea, bronchi, and lungs, it must be between 96.8 and 98.6 °F. The nose accomplishes this by passing the air over the turbinates. This large surface area, rich in blood supply, warms the air as it passes. Cold air stimulates swelling of the turbinates with more warm blood resulting in this warming effect. Air must also be humidified and conditioned by the time it arrives at the inner system. The nasal mucosa can add or remove moisture from the air to give a constant relative humidity of 75 to 80 percent by the time the air arrives in the nasopharynx. It is estimated that 1,000 ml of moisture is evaporated during the breathing that takes place in one day. A blanket of moisture covers the nasal cavity, sinuses, eustachian tube, and trachea. Bacteria and

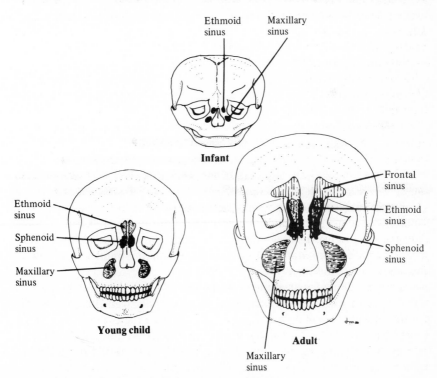

Figure 8-2 The sinuses in the infant, child, and adult.

foreign matter are deposited on this blanket and must be removed. A constant ciliary action moves this material to the nasopharynx and pharynx for swallowing and exiting through the stomach.

The nose is also used for *olfaction*. Although the sense of olfaction (smell) may not be needed for survival by the human being, it makes life much more pleasant. When the ability to smell is reduced, most people find a reduction in the taste of food.

HOW TO EXAMINE

As with other parts of the body, the examiner must observe, palpate, and percuss to gather adequate data about the nose. Auscultation is sometimes used as well.

The child is best approached when he is sitting—either on the table or on the mother's lap. For a very young infant, the examination can be done with the child lying on his back on the table. This part of the examination is usually done as part of the head.

To observe the inner nose most examiners use an otoscope with the very short, broad speculum which is gently inserted into the rim of the nares, although some examiners prefer using a head mirror and long-handled nasal speculum. To be useful, the mirror must be used regularly. It is attached to the examiner's head with a leather strap and is positioned over one eye, with both eyes remaining open for binocular vision. The focal length is usually 14 inches from the patient's face. In addition to the mirror, the examiner must obtain a good source of light, usually a moveable, gooseneck lamp that can be repositioned for the reflection.

The nose should be palpated along the ridge for the presence of bone and cartilage. The maxillary sinus may be palpated by holding the head steady with one hand while pressing on both cheeks simultaneously with the other hand (see Fig. 8-3). The frontal sinus can be palpated by placing two fingers below the eyebrows and pressing upward from the eye socket.

Percussion is usually reserved for the sinuses; both the maxillary and frontal sinuses may be lightly tapped with a forefinger to ascertain if the child feels pain. The sinuses may also be transilluminated. However, this procedure has its limitations. Only the maxillary and frontal sinuses can be transilluminated and the procedure is not highly successful in children. The examiner is looking for asymmetry of the illumination, but sometimes even normal sinuses will show different degrees of light. In transilluminating the frontal sinuses, a small light is placed firmly against the upper eye socket in a totally darkened room; for the maxillary sinuses a light is placed in the patient's mouth and the lips closed. In a darkened room the red pupillary reflexes will show with crescents of light under them.

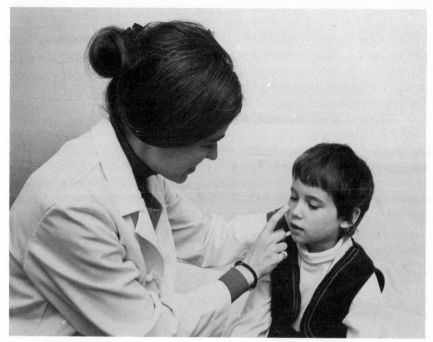

Figure 8-3 Palpation of the maxillary sinus.

WHERE TO EXAMINE

A complete examination of the nose includes the entire exterior nose and sinus areas and as much of the internal nose as can be seen with a nasal speculum.[1]

WHAT TO EXAMINE WITH

Either the otoscope with the nasal speculum attachment or the head mirror with the long-handled nasal speculum and gooseneck lamp are used in the examination of the nose. Their use has been discussed previously in this chapter. A flashlight to examine for perforated septum has also been explained. A stethoscope is sometimes used to be sure that each side of a child's nose is patent. The diaphragm is held over the naris (nostril) in question while the other naris is occluded by the examiner's finger. Breath sounds should be audible if the tested naris is open. Some condensation will also appear on the diaphragm.

[1] The checklist for the physical examination of the nose is combined with that of the mouth and throat and is found at the end of Chapter 9.

WHAT TO EXAMINE FOR

Before touching the child the examiner should observe the external nose. Does it have a straight shape? Are the nares symmetrical? Do they flare? Is there anything significant about the skin? Does it have milia, freckles, or acne? Is there any discharge? If so, is it purulent, watery, bloody, or crusty? How much is there?

The nurse should carefully examine the septum and the mucosa. Are there any polyps or tumors on the septum? Is it perforated? The easiest way to check for perforation is to shine the flashlight into one side of the nose while looking at the other side. Is the bright white light visible through to that side? If so, a perforation exists. Examine the color of the mucosa. Inflammation and erythemia indicate infection; pale, boggy mucose is typical of allergy, while swollen, gray mucose usually results from chronic rhinitis.

When looking through the otoscope the examiner should also be able to visualize the vestibule, septum, turbinates, and meatuses. The middle turbinate and meatus are most easily visualized because of their location.

GLOSSARY

antrum of Highmore   the maxillary sinus

conchae (turbinates)   the shell-shaped bones forming the lateral walls of the nasal cavities

depressor septi   the antagonist of the three muscles attached to the nose

epistaxis   bleeding from the nose

ethmoid sinuses   paranasal sinuses located behind the frontal sinus and near the superior part of the nasal cavities

frontal sinuses   paranasal sinuses located behind the superciliary arches of the frontal bone

Kiesselbach's triangle   a fine network of small blood vessels located near the tip of the nose

maxillary sinuses   the largest of the paranasal sinuses located along the lateral wall of the nasal cavity

meatus   an anatomic opening or passage

nares   orifices at the base of the nose; nostrils

nasalis muscle   one of the three muscles attached to the nose that aids in keeping the nares open

nasopharynx   the area where the nasal cavity enters the pharynx

procerus muscle   one of the three muscles attached to the nose that aids in wrinkling the nose

Chapter 9

The Mouth and Throat

WHY THE CHILD IS EXAMINED

Evaluation of the mouth and throat is an extremely important part of the physical examination of a child. A large majority of ambulatory illnesses in the pediatric age group focalizes in the mouth and throat. (Indeed, one of the major health problems of our civilization—dental disease— is found in this area). These areas are equally important as focal points in identifying certain systemic disease, for example, the Koplik spots of measles or the enlarged Stensen's duct in mumps.

WHAT TO EXAMINE: ANATOMY OF THE AREA

Anatomically, the mouth and throat are the beginning of the digestive tract, which continues throughout most of the body to terminate in the rectum and anus. Each part of this tract is highly specialized to perform some function in the utilization of food, but in this chapter only the mouth and throat and their structure and function will be considered.

137

The mouth is composed of a vestibule, the cavity proper, the lips, cheeks, labial glands, buccal glands, gums, and hard and soft palate; it contains the teeth, tongue, and salivary glands (see Fig. 9-1). The encasement of the mouth is a combination of hard and soft tissue—the floor and roof consisting of hard bone, and the lateral walls formed by soft, elastic muscles. The floor, although formed by the hard mandibular bone that supplies the needed firmness for tooth attachment, is covered by extremely loose, mobile tissue. The roof of the oral cavity is formed by the maxilla and divided into two parts: *the hard and soft palate.* The hard palate is anterior and separates the nasal and oral cavities. The soft palate is posterior continuing this separation between the nasal and oral cavities.

When in a relaxed position, the soft palate is concave as it leaves the hard palate and convex at the posterior edge, where the *uvula* hangs loosely from the midposterior border. The soft palate is a fold of muscular fibers; the hard and soft palates both are covered with mucous membranes. The lateral walls of the oral cavity are soft, mobile and composed of several muscle layers.

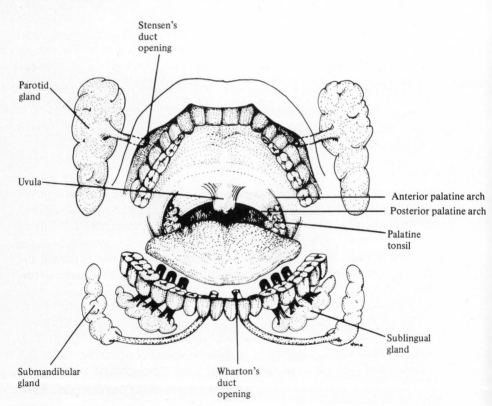

Figure 9-1   The internal structures of the mouth.

The muscles involved in the oral area are complex. Ten of them are intricately involved in controlling movement of the lips. One large muscle, the *orbicularis oris,* surrounds the entire lip area and controls closure of the lips. The *buccinator* is the deep muscle of the cheek and forms the lateral wall of the oral cavity. Trumpet players rely heavily on this muscle in forcing air out through the mouth. Four major muscles are involved in mastication; as a unit they control the opening and closing of the jaws. One of the most powerful muscles in the body is the *masseter.* The masseter muscle in an adult female can exert pressure up to 150 lbs/in^2, and the adult male can double that—a good reason for keeping fingers out of hostile mouths!

The *gingivae* (gums) are a dense fibrous tissue attached directly to the bony alveolar surface and covered with smooth, vascular mucous membranes, as are all the internal surfaces of the oral cavity.

The primary blood supply is the external carotid artery which supplies blood to the mouth through three main branches: (1) the facial branch which supplies the oral cavity itself, (2) the lingual branch which supplies the tongue, and (3) the maxillary branch which supplies the teeth and gum areas.

The lymphatic system in the oral cavity is profuse and drains into the lymph nodes along the neck. The gums drain into the submandibular nodes; the hard and soft palates drain into the deep cervical and subparotid nodes; and the floor of the oral cavity drains into the submandibular, superior deep cervical, or submental nodes. Knowledge of this drainage system is very useful when evaluating enlarged lymph nodes in the neck, a common finding in children.

Innervation of the oral cavity is supplied by two main nerves: the fifth cranial nerve (the trigeminal) and the seventh cranial nerve (the facial).

There are two important sets of nonsalivary glands located in the mouth. The *labial glands* are small, pea-sized glands situated in the orbicularis oris muscles; their ducts open directly into the mucous membranes. The *second group,* the buccal glands, are smaller and located between the buccinator and masseter muscles, with the ducts opening opposite the last molar tooth.

The posterior portions of mouth and nose join to form the throat or *pharynx.* The pharynx is a musculomembranous tube divided into three sections: the *nasopharynx,* the *oropharynx,* and the *laryngopharynx* (see Fig. 9-2). The nasopharynx is posterior to the nasal cavity above the soft palate; it always remains open. The posterior wall of this cavity contains the pharyngeal tonsil which, when enlarged during childhood, is called the *adenoid tissue.* The opening for the eustachian tubes is also found in this cavity.

The oral pharynx is posterior to the oral cavity. Along both lateral walls of this pharynx are two palatine arches and between them are lymph nodules called *palatine tonsils.* This tonsillar tissue enlarges until puberty and then shrinks back into the folds of the palatine arches.

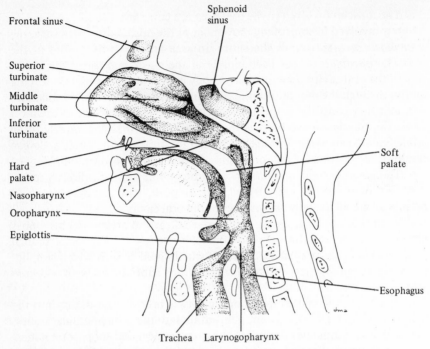

Figure 9-2 A side view of the nasopharynx, oropharynx, and laryngophargynx.

The most inferior part of the throat is the laryngopharynx which lies between the oropharynx and the cricoid cartilage and esophagus. It is in this section that the epiglottis is located.

There are three important related structures within the mouth: the salivary glands, the tongue, and the teeth. The *salivary glands* are exocrine glands which perform excretory and secretory functions in the first stages of digestion.

Secretions from three salivary glands—the parotid, submandibular, and sublingual—pour into the oral cavity. The largest of these is the *parotid* which lies in front of and below the external ear. The parotid (*Stensen's*) duct opens into the oral mucosa opposite the second upper molar, and is an important landmark for certain diagnoses. The *submandibular gland* is the size of a walnut and lies below and in front of the parotid deep within the lower cheek. Its duct, *Wharton's duct,* runs upward from the gland and opens at the side of the frenulum linguae which lies on the undersurface of the tongue. The *sublingual gland* is the size of an almond and lies on the floor of the mouth near the center of the underside of the tongue. Its ducts join with the openings from the submandibular ducts. These three glands produce saliva for the oral cavity. Depending upon age, diet, and exercise, they can produce an average of 1,500 ml of saliva per day. The glands are sensitive to touch, smell, sight, and thought. Saliva is a clear, colorless fluid that contains water, proteins, minerals, and certain enzymes. Salivation increases at 3 months of age and infants usually drool for several months until they learn how to swallow the saliva. This has nothing to do with teething, although many parents will expect their baby to get the first teeth soon after this drooling begins.

The tongue's function in taste, speech, and mastication makes it an extremely important organ in physical assessment. It is composed of a mass of muscles crossing each other at various angles. Posteriorly, the tongue is attached to the hyoid bone near the *epiglottis,* and anteriorly it swings loose and lies against the inner surfaces of the lower teeth. The crisscross effect of the muscles allows the tongue to alter its position, shape, and contour. The inferior surface of the tongue is also attached to the floor of the oral cavity by a central mucous membrane called the *frenulum linguae.* The dorsum or superior surface of the tonue is convex and covered with papillae. The four types of papillae (*papillae vallatae, papillae fungiformes, papillae filiformes,* and *papillae simplices*), give the tongue a rough appearance. Looking like 8 to 12 large mushrooms, the papillae vallatae form the letter V across the posterior surface of the tongue. Each of them contains many taste buds. The papillae fungiformes are large, deep red, and rounded. They are more numerous than the papille vallatae and are scattered over the sides and tip of the tongue. They contain fewer taste buds. The papillae filiformes are tiny, fringed, and cover the anterior two-thirds of the tongue, while the papillae simplices cover the entire surface of the tongue.

The teeth are extremely important in the physical examination. During life, two sets of teeth appear: the deciduous, or baby teeth, and the permanent teeth. Each tooth is divided into three parts: the crown, the neck, and the root. The crown is the exposed portion of the tooth composed of enamel. The neck of the tooth is the constricted connecting portion of the tooth between the crown and root. The root of each tooth is implanted in the alveoli of the mandibular and maxillary bones (see Fig. 9-3).

By the 6th week of fetal life, deciduous teeth are beginning to form. Each tooth erupts through the gums when calcification is sufficient to allow the pressure it must endure for chewing. Every child gets 20 deciduous teeth, each jaw containing 4 incisors, 2 canines, and 4 molars. Generally the lower incisors are the first to erupt, usually around 6 months of age; however, the first teeth may not erupt until 12 months and still be considered within normal limits. All 20 teeth should be present by $2\frac{1}{2}$ years of age.

The permanent teeth begin developing within the jaw during the first 6 months of life. A normal adult has 32 permanent teeth: 4 incisors, 2 canines, 4 premolars, and 6 molars in each jaw (see Fig. 9-4). Usually the

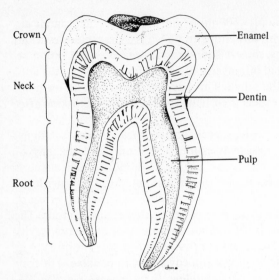

Crown

Neck

Root

Enamel

Dentin

Pulp

Figure 9-3 A tooth.

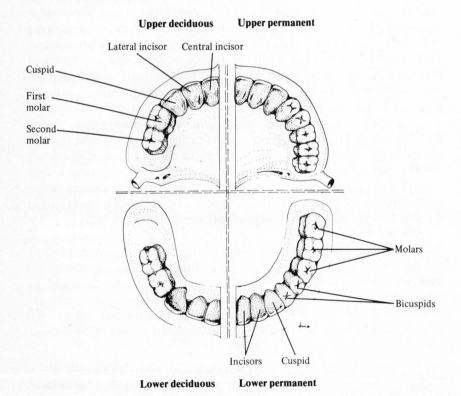

Upper deciduous   **Upper permanent**

Lateral incisor   Central incisor

Cuspid

First molar

Second molar

Molars

Bicuspids

Incisors   Cuspid

Lower deciduous   **Lower permanent**

Figure 9-4   The deciduous and permanent teeth.

lower incisors are shed around the end of the sixth year as the first molars begin erupting. The two central incisors erupt by the seventh year and the teeth are shed and erupt in an orderly fashion until the seventeenth to twenty-fifth year, when the third molars appear (see Table 9-1).

HOW TO EXAMINE

Because the mouth and throat can be a touchy area to examine, it may be wise to leave it for last. The position and the degree of difficulty depend on the age of the child. Since the infant does not need an explanation and will not open the mouth on command, it is best to examine the mouth and throat while the child is lying on his back on the examining table. The parent can hold his arms firmly over his head, and the examiner can use his or her body and arms to stabilize the rest of the child.

The older child might be shown the equipment, watch the examination of her mouth, and probably be held in position on the parent's lap. With her legs caught between the parent's knees, the child should be facing the examiner. The parent can place one arm around the child's chest to restrain her arms, and the other hand can hold the child's head firmly against the parent's chest. A school-age child is generally happy to show off her teeth and tongue if the examiner takes time to show her the light and the stick. This child can sit on the examining table in front of the examiner.

The only way to see all areas of the mouth and throat adequately is with a light. A small pencil-sized flashlight or an otoscope (minus the speculum) works well. The tongue blade is also helpful in pushing aside the tongue or gums for a better look. In infants, the tongue blade is essential for testing the gag reflex. In the older child, it may be needed for a better look at the uvula and tonsils. To avoid the feeling of gagging that children dislike, they should be instructed to pant like a puppy, and the tongue blade can be placed on the lateral portions of the tongue. Some children can easily stick their tongues out far enough for the examiner to get a good look at the throat without the tongue blade. The amount of salivation should be noted. If it is necessary to test for tenth cranial nerve funtion, an applicator stick should be brushed lightly along the lateral walls of the uvula. The uvula should respond by moving upward toward the stimulated side.

To examine the mouth the examiner uses the techniques of inspection and palpation. Percussion and auscultation are not used in this area.

WHERE TO EXAMINE

The entire mouth must be examined thoroughly. Inside and outside of the cavity itself, as well as all surfaces of the relevant structures, must be inspected carefully and where indicated, palpated.

Table 9-1 Chronology of the Human Dentition

Tooth	Hard tissue formation begins	Amount of enamel formed at birth	Enamel completed	Eruption	Root completed
Primary Dentition					
Maxillary					
Central incisor	4 mo in utero	Five-sixths	$1\frac{1}{2}$ mo	$7\frac{1}{2}$ mo	$1\frac{1}{2}$ yr
Lateral incisor	$4\frac{1}{2}$ mo in utero	Two-thirds	$2\frac{1}{2}$ mo	9 mo	2 yr
Cuspid	5 mo in utero	One-third	9 mo	18 mo	$3\frac{1}{4}$ yr
First molar	5 mo in utero	Cusps united	6 mo	14 mo	$2\frac{1}{2}$ yr
Second molar	6 mo in utero	Cusp tips still isolated	11 mo	24 mo	3 yr
Mandibular					
Central incisor	$4\frac{1}{2}$ mo in utero	Three-fifths	$2\frac{1}{2}$ mo	6 mo	$1\frac{1}{2}$ yr
Lateral incisor	$4\frac{1}{2}$ mo in utero	Three-fifths	3 mo	7 mo	$1\frac{1}{2}$ yr
Cuspid	5 mo in utero	One-third	9 mo	16 mo	$3\frac{1}{4}$ yr
First molar	5 mo in utero	Cusps united	$5\frac{1}{2}$ mo	12 mo	$2\frac{1}{4}$ yr
Second molar	6 mo in utero	Cusp tips still isolated	10 mo	20 mo	3 yr
Permanent Dentition					
Maxillary					
Central incisor	3–4 mo		4–5 yr	7–8 yr	10 yr
Lateral incisor	10–12 mo		4–5 yr	8–9 yr	11 yr
Cuspid	4–5 mo		6–7 yr	11–12 yr	13–15 yr
First bicuspid	$1\frac{1}{2}$–$1\frac{3}{4}$ yr		5–6 yr	10–11 yr	12–13 yr
Second bicuspid	2–$2\frac{1}{4}$ yr		6–7 yr	10–12 yr	12–14 yr
First molar	At birth	Sometimes a trace	$2\frac{1}{2}$–3 yr	6–7 yr	9–10 yr
Second molar	$2\frac{1}{2}$–3 yr		7–8 yr	12–13 yr	14–16 yr
Mandibular					
Central incisor	3–4 mo		4–5 yr	6–7 yr	9 yr
Lateral incisor	3–4 mo		4–5 yr	7–8 yr	10 yr
Cuspid	4–5 mo		6–7 yr	9–10 yr	12–14 yr
First bicuspid	$1\frac{3}{4}$–2 yr		5–6 yr	10–12 yr	12–13 yr
Second bicuspid	$2\frac{1}{4}$–$2\frac{1}{2}$ yr		6–7 yr	11–12	13–14 yr
First molar	At birth	Sometimes a trace	$2\frac{1}{2}$–3 yr	6–7 yr	9–10 yr
Second molar	$2\frac{1}{2}$–3 yr		7–8 yr	11–13 yr	14–15 yr

Source: After Logan and Kronfeld (slightly modified by McCall and Schour). From Finn, *Clinical Pedodontics*, W. B. Saunders Co., 1962.

WHAT TO EXAMINE WITH

The equipment needed to examine the mouth adequately is simple and inexpensive. A tongue blade and good light are essential. The batteries in the light, whether flashlight or otoscope light, must be new. It is easy to grow accustomed to a gradually fading light, but without realizing it, the examiner will greatly decrease his or her observational powers in this way. The nurse should make it a habit to change these batteries at least once a week (less often for the "long life" batteries). An applicator may be used to test the function of the tenth cranial nerve. Although it is not generally used, a postnasal mirror is recommended by many authors, as is a retractor to pull back the tonsillar pillar to view the complete tonsil behind it. Although helpful at times, these items are probably not absolutely necessary. A nasopharyngoscope, although used in certain types of specialized examinations of the nasopharynx, is not used in a routine examination, and the nurse-examiner need not be concerned with it.

WHAT TO EXAMINE FOR

The amount of salivation should be noted. The lips should be inspected for symmetry (any twisting, drooping, or clefts), for fissures, for color and for edema. They should be palpated for muscle tone.

The normal lips of infants are moist and pink-tinged, and the skin is fairly smooth. A *sucking tubercle* may be found in the middle of the upper lip of bottle- or breast-fed infants; this is normal, and the parent should be assured that it will disappear within a few weeks after weaning. Cracked, bleeding lips (*cheilitis*) may be due to wind and sun; protection from the elements will allow healing and the application of an ointment or cream may speed the process. Children with upper respiratory infections or any febrile illness may also exhibit cheilitis. Again, the application of a cream may help, but the parent must always be warned to apply only a thin covering, since there is a possibility that an excess amount might be aspirated. Some children have a habit of licking their lips until they are red, sore, and chapped. Usually, a coating of cream will help the child to remember not to lick and will also help to heal the chapping. Children with dry, scaly patches at the corners of the lips should be examined for nutritional deficiencies, and a careful history should be taken. The color of the lips is important. A gray cyanosis may mean the child has a congenital heart lesion, while a deep purple hue may indicate severe congenital heart disease. A child with pale lips and gums may be anemic. Bright cherry-red lips may be indicative of acidosis from aspirin poisoning, diabetes, or carbon monoxide poisoning.

The oral cavity itself must be examined thoroughly. The mouth is inspected for odor. *Halitosis* may be due to poor hygiene, a local or systemic infection, sinusitis, mouth breathing, or a foreign body (as a pea or bean) in the nose. The child who is brought in with a specific complaint or illness frequently has halitosis which clears up when he regains his health and begins to eat and drink normally. The amount of salivation should be noted.

Children with dehydration, malnourishment, or diabetic acidosis give off a sweet smell like acetone and need prompt referral.

Some diseases give off distinct odors. For example, diphtheria causes a mouselike odor; typhoid fever smells like decaying tissue; and uremic patients have ammoniacal breath.

The buccal mucosa may display several important physical signs: an enlarged Stensen's duct, often puffy and red, may accompany mumps or other infections of the parotid gland; *Koplik spots* indicate that the child is in the prodromal stage of measles. These spots are grayish in the center and are surrounded by a red, irregular areola. They first appear on the buccal mucosa opposite the lower molars, although they may later become much more widespread. A white raised line directly adjacent to the biting surface of the molars may be caused by sucking or biting on the cheek and is harmless unless very severe and painful. Brownish or blackish blue areas on the buccal mucosa may be a sign of Addison's disease or may appear in children suffering from intestinal polyposis. Blue translucent cysts that may block any mucous gland in the mouth are usually benign. The floor of the mouth should be palpated bimanually for neoplasms or calculi in the submaxillary glands. Tonsillar tissue, of course, must be examined for enlargement, erythema, and white or yellowish follicles filling the crypts. The size of the tonsils is usually estimated on a scale from $+1$ to $+4$. Tonsils that are recorded as $+1$ are usually those with barely visible edges; if they meet in the midline they are graded as $+4$. These signs, as well as general erythema of the posterior pharynx, will usually be present in varying degrees in *pharyngitis.*

The hard and soft palates should be inspected and palpated. *Epstein's pearls* (or Bohn's nodules) are frequently found along the alveolar ridge or bilaterally along the median raphe in the newborn. These represent an accumulation of epithelial cells and look like white glistening circular patches a few millimeters in diameter. The hard palate should be observed for color and shape, the presence or absence of jaundice or petechiae, and any cleft.

When a gag reflex is elicited or when the child says "ah," the soft palate should be observed for upward movement. The uvula should be midline and should not deviate with this movement. Its length should be noted and whether it is bifid; a finger should be inserted into the child's mouth to palpate the soft palate. If the soft palate is incomplete and a notch is felt at the junction of the hard and soft palate, the child needs further evaluation. If such a submucous cleft exists, it may lead to speech difficulties later.

Since it indicates a minor degree of penetrance for the genetic defect which causes cleft palate, it may be appropriate to refer such a family for genetic counseling.

Bednar's aphthae are reddish or yellow-gray patches of eroded tissue found posteriorly on each side of the midline of the hard palate. They are usually due to vigorous aspiration at birth or to trauma from sucking on a very hard nipple. The height of the palatal arch should also be evaluated. High palatal arches are normal in the new born (the so-called "infantile palate" which gradually recedes until it reaches adult proportion at 4 to 5 years of age), but very high narrow arches appear with several syndromes, such as Marfan's, Treacher Collins, Ehlers-Danlos, and Turner's, and are often present in children who constantly breathe through their mouths. Such an arch in an older child is frequently accompanied by orthodontia problems.

During examination of the mouth and throat, the size of the lower jaw should be considered. The mandible is excessively small in the birdface (vogelgesicht) syndrome and in juvenile rheumatoid arthritis; it is quite large in chondrodystrophy and in Crouzon's disease.

The teeth can easily give clues of health or illness. The delayed appearance of teeth after the first 12 months may be normal, due to genetic factors, but it should not be assumed to be normal until the child has been checked for signs of cretinism, rickets, and congenital syphilis, which may also cause the delay.

Bruxism is the grinding of the teeth. Infants often develop this habit as they acquire a few teeth, and older children will sometimes grind their teeth in their sleep, occasionally resulting in teeth with flattened edges. The cause is often tension, and this possibility should be explored with the child and parents. Checking for *malocclusion* is also important. Generally, teeth are not classified as malocclusive unless there is an interference with the ability to chew properly, or the condition presents a severe cosmetic problem. Children who continue to suck their thumbs after the age of 6 years are likely to push their jaws and teeth out of alignment, sometimes causing malocclusion.

Caries are a very common health problem and should be looked for at every visit. Generally only large surface cavities are detectable by the nurse. A dental visit is essential to find smaller cavities or those between tooth surfaces.

Discoloration of the teeth can be caused in several ways. Green and black teeth may be caused by iron ingestion and will disappear as soon as iron has been reduced in the child's diet. It is important to tell parents this so that they do not become upset when the teeth turn green. Children who have had jaundice at birth will also occasionally display green teeth.

Mottled and pitted teeth are seen in children who have been exposed to excess fluoride in the drinking water or to tetracycline treatment.

Just as important as evaluation of the teeth is an evaluation of the gums. The *alveolar frenulum,* a septum extending downward from the center upper gum line and causing a separation between the central incisors, is a common occurrence in children, and mothers should be assured that this will correct itself. Children who are taking Dilantin will frequently have gingival hypertrophy; however, meticulous attention to dental hygiene and digital pressure to the gums several times a day will usually help or completely eliminate the problem. A black line along the margin of the gums may be a sign of metal poisoning, but this should not be confused with the melanotic line along the gums normally seen in the black child. Purple, bleeding gums are seen with scurvy; leukemia and poor oral hygiene also cause bleeding gums. Children with hypertrophy around each tooth crown are usually mouth breathers or are taking Dilantin or are vitamin deficient. Normal infants have retention cysts in or near the midline of the gums. When on the gums, they are called Epstein's pearls, when on the midpalate, they are called Bohn's nodules. However, both types usually disappear in 2 to 3 months.

The tongue is observed for movement in all directions, for any coating, and for the size of the papillae and frenulum. A child is not "tongue-tied" (i.e., does not have a tight frenulum) if he or she can touch the tip of the tongue to the lips. Variations in the condition of the tongue can be very significant. A white, cheesy coating on the tongue often extending to the buccal mucosa is most likely to be *thrush,* caused by infection with *Candida albicans.* It is usually easy to identify microscopically, but if there is any doubt, a smear of the coating should be mixed with 10 percent potassium hydroxide. The hyphae of the organism will show up clearly under the microscope. The tongues of babies who have just taken a formula may have a coating similar to thrush, but the white patches can be brushed off easily with a tongue blade. Thrush patches, on the other hand, leave a red, bleeding spot when they are scraped off.

Geographic tongue is sometimes seen in children. In this condition, the tongue has irregular areas of differently textured papillae, which change from day to day, and usually cause no problems. *Macroglossia,* or large tongue, is a sign of cretinism, Down's syndrome, Hurler's syndrome, and many other syndromes. These children should be referred for further evaluation.

If a child presents with unexplained *dysphagia* and *stridor,* palpation of the base of the tonue is indicated. In rare situations there will be duplication of the alimentary canal, beginning at the level of the tongue.

Glossoptosis refers to a tongue whose attachment is more forward than usual. It is frequently accompanied by a small mandible which may create problems in feeding, as well as cause episodes of hypoxia, cyanosis, and dyspnea. Also, glossoptosis may be associated with cleft palate.

Protrusion of the tongue is frequently seen in children suffering from mental retardation. Rhythmic protrusion, however, has been implicated in intracranial hemorrhage and edema of the brain.

A *white strawberry tongue* consists of erythematous, swollen fungiform papillae intermingled with smaller white filiform papillae. This is the classic sign of scarlet fever, occurring on the second to third day of the illness, but it sometimes occurs in measles or other febrile diseases. *Raspberry tongue* refers to a condition in which the filiform papillae desquamate and take on a beefy-red appearance; the fungiform papillae appear quite large and erythematous. This occurs on the sixth to seventh day of scarlet fever and sometimes in other febrile conditions.

A beefy-red, swollen tongue may also be an indication of pellagra and necessitates a careful nutritional history.

Tremor of the tongue may be a sign of thyrotoxicosis.

Deviation of the tongue to one side may indicate an impairment of the twelfth cranial nerve or a neoplasm on one side of the tongue.

Fissures of the tongue should be inspected carefully. If the tongue has fissures that extend transversely, it is called *scrotal tongue* and is a normal variant. Longitudinal fissures, however, are more worrisome and may indicate syphilitic glossitis.

Glossitis in general may result from any type of infection, usually one extending from a pharyngitis. *Atrophic glossitis* looks like a smooth, glistening, erythematous tongue. The papillae are small and look like tiny pinpoints appearing randomly on the glistening surface.

Evaluation of the salivary glands is accomplished by means of inspection and palpation. Inflammation of the parotid gland is the most common finding. To be sure that the swelling is indeed due to the parotid gland, one must be familiar with the distribution of this gland. Swelling due to its inflammation usually will be found beginning in front of the tragus, extending downward to the angle of the jaw, and then up and behind the pinna, frequently pushing it outward to form an acute angle with the skull. Painful swellings with this distribution will be found in mumps. Similar but painless swellings can be found in several other conditions.

Purulent parotitis is sometimes encountered in the child. In this condition, the parotid gland is enlarged, often erythematous, and warm to the touch. Pus can be expressed through Stensen's duct. In infants, this problem seems to be associated with a general failure to thrive.

Calculi can at times be lodged in the ducts leading to the salivary glands. The most frequent site is the submaxillary gland. Swelling will often occur only with meals and will subside within an hour or two after eating.

GLOSSARY

atrophic glossitis   a smooth, glistening, erythematous tongue

bednar's aphthae   reddish or yellow-gray patches of eroded tissue found posteriorly on each side of the midline of the hard palate

bruxism   tooth grinding

buccal glands   nonsalivary glands located between the buccinator and masseter muscles of the mouth

caries   tooth decay leading to destruction of the tooth

cheilitis   cracked, bleeding lips

dysphagia   inability to swallow

epiglottis   the flap covering the superior opening of the larynx

Epstein's pearls   retention cysts found on the gums of newborns

frenulum   mucous membrane attaching the inferior surface of the tongue to the floor of the oral cavity

geographic tongue   irregular areas of differently textured papillae on the tongue

gingivae   the gums

glossitis   infection of the tongue

glossoptosis   a tongue whose attachment is more forward than usual

halitosis   foul-smelling breath

hard palate   the anterior portion of the maxilla bone dividing the nasal and oral cavities

herpes simplex (cold sore)   a viral infection causing inflamed, burning, itching vesicles on the lips, gums, palate, and tongue

Koplik spots   red, irregular spots with a grayish center seen on the buccal mucosa of children with measles

labial glands   small, pea-sized glands located in the orbicularis oris muscles

laryngopharynx   the lower end of the pharynx which opens into the larynx

occlusion   the normal relationship of the upper and lower teeth when the jaws are closed or when masticating

oropharynx   the junction between the oral cavity and the pharynx

papillae filiformes   tiny, fringed bumps covering the anterior two-thirds of the tongue

papillae fungiformes   large, deep-red, rounded bumps scattered over the sides and tip of the tongue

papillae simplices   small, rounded bumps covering the entire surface of the tongue

papillae vallatae   large, mushroom-like bumps forming a large V across the posterior surface of the tongue

parotid gland   a salivary gland located in front of and below the external ear on each side of the face

pharynx   the throat

raspberry tongue   a beefy-red tongue the appearance of which is caused by desquamation of papillae filiformes

salivary glands   exocrine glands which perform excretory and secretory digestive functions in the mouth

soft palate   the soft posterior roof of the mouth, separating the nasal and oral cavities

Stensen's duct the opening for the parotid gland which is located in the oral mucosa opposite the second upper molar tooth

sublingual glands a salivary gland the size of an almond, located on the floor of the mouth near the center of the underside of the tongue

submandibular gland a salivary gland the size of a walnut, located below and in front of the parotid and deep within the lower cheek

sucking tubercle a small, firm, rounded pad of skin seen in the middle of the upper lip in bottle- or breast-fed infants

thrush a fungal infection of the mouth caused by *Candida albicans*

tonsils the small, oval-shaped, lymphoid tissue between the anterior and posterior palatine arches

uvula a small tag of tissue hanging from the posterior edge of the soft palate

Wharton's duct the opening for the submandibular gland at the side of the frenulum linguae on the undersurface of the tongue

white strawberry tongue a tongue covered with erythematous, swollen fungiform papillae intermingled with smaller white filiform papillae

Inspection of the Nose, Mouth, and Throat*

Nose	Yes	No	Not appli-cable	Describe (where appropriate)	Significance
A. External nose 1. Skin normal					Same significance as elsewhere.
2. Normal shape					Abnormalities of shape may be due to congenital factors or trauma; if excessive, cosmetic plastic surgery is sometimes attempted.
B. Internal nose 1. Mucosa a. normal red color					
b. grey color					Usually indicates chronic allergy.
c. boggy					Same significance as B.
d. polyps					Same significance as B.
e. dry, cracked					May indicate chronic infection.
f. other					
2. Septum a. deviation					Often from trauma; needs no treatment unless it interferes with air passage.
b. perforation					Often from trauma; may need no treatment if air exchanged is not hampered.
3. Normal turbinate					
4. Drainage a. bleeding					Requires immediate attention—compression over the nostrils and ice over the bridge of the nose.

b. clear		Sometimes transient from sudden cold air; sometimes a sign of allergy or beginning cold.
c. white		May be a sign of upper respiratory infection or allergy and superinfection.
d. yellow		Indicates infection.
e. green		Indicates infection.

Mouth

A. Lips		
1. Normal color		Cyanosis may be most detectable in the lips.
2. Normal shape and fullness		Very thin-lined lips accompany several mental retardation syndromes.
3. Cracking		May indicate dry skin or vitamin deficiency, particularly at corners.
B. Gums		
1. Swollen		May indicate use of dilantin or gum disease; may occur in pregnancy.
2. Bleeding		Same as above.
3. Discolored		Blue "lead line" may indicate lead ingestion.
4. Other		

*This chart is meant to be used by beginning students as they perform their first physical assessments. Each item should be examined on the child and then checked off on the checklist. The significance of the items follows in the right-hand column.

153

Inspection of the Nose, Mouth, and Throat (*Continued*)

Mouth	Yes	No	Not appli-cable	Describe (where appropriate)	Significance
C. Teeth*					
1. Cavities					Require education and referral.
2. Malocclusion					Any severe degree requires referral.
3. Number of primary teeth					Average is the number of months minus 6 up to 20.
4. Number of secondary teeth					Should begin at about 7 years.
5. Number of missing teeth					Important to assess whether the teeth missing are expected to be missing at that age.
6. Normal color					Tetracycline taken during pregnancy or early childhood can discolor and mottle teeth; excessive fluoride intake can also mottle teeth; cavities may appear as brownish spots.
7. Other					
D. Buccal mucosa					
1. Stenson's ducts					May be enlarged in mumps.
2. Ulcerations					May be due to suction trauma in newborn, chewing on inner cheeks in childhood, herpes, or other infections.
3. Irritation					May be from biting cheeks, from dentures, etc., or sucking.
4. Other					
E. Palate					
1. Soft					Should be visible, but small indentation on phonation needs immediate attention.
2. Cleft (overt)					Needs immediate attention.

3. Submucous cleft		Probably indicates a genetic predisposition for cleft palate in the family; may need genetic referral, also needs careful speech evaluation.
4. Thrush		May be associated with vaginal monilial infection in mother if a new-born; can be associated with malnutrition or underlying poor health; often painful enough to interfere with eating.
5. Other		
F. Tongue		
1. Normal tongue movements within mouth		Important for sucking, eating, and later speech; indication of muscular and neurological functioning.
2. Movement outside mouth		If tongue can reach to gum line, tongue-tie does not exist; normal movements indicate intact muscular and neurological development.
3. Normal size		Macroglossia can be a sign of certain mental retardation syndromes; it can also be a cause of anoxia if it obstructs the posterior throat.
4. Normal shape		
5. Normal texture		Geographic tongue is a normal variant; furrows may indicate need to teach about tongue brushing.
6. White patches		May indicate thrush (if thrush, they cannot be manually removed).
7. Frenulum		If long enough to allow tongue to touch gums, it is not causing tongue-tie.
8. Wharton's ducts		Should be present and free of signs of infection.
9. Normal underside of tongue		Varicose veins may be apparent here indicating vascular obstruction.
10. Coating of tongue		May indicate digestive problem or mouth breathing.

*For charting purposes, primary teeth are identified by a letter starting with "A" as the second molar in the upper right jaw, proceeding across the upper jaw to "J" as the second molar in the upper left jaw. The lettering then proceeds to "K" as the second molar in the lower left jaw and ends with "T", the second molar in the lower right jaw. The system is the same for permanent teeth except numbers are used instead of letters (beginning with number 1, which indicates the upper right wisdom tooth and ending with number 32, which indicates the lower right wisdom tooth).

Inspection of the Nose, Mouth, and Throat (*Continued*)

Mouth	Yes	No	Not applicable	Describe (where appropriate)	Significance
G. Salivary glands					
1. Visible parotid glands					Visibility may indicate enlargement; enlargement occurs in mumps or parotitis.
2. Visible submandibular (submaxillary)					Visibility may indicate enlargement, usually secondary to infection.
3. Visible sublingual					Same as above.
Throat					
A. Uvula					
1. Bifid					Often associated with submucous cleft and speech defect; may also indicate nonpenetrant gene for cleft palate and have implications for genetic counseling.
2. Movement to each side					Movement with phonation indicates intact cranial nerve numbers nine and ten.
B. Palatoglossal arches					Should be inspected for signs of infection.
1. Normal color					Erythema may indicate infection.
2. Exudate					May indicate infection, particularly streptococcal infection.
3. Crypts					May indicate long-standing infection.
C. Palatopharyngeal arches					
1. Normal color					Same significance as in palatoglossal arches.
2. Exudate					
D. Palatine tonsils					
1. Enlarged					May indicate infection (present or past).

156

					Significance
2. Crypts					Indicates previous chronic infection.
3. Normal color					Same significance as in palatoglossal arches.
4. Exudate					
E. Wall of oropharynx					
1. Normal color					Same significance as in palatoglossal arches.
2. Exudate					

Palpation of the Nose and Mouth

Nose	Yes	No	Not appli-cable	Describe (where appropriate)	Significance
A. Skin texture					Same significance as elsewhere.
B. Bony structure					
Mouth					
A. Skin texture					Same significance as elsewhere.
B. Any palpable lesions					Same significance as listed under inspection.
C. Submucous cleft					

Source: These checklists are printed with permission from Blue Hill Videotape Incorporated and are part of a more complete programmed learning approach to the physical examination, which includes a workbook and series of videotapes. It can be purchased from Blue Hill Educational Systems, Inc., 52 South Main Street, Spring Valley, New York 10977.

157

Chapter 10

The Chest and Lungs

WHY THE CHILD IS EXAMINED

The condition of the chest and lungs in children is of vital importance. The cartilage and bones of the chest may give an early indication of nutritional problems, as well as clues to pathologic disturbances in the organs below or adjacent to them. The lungs are certainly the seat of one of the most common of childhood ailments, the upper respiratory infection, but also of many more serious problems, including respiratory distress syndrome, cystic fibrosis, asthma, and many others.

WHAT TO EXAMINE: ANATOMY OF THE AREA

The chest, or thorax, is the large cavity occupying the upper portions of the trunk, which contains the heart and lungs. It is enclosed in a bony, cartilaginous cage made up of 12 thoracic vertebrae, 12 ribs, the costal cartilages, and the sternum. The vertebrae are described in more detail in the

158

chapter, "The Skeletal System: Spine nd Extremities."

The majority of the bony thorax is composed of ribs. Each rib is a highly vascular structure covered with a small layer of dense bone. There are 12 ribs on each side. The 7 true, or vertebrocostal, ribs are attached posteriorly to the vertebrae and anteriorly through the costal cartilages to the sternum. Of the 5 false, or vertebrochondral, ribs the first 3 have cartilages that attach to the rib above them, while the remaining 2 are called *floating ribs,* because they do not attach to either the upper rib or the sternum. The anterior portion of all the ribs attaches to cartilage. These costal cartilages frequently become enlarged in rickets, causing the condition known as *rachitic rosary* which can be palpated as a series of small lumps running down each side of the sternum (see Fig. 10-1).

The sternum is a flat, narrow bone composed of highly vascular cancellous tissue enclosed by dense bone. The superior portion attaches to the first 7 ribs. It is composed of three parts: the manubrium, the body, and the xiphoid process. The *manubrium* is roughly triangular and attaches to the first and second ribs and provides a place of attachment for the *pectoralis major* and *sternocleidomastoid muscles.* The body of the sternum consists of four segments which become fused throughout life. The *xiphoid process* is the small, thin, long cartilaginous end of the sternum. It may remain cartilaginous throughout life or it may ossify around 30 to 40 years of age. There are great variations in the xiphoid: some are flat, some bifid, some curved, and some one-sided.

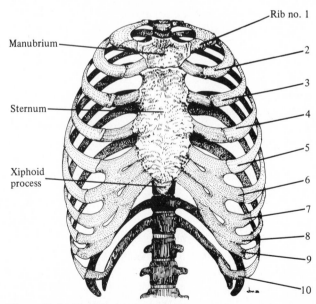

Figure 10-1 The rib cage and sternum.

The chest can assume several different shapes. Many of these are associated with disease. The normal shape is generally conical and slightly kidney-shaped. Various abnormalities will be discussed under the section "What To Examine For."

The thorax contains many muscles used in the movement of the upper extremities (which are further described in the section on extremities), as well as 8 thoracic muscles: the *intercostales externi, intercostales interni, subcostales, transversus thoracis, levatores costarum, serratus posterior superior, serratus posterior inferior,* and *diaphragm.* There are 11 intercostales externi muscles which extend from the dorsal sections of the ribs to the ventrocostal cartilages. These help in increasing the volume within the thoracic cage. The intercostales interni also number 11 and extend from the sternum to the vertebrae. They help to decrease the thoracic cavity volume. The subcostales attach the upper to the lower ribs and help in decreasing the thoracic volume. The transversus thoracis is a thin sheet of muscle and tendon fibers extending from the sternum to the costal cartilages. It also helps to decrease the chest volume. The 12 levatores costarum muscles extend from the cervical and thoracic vertebrae to the outer surfaces of the ribs. The thoracic volume is decreased and the vertebral column laterally curved by these muscles. The thin serratus posterior superior muscles extend from the spinous processes of the cervical and thoracic vertebrae to the upper borders of the second, third, fourth, and fifth ribs. The thoracic cage is increased in volume by this muscle. The broad serratus posterior inferior runs from the spinous processes of the thoracic and lumbar vertebrae to the lower edges of the last 4 ribs. It works as the antagonist to the diaphragm. The diaphragm is a large, musculofibrous membrane dividing the abdominal cavity from the thoracic cavity; its cranial surface is convex, while its caudal surface is concave. There are three parts to the diaphragm: the sternal portion, costal portion, and lumbar portion. The sternal portion lies near the posterior xiphoid process; the costal portion is near the rib cartilages, and the lumbar portion rests near the lumbar vertebrae. There are three large openings in the diaphragm which allow certain structures to pass from one cavity to the other. The *aortic hiatus* lies in a dorsal and lateral position and allows the aorta, azygos vein, and thoracic duct to pass. To the left of the aortic hiatus lies the *esophageal hiatus.* The esophagus, vagus nerves, and some esophageal blood vessels travel through this opening. The inferior vena cava and several branches of the right phrenic nerve pass through the third opening—the *foramen venae cavae.*

In examining the chest, the nurse must also be familiar with the anatomy of the mammary glands, or breast (see Fig. 10-2). These structures are situated on the anterior chest wall between the second and seventh ribs midway between the sternum and axilla. In adulthood the average female breast weighs between 150 to 200 g and the left is usually slightly larger than

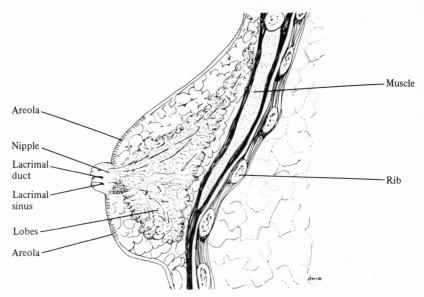

Areola
Nipple
Lacrimal duct
Lacrimal sinus
Lobes
Areola
Muscle
Rib

Figure 10-2 The mature breast.

the right. It is composed of glandular tissue, adipose tissue, and suspensory ligaments, which are situated within the subcutaneous fascia, as well as a nipple and areola on the cutaneous level. Between 15 to 20 lobes make up the glandular tissue which encircles the nipple. Adipose tissue is found interspersed among these lobes and between them and the skin. The suspensory ligaments (*Cooper's ligaments*) are fibrous bands which run vertically throughout the breast and attach the deep subcutaneous tissue to the skin. The nipple (or *mammary papilla*) is the rough, wrinkled, pigmented projection slightly below the center of the breast and at the fourth intercostal space. From 15 to 20 lactiferous ducts open into the tip of the nipple. The rough, pigmented area surrounding the nipple is called the *areola.* The areolar (*Montgomery's glands*) are large sebaceous glands distributed throughout the areola. These glands secrete a substance for lubrication and protection during lactation. The areola also contains smooth muscle fibers which can cause the nipple to become erect with stimulation. At birth the lactiferous ducts within the nipples may be the only breast structures that are present. At puberty the glandular tissue increases as the ducts and the amount of adipose tissue increases.

Basically the thorax is innervated by the intercostal, thoracic, phrenic, and cervical nerves.

Blood supply to the chest comes from the thoracic branch of the descending aorta. The thoracic aorta has 7 branches (pericardial, bronchial, esophageal, mediastinal, posterior intercostal, subcostal, and superior phrenic) to carry blood to the thorax. Blood is carried from the thorax via the azygos veins and tributaries which pour into the superior vena cava.

The chest contains several important organs: the heart and great vessels, as well as the organs of the lower respiratory tract. (The heart will be described elsewhere.) (see Fig. 10-3).

The chest cavity is divided into halves, with a middle portion known as the *mediastinum.* The superior portion of the mediastinum is divided into the anterior mediastinum, middle mediastinum, and posterior mediastinum.

The lower respiratory trace consists of the trachea, the bronchi, the pleura, and the lungs. The *trachea,* or windpipe, is a 2-cm, almost cylindrical cartilaginous tube that connects the larynx and the bronchi. In children it is quite mobile and lies deep within the neck musculature. The trachea contains between 16 and 20 cartilages, some of which form the *larynx,* or voice box. As the trachea extends downward towards the bronchi, its ventral surface passes behind the isthmus of the thyroid, several neck muscles, cervical fascia, the manubrium of the sternum, the *thymus,* the left brachiocephalic vein, the aortic arch, and the common carotid arteries. The dorsal side of the trachea lies against the esophagus.

The trachea bifurcates at the fifth thoracic vertebra to form the right and left *bronchi.* The right bronchus is broad and short and curves gently to the right. It subdivides into three smaller bronchi, each one entering one lobe of the lung. These again divide into smaller and smaller bronchi within

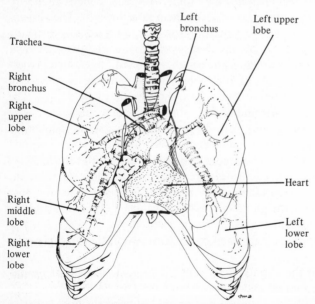

Figure 10-3 The structures within the chest.

the lung. The left bronchus is narrower but longer than the right. It divides into two smaller bronchi, going to the lung lobes.

Each lung is covered with a single layer of serous membrane called the *pleura*. Different portions of the membrane are given different names. Between the pulmonary pleura (which covers the surface of the lungs) and the parietal pleura (which covers the diaphragm and inner surface of the chest wall) lies the pleural cavity. In the healthy person, these two membranes lie together. In illness, air or fluid may separate the membranes.

The lungs are two spongy sacs in the lateral aspects of the thorax separated by the heart and other mediastinal contents. The lungs are composed of serous tissue, subserous areolar tissue, and parenchyma (small lobules). An infant's lungs are pink and white, but by adulthood carbon granules deposited on the areolar tissue give the lungs a gray–black color.

Each lung is divided into an apex, which is the rounded, blunt top reaching above the first rib, a base, which is the wide, concave bottom that lies on the diaphragm, and two surfaces: the costal surface which faces the chest walls, and the mediastinal surface which faces the mediastinal area. The lungs are divided into lobes. The right lung is heavier, shorter, and has a larger total capacity than the left lung. It contains three lobes, while the left lung has only two lobes. Entering the lungs are many subdivisions of the bronchi. After the trachea bifurcates to form two bronchi, each bronchus divides to form secondary multiple bronchi which enter the lobes of the lung. These multiple bronchi continue to divide into smaller branches called *bronchioles* and finally become microscopic tubules called *respiratory bronchioles*. Well within the lung, the respiratory bronchioles divide into many alveolar ducts, which connect to the atria, and contain alveolar sacs. The *alveoli* are tiny areas 0.25 mm in diameter, lined with pulmonary alveolar epithelium. Its walls contain blood capillaries and collagenous, reticular, and elastic connective tissue fibers. In this area the exchange of gases from the air to the blood takes place.

Respiration is the exchange of gases between the air and bloodstream. This is performed by coordinated efforts of the chest muscles to expand and decrease the volume of the chest cavity.

After the deepest inspiration, the largest amount of air that can be exhaled (*vital capacity*) is about 3,700 ml for an adult male. An adult male can exchange about 500 ml of air during quiet, normal respiration while the infant exchanges around 20 ml. This is called *tidal air*. Normal respiration may be diaphragmatic (abdominal) or costal (thoracic). Costal breathing is more predominant in the adult and abdominal breathing is predominant in infants and young children.

During inspiration the diaphragm contracts and pulls away from the thoracic cage into the abdominal cavity. This decreases the pressure within the thorax and draws air into the lungs. It also increases the pressure within the abdominal cavity. During expiration the diaphragm relaxes and rises to its original position. This increases the pressure in the thoracic cage and forces the gases into the bloodstream or out through the upper respiratory tract. The relaxed diaphragm decreases the pressure in the abdominal cavity.

HOW TO EXAMINE

For examination of the chest and lungs, all four basic methods of assessment are utilized: inspection, palpation, percussion, and auscultation.

WHERE TO EXAMINE

The entire chest from neck to abdomen and from front to back must be thoroughly examined. The sides under the arms must not be forgotten.

WHAT TO EXAMINE WITH

Besides inspection, palpation, and percussion, for which no specialized instruments are needed, examination of the lungs entails thorough auscultation. For this a stethoscope is necessary; the details of the stethoscope are discussed in the chapter "The Heart."

WHAT TO EXAMINE FOR

In examining the chest, all the anatomical structures must be considered and assessed. The skin in this area is examined in much the same way as skin on any other part of the body. There are a few skin manifestations, however, which are peculiar to this area. The spider nevi of liver disease, for instance, will frequently occur only on the chest and shoulders. The nipples are a cutaneous structure which deserve special attention. Supernumerary (extra) nipples will occasionally be found and should be considered normal. If found, they are usually about 5 to 6 cm below the normal nipple; however, they can be located anywhere on the milk line which extends on a diagonal from the upper outer shoulders, cutting through the true nipples and continuing to the medial pubic bone. Supernumerary nipples which are located at a lateral, superior position on this line are more likely to be large and to lactate during pregnancy. Extra nipples are more common on black women. Nipple color must also be checked; particularly dark nipples may indicate adrenocorticosteroid problems. Spacing is also important. Wide-set nipples (the condition in which the distance between the outside areolar edges is more than $\frac{1}{4}$ of the chest circumference) can be a sign of Turner's syndrome.

Nipples should also be checked for fissures, inversions, secretions, scaling, and lumps. These conditions are uncommon in children.

The muscles of the chest must be assessed next. Atrophy or agenesis of the pectoralis major muscle is an infrequent, but possible, finding as is pseudohypertrophy of the chest muscles.

The cartilage must be carefully inspected and palpated. Rachitic rosary at the *costochondrial junction* may be an indication of vitamin D deficiency. These sharp, angular bumps in this area give the examiner a clue to search for further signs of rickets, although hypophosphatase and chondrodystrophy may also cause these bumps. Painful swellings of the first 4 costochondral junctions may be an indication of the *Tietze's syndrome.* In this case, the nodules are firm but tender on palpation; this tenderness and at times actual pain may radiate the length of the rib. Usually, it subsides spontaneously in 4 to 5 months. It is uncommon in children at this age.

The bones are another chest structure which must be evaluated (see Fig. 10-4). Shape of the individual bones and the general bony configuration must be assessed through inspection and palpation. *Pigeon chest* is the condition in which the sternum protrudes from the chest wall and a series of vertical depressions along the costochondral junction appear. This can accompany rickets, Marfan's syndrome, Morquio's disease, and any type of chronic upper respiratory obstruction.

Funnel breast (pectus excavatum) is a condition most obvious on inspiration. It begins with a mild oval pit at the sternal notch and progresses

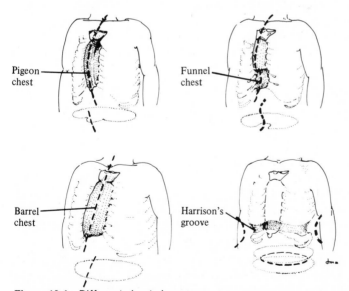

Figure 10-4 Different chest shapes.

to form an indentation in the sternal area. Mild degrees of funnel breast are usually normal. More severe forms can be seen in rickets and Marfan's syndrome.

Barrel chest refers to the condition in which the ribs form perfect circles. This is usually accompanied by kyphosis and may be an indication of pulmonary emphysema or such chronic lung problems as asthma and cystic fibrosis. Although mild degrees of barrel chest can be normal in the elderly, this is never true in children.

Localized bulges may also occur from underlying pressure. Cardiac enlargement and aneurysms are two examples of such conditions.

Spinal deformities, such as *kyphosis* (humpback), *gibbus* (angular humpback), and *scoliosis* should also be evaluated. Scoliosis is considered functional if there is only one curve present. In this situation the curve of the back resembles the letter C. If a compensatory curve has appeared forming an S shape, it is considered organic. The best test for scoliosis is to have the child bend forward toward his toes. A functional scoliosis will disappear with this maneuver, and organic scoliosis will not disappear.

Harrison's groove is a horizontal groove at the level of the diaphragm, with some flaring of the rib cage below the groove. This sign may indicate rickets or congenital syphilis. A very mild degree is present in newborn infants, and some young thin children, and should be considered normal.

The nurse-examiner should be familiar with accepted anatomical landmarks in this area of the body in order to be able to coherently convey the findings to other clinicians (see Fig. 10-5).

Some rib locations are useful to know: the last rib which attaches directly to the sternum is the seventh rib, the lowest floating rib which can be felt laterally is the eleventh rib; the twelfth floating rib can usually be palpated posteriorly; the rib directly below the scapula posteriorly is the seventh rib.

The nipple is usually considered inadequate as a landmark because its placement is so inconsistent. The anterior landmarks most commonly used are the midsternal line (a line bisecting the sternum) and the right and left midclavicular lines (a line drawn from the middle of the clavicle straight down).

The angle of Louis or *sternal angle* is the most prominent projection on the upper sternum and marks the point where the second rib joins the sternum. Palpation of this landmark is helpful when counting ribs.

The sternal notch refers to the notch located at the most superior part of the manubrium. The costal angle refers to the angle formed where the right and lower rib borders meet at the xiphoid process.

Laterally the *anterior axillary line* originates at the anterior axillary fold (the fold formed when the arm is abducted to a 90° angle) and proceeds downward; the *posterior axillary line* originates at the posterior axillary fold

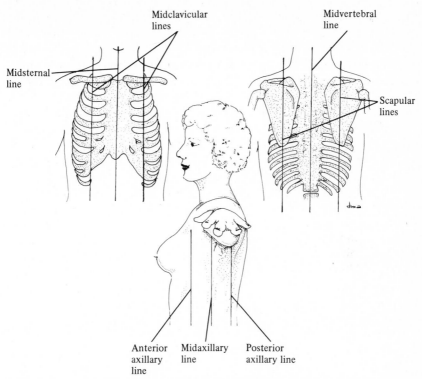

Figure 10-5 Accepted anatomical landmarks of the chest.

and proceeds downward; and the *midaxillary line* begins at the apex of the axilla and proceeds downward.

There are three landmarks posteriorly. The first is the midspinal or *vertebral line,* which is down the center of the vertebral column. The other two are not often used because they are somewhat less exact. They are the right and left *scapular lines* which begin at the inferior angle of the scapula, as the patient stands erect with arms at the sides, and proceed straight downward. The most prominent spinous process is usually C7; occasionally it is T1.

The next structure in the chest to be evaluated are the lungs. It is important to have some idea of the anatomical relation of the ribs to the lungs. The apex of each lung is found about 2 to 4 cm above the inner third of the clavicle. The trachea bifurcates into the two large bronchi at the level of the sternal angle anteriorly and the fourth thoracic spine posteriorly.

The rib overlying the inferior border of the lungs in the midclavicular line is the sixth rib; at the midaxillary line it is the eighth rib.

The anterior horizontal fissure that separates the upper from the middle lobe of the right lung lies at the fourth rib in the midclavicular line and the fifth rib in the midaxillary line. The oblique fissure separating the upper from the lower lobes posteriorly begin at the third thoracic process and run obliquely down the inferior border of the scapulae at the position they would be when the child's arms are raised.

In observing the lungs the nurse must first evaluate their expansion. This is best observed if the nurse holds the palms of the hands flush against the patient's chest and with the fingers spread out. Hands should be held in symmetrical areas of the chest. As the chest expands, it will push the fingers further apart; in this way the nurse can easily observe whether both sides are expanding to the same degree (see Fig. 10-6).

Retractions of the chest are also important. Any intracostal, subcostal, or suprasternal retractions indicate abnormally labored breathing; these cases should be referred. They usually occur in pneumonia and other abnormal conditions.

Respiration must be assessed with regard to rate, quality, and depth. Normal rates vary, of course, with the age of the individual, and a chart, such as the following, should always be easily accessible to the nurse-examiner.

Age	Respiration rate
Newborn	30–50
6 months	20–30
2 years	20–30
Adolescent	12–20

Bradypnea, or a slow rate of breathing, is a cause for concern, since this may be due to brain tumors or opiate poisoning. *Tachypnea,* or a very fast rate of breathing, can be equally alarming and may indicate pneumonia, fever, heart failure, meningitis, shock, anxiety, salicylate poisoning, alkalosis, or pleurisy. The ratio of respiration to pulse should be 1:4, and the ratio of respiration to temperature should be 4:1 (4 respirations for every 1°F of fever over normal). *Apnea,* or temporary cessation of breathing, is also a cause for concern if it continues for extended periods of time. Very short periods of apnea may occasionally be normal in the neonatal period.

The quality of respiration is also important. Respiration is basically abdominal in infancy, and the transition to costal respiration is gradual until about 7 years of age, at which time it should be predominantly costal. A very young child who breathes costally or an older child who breathes abdominally should be watched for *dyspnea.* There is probably some truth to the fact that males tend to breathe more abdominally than females. All accessory muscles should be checked to see if the child is using them to help in the breathing process. A child who is actively using his neck or shoulder muscles to help him breathe is in respiratory difficulty, and should be referred.

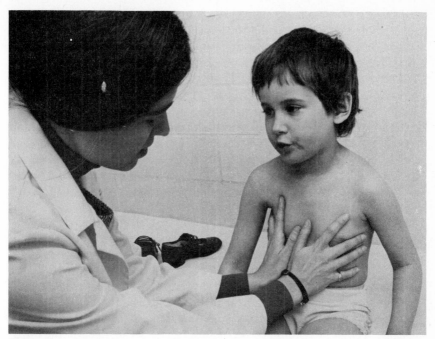

Figure 10-6 Proper placement of hands for ease in observing chest expansion.

Expiratory grunts are another respiratory quality which is worrisome; this occurs in pneumonitis, respiratory distress syndrome, and left-sided heart failure. Two rather serious patterns of respiration are *Biot's breathing,* which is a rapid, irregular breathing, first shallow and then deep, and *Cheyne-Stokes respiration,* which is a regular predictable pattern of several breaths followed by a pause and again by several breaths.

Depth of respiration, or *hyperpnea,* must also be assessed. Hyperpnea is a deep, gasping kind of breathing such as occurs in metabolic acidosis, when it is called *Kussmaul breathing. Alkalotic breathing* is diminished in depth; it is slow and shallow. Shallow breathing may also be present in pleuritis or pleural effusion, in a child with broken ribs, or in any condition in which breathing causes pain.

The nurse must be familiar with such signs of dyspnea as restlessness, apprehension, retractions, nasal flaring, and cyanosis. If these signs occur primarily on inspiration there is usually an obstruction of the larger tubes, such as the trachea and mainstem bronchi, a tumor or foreign body. If these signs occur primarily on expiration, there may be an obstruction of the small bronchi or bronchioles, often associated with asthma, bronchitis, or emphysema.

After a thorough inspection, the examiner proceeds to palpate the thorax. Palpation will reveal only those abnormalities that are within 4 to 5 cm below the surface; consequently the nurse should expect to pick up only gross or superficial pathologic conditions.

Fremitus is the procedure by which the examiner palpates the conduction of voice sounds through the thorax. The nurse does this by placing the hands in much the same way as was done for testing expansion, palm down on the chest in symmetrical bilateral positions. The nurse begins at the top of the chest and slowly inches down, first in front and then in back. Each time the hands are moved further down, the patients are instructed to say "99" or "blue moon"; the vibrations of the vocalization should be felt.

The vibrations should be felt by the fingertips in areas such as the trachea and bronchi, where the tubes are bigger and closer to the surface. They will be absent or decreased in situations of bronchial blockage, emphysema, asthma, pneumothorax, pleural effusion, or pleural thickening. The sensation will be increased in conditions where a solid mass is present, such as pneumonia, atelectasis, or other types of consolidation.

The chest should also be palpated for pleural friction rubs and crepitation caused by the escape of air into the subcutaneous fat.

Percussion is the third method of examination utilized in evaluation of the chest. The basic method of percussion has been explained in the introductory section and only the specifics which refer to the thoracic region will be discussed here (see Fig. 10-7).

At the fourth or fifth interspace on the right in the midclavicular line, percussion can be expected to turn dull; this is where the liver begins. A few centimeters further down, where the lung ends and the liver alone remains, the percussion note should become flat.

Tympany can occur at the sixth interspace and below on the left side; this is due to the air-filled stomach and bowel. Its absence is normal, merely indicating that the stomach is not filled with air.

Dullness encountered in areas where it would not normally be expected may be a sign of lobar pneumonia during the consolidation phase, atelectasis, pleural effusion, empyema, pleural thickening, intrathoracic neoplasms, or a diaphragmatic hernia.

Hyperresonance in unexpected areas may indicate pneumothorax, lobar emphysema, asthma, or pneumonia. Percussion can also be used to estimate diaphragmatic excursion. The child is asked to hold the breath in full inspiration, while the level of the diaphragm is percussed. He or she is then asked to hold the breath in full expiration and the level of the diaphragm is again percussed. The difference between the two levels is then compared. The diaphragm should move several centimeters. If it does not, or if it moves more on one side than the other, pleurisy or consolidation is suspected.

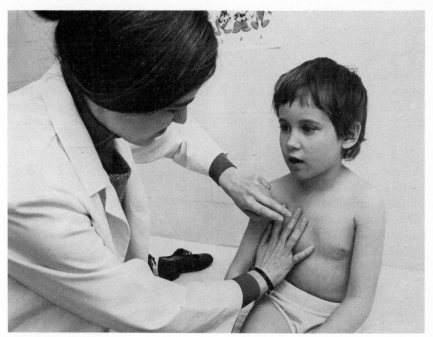

Figure 10-7 Percussion of the chest.

Auscultation is the final method of evaluation utilized in the physical examination of the chest. The diaphragm, rather than the bell, should be used since most of the important sounds will be of high frequency. The nurse should begin at the top, inching the stethoscope from side to side, covering all areas of the lung, including the region under the arms. Gradually he or she should work down, listening to breath sounds, voice sounds, and adventitious sounds.

Breath sounds should always be evaluated as to pitch, intensity, quality, and duration. Although they are expected to be louder in infants and very young children (under about 6 years of age), the nurse will find three basic categories of breath sounds in children of all ages. The first category is *vesicular breath sounds*. These breath sounds are characterized by having a louder, longer, and higher-pitched inspiration and a shorter, softer, and lower-pitched expiration. The ratio of the length of inspiration to expiration is about 5:2. They would be diagrammed like this: ⟋⟍ (the thick long upstroke indicates a loud, long inspiration; the short thin downstroke indicates a softer, shorter inspiration; the small angle between the two indicates a relatively high pitch; there is no pause between inspiration and expiration, as indicated by the continuity of the two lines). Vesicular sounds should normally be found all over the chest except in the areas of the manubrium and the upper interscapular area. They may be exaggerated in tuberculosis, emphysema, and late stages of pneumonia, but diminished during the early stages of pneumonia.

Bronchial or tubular breath sounds have a shorter inspiratory phase and a longer expiratory phase; they are usually louder than other types of breath sounds. There is a pause between inspiration and expiration. They are diagrammed like this: ╱╲ They should never be considered normal except over the tracheal area; if they are found elsewhere, they may indicate atelectasis or consolidation.

Bronchovesicular breath sounds are a combination of both bronchial and vesicular breath sounds; they can be recognized by the fact that inspiration is louder and higher in pitch than vesicular breath sounds, and inspiration and expiration are equal in quality, intensity, pitch, and duration. There is no pause between inspiration or expiration. They are diagrammed like this: ╱╲ These sounds are normal at the manubrium and upper intrascapular area; if found in other areas they should be suspect, since they may indicate an abnormality such as consolidation.

There are also several types of abnormal or unusual types of breathing. *Amphoric breathing* produces a hollow, low-pitched sound which resembles that produced by blowing over a bottle. The expiratory phase is lower in pitch than the inspiratory phase. Amphoric breathing may indicate pneumothorax, pleural effusion, or a broncho-pleural fistula.

Cogwheel breath sounds are an unusual, but not abnormal, type of breathing that may be encountered occasionally. They are very similar to vesicular breath sounds except that the inspiratory phase is quite jerky, being broken by short pauses.

The nurse-examiner must also pay attention to absent or decreased breath sounds. These may indicate a diaphragmatic hernia, fluid or air in the pleura, a thickened pleura, bronchial obstruction, or any condition that might cause shallow breathing, such as painful pleurisy.

After breath sounds, the nurse must evaluate voice sounds. Three types of voice sounds will be discussed here. The first is *whispered pectoriloquy.* This refers to the procedure in which the child is asked to whisper several words while the nurse listens to the chest through the stethoscope. The nurse should not be able to understand the syllables. If the syllables are clearly distinguishable, an abnormality should be suspected.

Bronchophony is similar to whispered pectoriloquy and is similarly abnormal. In bronchophony, however, the child is asked to speak rather than whisper. The intensity of the sounds should be increased as the nurse listens through the stethoscope, but again, the syllables should not be understood.

Egophony is a type of bronchophony in which a particularly nasal quality is heard through the stethoscope. When the child makes the sound "eeee," it is heard through the stethoscope as a nasal "aaaa." This also indicates an abnormality.

Table 10-1 Types of Rales

1. *Musical rales* (dry rales)—continuous, noninterrupted adventitious sounds.
   a. Sibilant (wheeze)—a high-pitched, squeaking sound that is produced when air passes through narrowed, small airways.
   b. Sonorous (snore)—a low-pitched, snoring sound that is produced when air passes through narrowed, larger airways.
2. *Crepitant rales* (fine moist rales)—high-pitched, crackling series of discreet sounds heard on inspiration thought to be a result of the separation of alveolar walls that are stuck to each other.
3. *Subcrepitant rales* (medium moist rales)—medium-pitched, noncrackling series of discreet sounds heard on inspiration thought to arise from the separation of adherent bronchiolar walls.
4. *Bubbling rales* (coarse moist rales; rhonchi)—low-pitched, loud series of discreet sounds with a bubbling quality to them. They are produced when air passes through fluid in the larger airways.
5. *Gurgling rales* (death rattle)—very low-pitched, loud, wet-sounding discreet sounds. They are produced when air passes through large amounts of secretions in the trachea.

George Druger: *The Chest: Its Signs and Sounds,* Humetrics Corporation, a subsidiary of Thiokol Chemical Corporation, Los Angeles, 1973, p. 58.

Adventitious sounds must also be evaluated. These are any sounds heard in the chest which would not be considered breath sounds or voice sounds. They can be classified in a variety of ways. Textbooks and clinicians differ widely in how these sounds are classified, but probably the best classification available at this time is one devised by Druger (see Table 10-1).

In the early stages of learning physical assessment, it is not necessary to be able to differentiate these abnormalities. With practice and increased proficiency, the nurse will learn to distinguish them and make appropriate decisions about them.

The final adventitious sound to be discussed in this chapter is the *pleural friction rub.* It is caused by the lung wall scraping against the pleura. Its sound can be simulated by cupping the hand to the ear and rubbing a finger of the other hand on the cupped one. Although pleural friction rub can occur during both phases, it is usually loudest at the end of inspiration. To differentiate it from cardiac friction rub, the examiner should ask the child to hold his or her breath. A pleural friction rub will disappear, but a cardiac friction rub will continue.

BIBLIOGRAPHY

Fuhs, Margaret, and Alice Stein: "Postural Drainage, Percussion and Vibration," *Nursing '76,* vol. 6, no. 2, pp. 36–38, February 1976.

Sweetwood, Hannelore: "Bedside Assessment of Respirations," *Nursing '73,* vol. 3, no. 9, pp. 50–52, September 1973.

GLOSSARY

alkalotic breathing slow, shallow breathing heard in systemic alkalosis

amphoric breathing a hollow, low-pitched type of breathing resembling the noise produced by blowing over a bottle, the expiratory phase being pitched lower than the inspiratory phase

anterior axillary line a thoracic landmark consisting of an imaginary line which originates at the anterior axillary fold and proceeds downward

aortic hiatus an opening in the dorsal lateral portion of the diaphragm, allowing the aorta, azygos vein, and thoracic duct to pass through

areola the circular pigmented area surrounding the nipple

barrel chest a condition in which the ribs form perfect circles rather than the usual ellipse

Biot's breathing rapid irregular breathing, first shallow and then deep

bradypnea slow breathing

bronchial (tubular) breathing sounds breath sounds which have a shorter inspiratory than expiratory phase and are loud compared to other types of breath sounds; considered normal over the trachea

bronchophony the abnormal phenomenon in which an examiner, listening through a stethoscope to the lungs, will hear not only an increase in the intensity of words, but will also be able to identify syllables

bronchovesicular breath sounds a combination of both bronchial and vesicular breath sounds in which inspiration and expiration are equal in quality, intensity, pitch, and duration; considered normal at the manubrium and upper intrascapular area

Cheyne-Stokes respiration an abnormal, regular, predictable pattern of several breaths followed by a pause and again by several breaths

cogwheel breath sounds an unusual, but normal breath sound with an inspiratory phase which is quite jerky and broken by short pauses

Cooper's ligaments suspensory ligaments formed from fibrous bands running vertically throughout the breast which attach the deep subcutaneous tissue to the skin

costochondral junction the cartilaginous juncture between the ribs and the sternum

crepitation the crackling feel caused by the escape of air into the subcutaneous fat

diaphragm a large, musculofibrous membrane dividing the abdominal cavity from the thoracic cavity

dyspnea difficult breathing

egophony an abnormal voice sound in which a particularly nasal quality is heard through the stethoscope as the patient speaks; when the child says "eeee" the sound heard through the stethoscope is "aaaa"

esophageal hiatus an opening in the diaphragm lying to the left of the aortic hiatus which allows the esophagus, vagus nerves, and several blood vessels to pass between the thoracic and abdominal cavity

foramen venae cavae an opening in the diaphragm through which pass the inferior vena cava and several branches of the right phrenic nerve

fremitus the conduction of voice sounds through the thorax in such a way that a vibration is palpable when the examiner places his hands flush against the child's chest

funnel breast an abnormal structure of the thoracic cage in which there is an indentation of the sternal area

gibbus angular humpback

Harrison's groove a horizontal depression formed around the chest at the level of the diaphragm; normal in infants, but may indicate rickets in older children

hyperpnea increased depth of respiration

intercostales externi the 11 muscles extending from the dorsal section of the ribs to the ventral costal cartilages which help in increasing the volume of the thoracic cavity

intercostales interni the 11 chest muscles extending from the sternum to the vertebrae which help to decrease the volume of the thoracic cavity

Kussmaul breathing the deep breathing characteristic of metabolic acidosis

kyphosis humpback

levatores costarum the 12 chest muscles extending from the cervical and thoracic vertebrae to the outer surfaces of the ribs which help decrease the thoracic volume and bend the vertebral column laterally

manubrium the uppermost triangular portion of the sternum which attaches to the first and second ribs and provides a place of attachment for the pectoralis major and sternocleidomastoid muscles

midaxillary line an anatomical landmark beginning at the apex of the axillary line and proceeding directly downward

Montgomery's glands (areolar) large sebaceous glands distributed throughout the areola which secrete a substance for lubrication and protection during lactation

pectoralis major the large triangular muscle of the upper chest which raises and lowers the humerus

pigeon chest the condition in which the sternum protrudes from the chest wall and a series of vertical depressions along the costochondral junction appear

posterior axillary line a thoracic landmark consisting of an imaginary line from the posterior axillary fold downward

pleural friction rub a grating sound caused by the lung wall scraping against the pleura

rachitic rosary an inflammation of the costochondral junction, forming a series of palpable bumps similar to rosary beads; usually an indication of vitamin C deficiency

rales discrete abnormal sounds (usually classified as fine, medium, or coarse) best heard during forced respiration, primarily at the end of inspiration

rhonchi loud gurgling noises transmitted from secretions in the pharynx

scapular line an anatomic landmark consisting of an imaginary line beginning at the inferior angle of the scapula and proceeding directly downward

scoliosis a lateral curvature of the spine

serratus posterior inferior a chest muscle which runs from the spinous processes of the thoracic and lumbar vertebrae to the lower edges of the last 4 ribs and acts as an antagonist to the diaphragm

serratus posterior superior a group of muscles extending from the spinous processes of the cervical and thoracic vertebrae to the upper borders of the second, third, fourth and fifth ribs which increase the chest volume

sonorous rhonchi low-pitched rhonchi originating in the larger bronchi and trachea, characterized by their moaning snoring quality

sternocleidomastoid muscle one of the major muscles of the neck, used to rotate and lower the head

subcostales chest muscles which attach the upper to the lower ribs and help in decreasing the thoracic volume

tachypnea rapid breathing

thymus a small organ found in the mediastinal cavity anterior and superior to the heart, important in the immune response in infants and young children

tidal air the amount of air exchanged during a normal respiratory cycle

Tietze's syndrome painful swellings of the first 4 costochondral junctions

transversus thoracis a thin sheet of muscle and tendon fibers which extends from the sternum to the costal cartilages and helps to decrease the chest volume

tympany a clear, hollow note obtained by percussion

vital capacity the total amount of air that can be expelled after a full inspiration

whispered pectoriloquy the normal phenomenon in which the examiner is unable to distinguish the syllables whispered by the patient when listening to the chest with a stethoscope

Inspection of the Respiratory System (Anterior View)*

General	Yes	No	Not appli-cable	Describe (where appropriate)	Significance
A. Nose					
1. Flaring					A serious sign of air hunger.
2. Bilateral air exchange					Visible air passage through both nostrils indicates lack of major obstruction.
3. Other					
B. Fingers					
1. Clubbing					Indicates long term air hunger; can result from respiratory, cardiac, or neurological pathology.
C. Skin (on areas other than chest)					
1. Cyanosis					Same significance as elsewhere.
2. Other					
Chest					
A. Skin					
1. Spider nevi					Same significance as elsewhere.
2. Supernumerary nipples					Those above the nipple line are more likely to lactate; more common in black children; not pathological.
3. Dark nipples					May be variant of normal; may reflect adrenal problems.

*This chart is meant to be used by beginning students as they perform their first physical assessments. Each item should be examined on the child and then checked off on the checklist. The significance of the items follows in the right-hand column.

177

Inspection of the Respiratory System (Anterior View) (Continued)

Chest	Yes	No	Not appli-cable	Describe (where appropriate)	Significance
4. Widely spaced nipples					May indicate Turner's syndrome.
5. Nipple fissures					Dry skin; likely in adolescent girls nursing babies; indicates need for help in nursing technique and nipple care.
6. Nipple inversions					Normal variant; may need help in everting them during a pregnancy if planning to nurse.
7. Nipple secretions					Normal during pregnancy or sexual arousal or nursing; otherwise requires further investigation.
8. Nipple scaling					Rare; may indicate Paget's disease.
9. Other					
B. Cartilage 1. Rachitic rosary					Indication of rickets.
2. Tietze's syndrome					Fairly common in young women; etiology and treatment unknown.
3. Other					
C. Muscle 1. Atrophy					May indicate local or generalized muscle or neurological pathology such as muscular dystrophy.
2. Hypertrophy					Same as above.
3. Harrison's groove					Normal variant.
4. Suprasternal retractions					Serious sign of air hunger.
5. Subcostal retractions					Same as above.
6. Intracostal retractions					Same as above.
7. Other					

D. Bones			
1. Palpable fracture			Needs referral.
2. Pigeon chest			Can accompany rickets, Marfan's syndrome, Morquio's disease, or chronic upper respiratory disease.
3. Funnel breast			Can accompany rickets or Marfan's syndrome.
4. Barrel chest			May accompany pulmonary emphysema or chronic lung pathology such as asthma and cystic fibrosis.
5. Localized bulges			May indicate cardiac enlargement or local pathology.
6. Other			
E. Respirations			
1. Normal rate for age?*			Bradypnea may indicate brain tumor or opiate poisoning, tachypnea may indicate pneumonia, fever, heart failure, meningitis, shock, anxiety, alkalosis, pleurisy, or salicylate poisoning.
2. Abdominal			If this occurs past the age of about 7 years, it may indicate chest pathology, such as pleurisy.
3. Costal			If this occurs below about 7 years, it may indicate abdominal pathology, such as peritonitis.
4. Hyperpnea			May indicate metabolic acidosis Kussmaul breathing.
5. Shallow breathing			May indicate alkalosis, broken ribs, or pleuritis.
6. Dyspnea			Serious indication of air hunger.
7. Expansion normal			Restriction may indicate lung pathology.
8. Use of accessory muscles			Indicates air hunger.
9. Other			

*Normal respiratory rates for (a) newborn: 30–50, (b) 6 months: 20–30, (c) 2 years: 20–30, (d) adolescent: 12–20.

179

Palpation of the Respiratory System (Anterior View)

General	Yes	No	Not appli-cable	Describe (where appropriate)	Significance
A. Fingers					
1. Clubbing					Same significance as under inspection.
Chest					
(Skin within normal range)					Same significance as elsewhere.
A. Cartilage					
1. Rachitic rosary					Indication of rickets.
2. Tietze's syndrome					Fairly common in young women; etiology and treatment unknown.
3. Other					
B. Muscle					
1. Atrophy					May indicate local or generalized muscle or neurological pathology such as muscular dystrophy.
2. Hypertrophy					Same as above.
3. Harrison's Groove					Normal variant.
4. Suprasternal retractions					Serious sign of air hunger.
5. Subcostal retractions					Same as above.
6. Intracostal retractions					Same as above.
7. Other					
C. Bones					
1. Palpable fracture					Needs referral.

	Significance
2. Pigeon chest	Can accompany rickets, Marfan's syndrome, Morquio's disease, or chronic upper respiratory disease.
3. Funnel breast	Can accompany rickets or Marfan's syndrome.
4. Barrel chest	May accompany pulmonary emphysema or chronic lung pathology such as asthma and cystic fibrosis.
5. Localized bulges	May indicate cardiac enlargement or local pathology.
6. Other	
D. Respirations	
1. Normal respiratory fremitus	Any respiratory fremitus indicates underlying congestion.
2. Normal vocal fremitus	Decreased vibrations due to bronchial blockage, emphysema, asthma, pneumothorax, pleural thickening, or effusion; increased vibrations due to pneumonia, atelectasis, or other types of consolidation.
3. Other	

Percussion of the Respiratory System (Anterior View)

General	Yes	No	Not appli- cable	Describe (where appropriate)	Significance
Normal cardiac dullness					See cardiovascular check list.
Normal liver dullness					Fifth interspace in midclavicular line and below.
Normal spleen dullness					About the ninth interspace in the midaxillary line.
Normal stomach tympany					Sixth interspace and below (only if stomach is filled with air).
Normal lung resonance					Expected in all other areas.
Diaphragmatic excursion					About 3 to 6 cm; less movement indicates consolidation.

181

Auscultation of the Respiratory System (Anterior View)

General	Yes	No	Not appli-cable	Describe (where appropriate)	Significance
1. Bronchial sounds in appropriate locations only (i.e. overlying bronchi)					If found in other places, may indicate lung pathology.
2. Vesicular sounds in appropriate areas only (i.e., overlying alveoli)					Same as above.
3. Bronchovesicular sounds in appropriate areas only (i.e. between bronchial and vesicular areas)					Same as above.
4. Adventitious sounds					Indicate some type of lung pathology.
5. Other					

Inspection of the Respiratory System (Posterior and Lateral Views)

General	Yes	No	Not appli-cable	Describe (where appropriate)	Significance
A. Skin					
1. Abnormal color					Same significance as elsewhere.
2. Abnormal markings					Same significance as elsewhere.
3. Other					

B. Muscles		
1. Atrophy		Same significance as anterior chest.
2. Hypertrophy		Same significance as anterior chest.
3. Retractions		Same significance as anterior chest.
4. Other		Same significance as anterior chest.
C. Bones		
1. Barrel chest		Same significance as anterior chest.
2. Bulges		Same significance as anterior chest.
3. Scoliosis		If the child bends over to touch toes without bending knees, a functional scoliosis will correct itself; an organic scoliosis will not.
4. Kyphosis		Needs treatment.
5. Lordosis		Excessive degree needs referral; common in black children.
6. Unequal scapulae		May indicate scoliosis
7. Localized bulges		May indicate underlying pathology such as fractures, tumors, cardiac enlargement, etc.
8. Other		
D. Respirations		
1. Expansion		Same significance as anterior chest.
2. Other		

183

Palpation of the Respiratory System (Posterior and Lateral Views)

General	Yes	No	Not appli-cable	Describe (where appropriate)	Significance
A. Skin					
1. Normal texture					Same significance as elsewhere.
2. Nodules					Same significance as elsewhere.
3. Other					
B. Bones					
1. Palpable fracture					Same significance as anterior chest.
2. Pigeon chest					Same significance as anterior chest.
3. Funnel breast					Same significance as anterior chest.
4. Barrel chest					Same significance as anterior chest.
5. Localized bulges					Same significance as anterior chest.
6. Other					
C. Muscles					
1. Atrophy					Same significance as anterior chest.
2. Hypertrophy					Same significance as anterior chest.
3. Other					Same significance as anterior chest.
D. Respirations					
1. Respiratory fremitus					Same significance as anterior chest.
2. Vocal fremitus					Same significance as anterior chest.
3. Other					

Percussion of the Respiratory System (Posterior and Lateral Views)

General	Yes	No	Not appli-cable	Describe (where appropriate)	Significance
1. Kidney dullness on left at eleventh rib					A higher level of dullness may indicate enlargement.
2. Kidney dullness on right eleventh intercostal space					Same as above.
3. Spleen (laterally) ninth to eleventh rib					Same as above.
4. Other					

Auscultation of the Respiratory System (Posterior and Lateral Views)

General	Yes	No	Not appli-cable	Describe (where appropriate)	Significance
1. Bronchovesicular sounds in appropriate areas only (i.e., over top of chest between scapulae)					May indicate lung pathology if found in other areas.
2. Vesicular sounds in appropriate areas only (i.e., over alveoli)					May indicate lung pathology if found in other areas.
3. Adventitious sounds					Indicates pathology.

Source: These checklists are printed with permission from Blue Hill Videotape Incorporated and are part of a more complete programmed learning approach to the physical examination, which includes a workbook and series of videotapes. It can be purchased from Blue Hill Educational Systems, Inc., 52 South Main Street, Spring Valley, New York 10977.

185

Chapter 11

The Heart

WHY THE CHILD IS EXAMINED

Careful examination of the heart and circulatory system is essential; it will assure the clinician that the patient is not endangered from the two most common cardiac problems of childhood: congenital heart problems and rheumatic fever. Congenital heart defects have their highest incidence of morbidity and mortality in infancy. Five of every thousand infants are born with a congenital heart defect (the incidence is two to three times higher in premature infants). Most of the deaths from congenital heart defects occur within the first week of life, and of these about half would have been eligible for surgery if the defect had been recognized early. Transposition of the great vessels, coarctation of the aorta, aortic atresia, and pulmonary atresia are the most common causes of these early deaths.

Rheumatic fever and its sequelae are the second largest causes of cardiac problems in the pediatric age group, and one reason a careful heart evaluation should always be done on the 2-week follow-up visit after a

186

streptococcal infection. The peak age of incidence for this disease is from 5 to 15 years.

WHAT TO EXAMINE: ANATOMY OF THE AREA

The heart is a muscular, four-chambered organ located between the lungs and above the diaphragm (see Fig. 11-1). It is shaped like a blunt, inverted cone with the apex pointed downward and posteriorly and the broad base directly upward and anteriorly. By the eighth year of life, the tip of the apex reaches the left fifth intercostal space. The size of the heart approximates an individual's doubled fist. Its walls are constructed of outer *epicardium,* middle *myocardium,* and inner *endocardium,* and it is covered by a membranous sac called the *pericardium.* There are four chambers divided into two strongly muscular chambers called *ventricles* and two smaller chambers called *atria.* The right atrium contains the openings for the superior vena cava, inferior vena cava, coronary sinus, and smaller minor vessels. The right ventricle is larger and lies beneath the right atrium; it contains the opening for the pulmonary artery. The left atrium is smaller than the right atrium, but its walls are much thicker. It contains openings for the four pulmonary veins and the remnant of the closing of the foramen ovale which fuses at birth. The left ventricle lies below the left atrium and has the thickest walls of the heart. This chamber empties into the aorta.

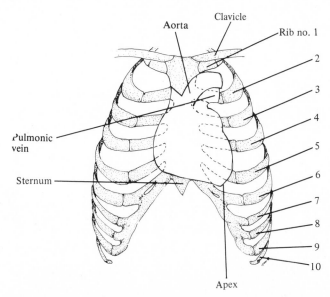

Figure 11-1 Position of the heart within the chest cavity.

The heart is fitted with a system of valves to control the flow of blood from chamber to chamber. The opening between the right atrium and ventricle is called the *tricuspid valve*. The three flaps (or cusps) of the valve are held in place by the chordae tendineae. The opening to the pulmonary artery in the right ventricle is guarded by the pulmonary valve. The left atrium and ventricle are separated by the *bicuspid (mitral) valve* which contains only two cusps; the pulmonary veins leaving the left atrium have no valves. The aortic opening from the left ventricle is regulated by the aortic semilunar valves composed of three strong cusps (see Fig. 11-2).

The conduction system of the heart is complex, and only a brief description of it will be given here. The interested reader is referred to a good physiology book for a more complete discussion. The heart muscle has an innate ability to produce spontaneous contractility as well as a conduction system which controls the rhythm of this contractility. The system consists of a *sinoatrial node* ("the pacemaker") located in the right atrium; an *atrioventricular node* in the septal wall of the right atrium; an atrioventricular bundle (*bundle of His*) which begins at the atrioventricular node and travels toward the apex and ventricles; and a terminal conducting fiber (*Purkinje fiber*) which runs throughout the musculature of both ventricles.

One of the most important things the nurse-examiner must remember when evaluating the heart and cardiovascular system of a child is that a great deal more than just the heart itself should be examined. There are some measures with which the nurse has long been familiar and which are

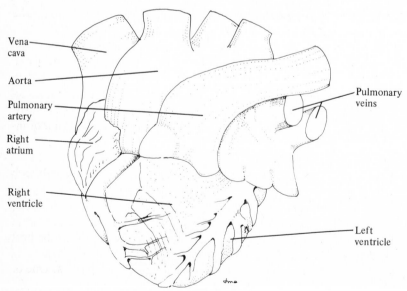

Figure 11-2 The chambers of the heart and vessels.

extremely important in this evaluation. It is easy to slight a pulse and blood pressure just because they are such common measurements, but the fact is that the reason these measures are so commonly taken is because they are so useful. Pulse rates are very helpful in determining the health of the child in general and the cardiovascular system in particular. It is very important to know, or at least be able to find, the normal rates for particular ages. The following chart should be easily accessible during every examination.

Age	Pulse rates
Newborn	70–170
11 months	80–160
2 years	80–130
4 years	80–120
6 years	75–115
8 years	70–110
10 years	70–110

An increase in rate may indicate many things. Excitement, hyperthyroidism, heart disease, severe anemia, or fever are all manifested in increased pulse rates. *Tachypnea* is particularly significant if it persists during sleep. In fever there is usually an increase of 8 to 10 pulse beats for every degree of fever. An increase higher than this ratio needs an explanation and may indicate rheumatic fever. A child who has a fever accompanied by a slow pulse may have a *Salmonella* infection. Rhythm of the pulse is also important and usually corresponds to the rhythm heard while auscultating the heart. This will be discussed further under the discussion of auscultation. The character of the pulse is also important. There are several characteristic types which are common enough to be given names. *Pulsus alternans* is one that consists of one strong beat followed by a weak one. This can be a sign of myocardial weakness. A *Corrigan's pulse* (water-hammer) is a very forceful bounding pulse felt best at the radial and femoral areas and accompanied by an increase in pulse pressure. This is often accompanied by capillary pulsations of the fingernail. This usually indicates some kind of insufficiency and can be a symptom of patent ductus arteriosus or aortic regurgitation. *Pulsus bisferiens,* or dicrotic pulse, is a double radial pulse for every apical beat. It can be auscultated over the brachial artery or felt with light palpation over the carotid. It can be a sign of aortic stenosis, hyperthyroidism, or other diseases. A *plateau pulse,* or pulsus torlus, is characterized by a normal upstroke and downstroke, but with an elongated peak, forming a plateau. *Pulsus bigeminus* is a coupled rhythm in which the beat is felt in pairs. *Pulsus paradoxus* is a pulse characterized by exaggerated waxing and waning. It is sometimes found in children with asthma. One of the most important parts of evaluating the pulses and the cardiac status of a young child is to compare the radial and femoral pulses. Normally these should be felt at essentially the same time. A time lag between the beat felt at the radial artery and that at the femoral artery may be a sign of coarctation, and a blood pressure reading should be obtained.

Blood pressure reading is another common procedure which many nurses underrate. The technique of taking a blood pressure is very important. The cuff size is essential to the accuracy of the reading. It should be not more than two-thirds nor less than one-half the length of the upper arm. A recent study[1] indicates that the recommendation of choosing a cuff which is 20 percent wider than the diameter of the arm may be more relevant. This recommendation has not yet been made officially by the American Heart Association, however. In a pediatric facility where many ages of children are seen, standard cuff sizes of 2.5 in, 5 in, 8 in, and 12 in should be available. The child should be sitting, and the arm should be at heart level. There are actually five sounds in a blood pressure reading, but most clinicians cannot accurately hear them all. At least three should be noted and recorded; these include the point at which the sounds are first heard, the point at which these sounds become muffled, and the point at which they disappear. The American Heart Association says that the muffling should actually be considered the diastolic in children; there is still some controversy over whether it is the muffling or the disappearance of sound which should be considered the diastolic in adults. To avoid confusion all three readings should be recorded (e.g., 120/80/60).

Thigh blood pressures can also be important. In a child under 1 year of age, the systolic pressure in the thighs should be equal to that in the arms. After that age it may be 10 to 40 mm Hg higher; the diastolic, however, should always be the same. If it is lower, the nurse-examiner should suspect coarctation. In children under 1 year of age, the blood pressure is inaudible, and the flush technique should be used. The nurse elevates the arm, draining the blood from it. Wrapping it in an Ace bandage may help drain it. The blood-pressure cuff is then applied and inflated, and the arm is lowered. The cuff is then gradually deflated, while the examiner observes the point at which the arm distal to the cuff flushes with color. This point is considered the median between the systolic and diastolic readings. Some clinics now have either an *oscillometer* or a *doppler* available. Both of these are mechanical devices which are more accurate than the flush technique. Again, it is important that the nurse have easy access to a chart of normal blood pressure readings for different ages (see Table 11-1).

A very important part of the blood pressure that is sometimes ignored by examiners is the pulse pressure or difference between systolic and diastolic readings. Normally this is about 20 to 50 mm Hg throughout childhood. An unusually wide pulse pressure may be due to an abnormally high

[1]Myung Park, I. Kawapowi and W. Guntheroth, "Need for an Improved Standard for Blood Pressure Cuff Size," *Clinical Pediatrics,* vol. 15, no. 9, pp. 784–787, September 1976.

Table 11-1 Normal Blood Pressure for Various Ages

Ages	Mean systolic $\pm$ 2 S.D.	Mean diastolic $\pm$ 2 S.D.
Newborn	80 ± 16	46 ± 16
6 months–1 year	89 ± 29	$60 \pm 10^*$
1 year	96 ± 30	$66 \pm 25^*$
2 years	99 ± 25	$64 \pm 25^*$
3 years	100 ± 25	$67 \pm 23^*$
4 years	99 ± 20	$65 \pm 20^*$
5–6 years	94 ± 14	55 ± 9
6–7 years	100 ± 15	56 ± 8
8–9 years	105 ± 16	57 ± 9
9–10 years	107 ± 16	57 ± 9
10–11 years	111 ± 17	58 ± 10
11–12 years	113 ± 18	59 ± 10
12–13 years	115 ± 19	59 ± 10
13–14 years	118 ± 19	60 ± 10

*In this study the point of muffling was taken as the diastolic pressure.

Adapted from data in the literature. Figures have been rounded off to nearest decimal place.

Source: R. J. Haggerty, M. W. Maroney, and A. S. Nadas, "Essential Hypertension in Infancy and Childhood," *A.M.A.J. Dis. Child.* **92**:536, 1956. Copyright 1973, American Medical Association.

systolic reading or an abnormally low diastolic reading. Of these two, the diastolic reading is the more important. If a widened pulse pressure is due to an unusually high systolic reading, it may indicate exercise, excitement, or fever. If, however, it is due to an abnormally low diastolic reading, the probability of patent ductus arteriosus, aortic regurgitation, or other serious heart disease should be raised. An abnormally narrow pulse pressure may indicate aortic stenosis.

The skin and mucous membranes can be another sensitive indicator of the health of the cardiovascular system. Pallor can be a sign of anemia in the older child or severe heart problems in the infant. Cyanosis will usually appear first in the lips, nail beds, or earlobes; it is often associated with polycythemia (usually considered when a hematocrit is over 70). Any persistent cyanosis is a matter of concern. Minor cyanosis in a neonate can be normal, but even then it must be evaluated carefully. Cyanosis should not be excessive or persistent; it should not cover the entire body, and it should not be darker in the upper extremities than in the lower. Any child with these conditions should be referred to the physician. They can be a symptom of either cardiovascular or respiratory difficulties. Edema of any part of the body, but particularly of the eyelids in the neonate, can be another cutaneous manifestation of cardiovascular problems.

Respiratory symptoms, while sometimes a sign of respiratory difficulties, can also reflect cardiovascular insufficiency. Symptoms like *dyspnea, orthopnea,* and frequent upper respiratory infections should be evaluated with this fact in mind. Other miscellaneous symptoms should also alert the practitioner to cardiovascular origins. Continuous squatting and sleeping in the knee-chest position is almost diagnostic of cardiac difficulty. An older child who is easily fatigued or an infant who takes only 2 to $2\frac{1}{2}$ oz of milk and falls asleep immediately or who manifests excessively labored breathing during defecation may be suffering from heart disease. Anorexia, vomiting, profuse sweating, or delays in growth and development, especially in infants, may be symptoms of heart problems. Enlarged liver, clubbing of the digits, enlarged heart, pulsating neck vessels, and tachypnea without retractions can be further symptoms.

HOW TO EXAMINE

Most of the cardiovascular examination depends not on instruments, but on the observation of the clinician. However, some specialized equipment is used in this part of the examination. The blood pressure cuff and its requirements have already been discussed. The stethoscope is also important (see Fig. 11-3). There are many types available. When choosing one, the nurse should remember a few important points. The earpieces should fit comfortably; this means both the size and angle must be correct. The

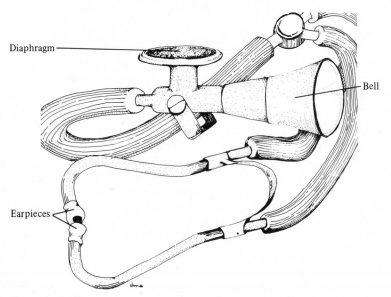

Figure 11-3 The stethoscope.

American Heart Association recommends that the tubing be as short as possible and that the diameter of the tubing be $\frac{1}{8}$ in. Both the bell and diaphragm should be available, since the bell is constructed to pick up low-frequency sounds and the diaphragm, high frequencies. This is important since some significant cardiac sounds are low-pitched and some are high-pitched. In using the bell, however, the examiner must be careful that the entire circumference of it touches the skin very lightly. If too much pressure is exerted, the surrounding skin will be flattened and will act like a diaphragm, blocking out low-frequency sounds.

WHERE TO EXAMINE

There are seven areas which the clinician may examine when evaluating heart function (see Fig. 11-4). Each has a specific name, and that name should be used when recording any abnormal sounds, murmurs, or thrills found in that location. The first is the *sternoclavicular area,* which extends to the right side, left side, and directly over the sternoclavicular junction. The second, or *aortic area,* is located at the second right intercostal space immediately adjacent to the sternum. Next is the *pulmonic area* which is found in the second and third left intercostal space near the sternum. The

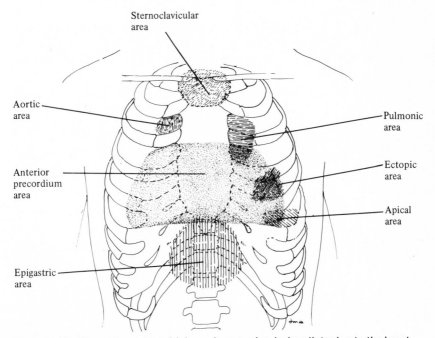

Figure 11-4 The seven areas which can be examined when listening to the heart.

tricuspid area consists of the third, fourth, and fifth intercostal space to the right, left and directly over the sternum. The *apical area* is a very important one. In adults and children over about 8 years of age, this area is located at the fifth intercostal space in the midclavicular line. In younger children, it is usually higher and more medial. Pregnancy or anything causing a high diaphragm may cause it to be higher and more lateral. This is not necessarily the *point of maximal impulse (PMI)* but it usually is. The sixth area is the epigastric area; any other areas are called the ectopic areas; usually the ectopic area refers to a space between the pulmonic and apical areas.

WHAT TO EXAMINE

Inspection, palpation, percussion, and auscultation are all important in the examination of the heart. Inspection and palpation are best done with the patient flat on his back with his chest elevated to a 45° angle. Tangential lighting is best. The most accurate assessments can be obtained at the end of expiration. The examiner must be aware that deformities of the shape of the chest may alter the position of the heart; some deformities, as in Marfan's syndrome, are associated with heart problems, but others which are not may give the appearance of heart problems just because of the alteration in position of the heart. The process of auscultation is very important. The nurse must develop a personal system and inch the stethoscope around all seven areas of the heart, first with the bell and then with the diaphragm. This should routinely be done with the child sitting straight, and lying flat on his back. In certain circumstances the examination should be repeated with the child lying on his left side (particularly the apical area), sitting leaning forward (particularly the aortic and pulmonic area) and standing. Percussion is the least useful, but can be performed to outline the border of the heart. The important findings from percussion would be enlargement or displacement of the heart.

WHAT TO EXAMINE FOR

Basically the nurse is examining for visible, palpable, and auscultatory indications of normal or abnormal heart functioning. Th signs the nurse is examining for by inspection and palpation are similar. In the aortic area a *thrill* (a feeling similar to that felt when you hold your hand on a purring kitten's stomach) that radiates to the right side of the neck may be indicative of aortic stenosis and should be investigated. Vibrations of aortic closure may be felt in individuals with hypertension in this area, as may some pulsations of patent ductus arteriosus.

In the pulmonic area the nurse should note any thrill radiating to the left side of the neck, as this may be a symptom of pulmonary stenosis. A slight, brief pulsation is normal in this area if the child has a thin chest, but it can also be a sign of anemia, fever, exertion, hyperthyroidism, or pregnancy. A stronger pulsation may exist with mitral stenosis or hypertension.

The tricuspid area should also be carefully inspected and palpated. A systolic thrill in this area may indicate ventricular septal defect, and a pulsation may be seen or felt with any condition that causes increased pressure in the right ventricle. Some of these causes could be mitral stenosis, pulmonary stenosis, pulmonary hypertension, atrial septal defect, or ventricular septal defect. A slight retraction in this area will be seen in many children and can be considered normal. Slight outward pulsation may be seen in children with thin chests or may indicate anxiety, anemia, fever, pregnancy, or hyperthyroidism.

In the apical area, the nurse may encounter a systolic thrill from mitral regurgitation or a diastolic thrill from mitral stenosis. Increased amplitude in this area may be due to a thin or flat chest, or a depressed sternum. If the apical area is displaced to the left, enlargement of the heart usually exists. If the heartbeat is very prominent, it may be associated with a gallop rhythm; sometimes the actual rhythm can be felt.

Pulsations in the epigastric area are often normal, particularly in children with anemia or fever, but can sometimes be abnormal, as in the case of thyrotoxicosis, tricuspid stenosis, or regurgitation. These possibilities should be investigated.

Pulsations in the ectopic area are rare in children and usually indicate ischemic heart disease.

The auscultatory evaluation should begin by determining whether the heart sounds are normal. There are four possible heart sounds. The first is designated S_1 (systolic) and indicates the systolic part of the cardiac cycle; it is the "lub" of the "lub-dub." Generally it is louder than the second heart sound at the apex and is longer and pitched lower than the second sound in all areas. It is synchronous with the carotid pulse, and when first beginning to auscultate hearts, it often helps to time the heart sounds by simultaneously feeling the carotid pulse. The first heart sound is caused by the closure of the mitral and tricuspid valves.

The second heart sound (S_2) is caused by the closure of the semilunar valves (both the aortic and pulmonary). It is shorter and pitched higher than S_1 and is louder than S_1 at the base. It reflects diastole and is the "dub" of the "lub-dub."

A third heart sound (S_3) is occasionally heard. S_3 is a low-pitched, early diastolic sound due to blood rushing through the mitral valve and hitting an empty ventricle. When heard, it is best heard at the apex. This sound is sometimes normal in a child, but it is almost never normal in an adult.

A fourth heart sound (S_4) is also possible, although almost never normal. It is caused by an audible atrial contraction at the very end of diastole and is heard best at the apex.

In evaluating the degree of normality of heart sounds, the practitioner should concentrate on four characteristics: rate, intensity, rhythm, and abnormal or unusual sounds.

The rate should be evaluated in the same manner as the rate of a peripheral pulse (i.e., the pulse palpated in an extremity) as was discussed previously. The apical and radial pulse should be the same, and there should be no significant lag between the two.

Intensity of heart sounds is also important. As mentioned before, the intensity of S_1 is normally greated than that of S_2 at the apex, while that of S_2 is greated than S_1 at the base. An increase in the intensity of S_1 may indicate anemia, fever, exercise, or *tachycardia;* a decrease in the intensity of S_1 is usually more serious and can accompany an infarction. If the S_1 is increased in the presence of *bradycardia* (a rate of 60 to 80 beats/minute, for instance), the examiner might consider the possibility of mitral stenosis, heart block, or atrial flutter. If S_1 is constantly changing in intensity and is accompanied by bradycardia, the possibility of heart block should be considered. An increase in S_2 may be normal or may indicate coarctation or arterial hypertension.

The nurse-examiner must evaluate carefully the rhythm of the heart sounds. The examiner must listen for irregularity and then decide if the irregularity follows any pattern. It may be either a *disordered arrhythmia* or an *ordered arrhythmia.* There are two types of disordered arrhythmia, both very serious and usually heard only in hospitalized individuals. The first is *atrial fibrillation.* At first this sounds very fast but regular; but if the examiner listens more carefully, he or she realize that a few beats are being dropped. This is always abnormal and can be from organic heart disease, rheumatic fever, thyrotoxicosis, or other serious illnesses. *Ventricular fibrillation* is the second disordered arrhythmia; it is grossly arrhythmic, always abnormal, and almost always fatal.

There are several types of ordered arrhythmias. The most common is *sinus arrhythmia*—an arrhythmia in which the heart speeds up with inspiration and slows down with expiration. This arrhythmia is found in normal children and should cause no concern. The problem is differentiating it from abnormal rhythms. In an older child, this can be done by asking her to hold her breath. When she does so the arrhythmia should disappear if it is sinus arrhythmia. In an infant, the examiner must observe very closely to see if the arrhythmia fluctuates with respiration.

There are other types of ordered arrhythmias. *Bigeminy* or coupled rhythm consists of a normal beat followed by a premature contraction. This can be normal in some children, but can also indicate organic heart disease. Another type of ordered arrhythmia is composed of three normal-sounding beats (some are actually premature contractions) followed by a pause. Again, this can be normal but can also be a sign of organic heart disease.

Dropped heart beats constitute another ordered arrhythmia and can be an indication of rheumatic heart fever or organic heart disease. Atrial or ventricular premature beats can be either normal or a result of organic heart disease. Gallop rhythms are combinations of extra sounds. An atrial gallop is the addition of an abnormal S_4; a ventricular gallop is the addition of an abnormal S_3; and a summation gallop is a combination of all four beats. All persons with gallop rhythms should be referred to a doctor.

The fourth category of things the nurse-examiner is listening for while evaluating the heart sounds is a series of abnormal or unusual sounds. S_3 has already been discussed. It is best heard at the apex in a child. Sometimes in a child and almost always in an adult, this is not just an S_3, but really a pathologic gallop rhythm. S_4 is also heard best at the apex. It is much more rare than S_3 and is always abnormal. It can be a sign of aortic stenosis, hypertension, anemia, hyperthyroidism, or other diseases. Its addition to S_1 and S_2 forms the atrial gallop.

A *pericardial friction rub* is also always abnormal. It is a scratchy high-pitched, grating sound not affected by changes in respiration (as is the pleural friction rub which has a similar sound). It extends through both systole and diastole and is best heard with the child leaning forward in deep expiration.

A *mediastinal crunch* (Hamman's sign) is a randomly distributed crunching noise resulting from air in the mediastinum. It is rare, but should always be referred when found.

Clicks (ejection sounds) form another group of unusual sounds. A pulmonary ejection click is a click localized at the pulmonic area which decreases during inspiration. It can be caused by pulmonary stenosis or hypertension. An aortic ejection click occurs in early systole at the base and apex of the heart. It exhibits no change with respiration. It can be caused by aortic valve stenosis, coarctation, or aneurysm.

An *opening snap* is similar to the click sounds but has a different quality. It occurs soon after S_2 in the third to fourth left intercostal space. Mitral stenosis and atrial tumors may cause this type of snap.

There are two types of *splits* which may occur. The first is a split of the first heart sound (S_1). The reader will remember that the first heart sound is caused by the closure of the tricuspid and mitral valves. Generally the mitral valve closure precedes the tricuspid closure by a small fraction of a second; however, the timing is usually so close that the two closures seem to produce one sound. There are times, particularly in children, when this double sound will be normally audible over the left lower sternal border in the tricuspid area. This is because the tricuspid closure is the softer of the two, and it is only when the stethoscope is immediately next to it that it can be heard clearly enough that the split or lag between it and the mitral valve can be heard. Whenever there is a wide split or the split is heard in other areas, particularly at the apex, it should be considered abnormal and referred. A split of the second sound (S_2) is also possible, and, in fact, more common. S_2 is caused by the closure of the two *semilunar valves,* the aortic and pulmonary valves. The aortic valve closes slightly ahead of the pulmonic valve, but again, this slight difference in timing is often not detectable. When it is, it is called a split. It is best heard at the pulmonic area (the third left intercostal space) again because the sound of pulmonic closure is softer than that of aortic closure and is normally wider on inspiration than on expiration. If the width of the split does not vary (a "fixed split") with respiration or if it is wider on expiration than on inspiration (paradoxical splitting), the child should again be referred for a further cardiac evaluation.

Another sound the nurse-examiner may occasionally encounter is a *venous hum.* This is a continuous low-pitched hum heard throughout the cardiac cycle, but loudest during diastole. It is heard most clearly at the supraclavicular fossae, but also in the second to third interspace on both sides of the sternum. It is not usually affected by respiration and may be louder when the child is standing. Its most distinguishing quality is the fact that it can be obliterated by turning the neck of the child or occluding the carotid pulse with your fingers. It is almost always normal, although it sometimes occurs in thyrotoxicosis and anemia.

There is one final classification of abnormal or unusual sounds which may be heard during auscultation. These are murmurs. All murmurs should be evaluated carefully and recorded with regard to their timing, location, radiation, intensity (grade I being the softest possible to grade VI being the loudest possible, i.e., a murmur which can be heard without a stethoscope), pitch, and quality (musical, blowing, rasping, harsh, or rumbling). There are two kinds of murmurs: *innocent,* or functional, and *organic.* Unless the nurse-examiner is very sure of his or her auscultatory skills, all murmurs should be referred to the physician who should distinguish between innocent and organic types. There are some clues which the examiner should keep in mind regarding this distinction, however. Innocent murmurs are usually systolic, grade I or II, of short duration, have no transmission, do not affect growth and development, and are usually located at the pulmonic area. These clues are not foolproof, however, so that the examiner will probably want to have all murmurs checked. For those who are beginning to learn auscultation, there are several recordings of heart sounds and heart murmurs available commercially which may be useful.

BIBLIOGRAPHY

Dessertine, Pauline S: "Those Neglected Heart Sounds," *Pediatric Nursing,* vol. 3, no. 1, pp. 18–20, January–February 1977.

Mechner, Francis: "Patient Assessment: Examination of the Heart and Great Vessels, Part I," *American Journal of Nursing,* vol. 76, no. 11, pp. 1–24, November 1976.

_____: "Patient Assessment: Auscultation of the Heart, Part II," *American Journal of Nursing,* vol. 77, no. 2, pp. 1–24, February 1977.

Park Myung, Kawapowi, I., and W. Guntheroth: "Need for an Improved Standard for Blood Pressure Cuff Size," *Clinical Pediatrics,* vol. 15, no. 9, pp. 784–787, September 1976.

GLOSSARY

apical area   an area of the chest overlying the apex of the heart and one of the classic areas for auscultation of the heart, located at the fifth intercostal space in the midclavicular line in adults and children over 8 years of age, but in younger children, higher and more medial

arrhythmia   a variation of the normal heart rhythm

atria (auricles)   the two superior, smaller chambers of the heart

atrial fibrillation   a very irregular rhythm caused by rapid, uncoordinated contractions of the atria

bradycardia   a slow pulse

bundle of His   a bundle of nerve fibers traveling from the atrioventricular node to the apex, which transmits impulses controlling the heartbeat

clicks (ejection sounds)   sharp "clicking" heart sounds considered abnormal

Corrigan's pulse (water-hammer pulse)   a forceful bounding pulse, best felt at the radial and femoral areas and accompanied by an increase in pulse pressure

disordered arrhythmia   a variation of the normal heart rhythm in which no repeated pattern can be discerned

dyspnea   difficult breathing

endocardium   the membrane lining the inside of the myocardium

epicardium   the visceral layer of the pericardium, surrounding and closely covering the myocardium

innocent murmur (functional murmur)   the type of heart murmur that does not indicate a pathologic condition

mediastinal crunch (Hamman's sign)   a randomly distributed crunching heart sound resulting from air in the mediastinum

myocardium   the muscular layer of the heart

opening snap   an abnormal heart sound similar to a click which occurs soon after S_2 in the third to fourth left intercostal space, often due to mitral stenosis

ordered arrhythmia   a variation of the normal heart rhythm in which a repeated pattern can be discerned

organic murmur   a heart murmur indicating an underlying pathologic condition of the heart

orthopnea   difficulty in breathing in any but an upright position

pericardial friction rub   a scratchy, high-pitched grating heart sound caused by the myocardium rubbing against the pericardium during the cardiac cycle

plateau pulse (pulsus torlos)   a pulse consisting of a normal upstroke and a normal downstroke, but which is characterized by an elongated peak forming a plateau

point of maximal impulse (PMI)   the cardiac area at which the strongest beat can be felt; most often at the apex

precordial area   the area of the chest overlying the precordium and one of the classic areas for auscultation of the heart, located at the third, fourth, and fifth intercostal spaces

pulmonic area   an area of the chest that is one of the classic areas for auscultation of the heart, located in the second and third left intercostal space near the sternum

pulsus alternans   a pulse consisting of one strong beat followed by one weak beat; it can be a sign of myocardial weakness

pulsus bigeminus   a coupled pulse in which the beats are felt in pairs

pulsus bisferiens (dicrotic pulse)   a double pulse in which two beats are felt in the radial area for every one beat at the apex

Purkinje fiber   a group of nerve fibers distributed throughout the musculature of both ventricles, which conduct nervous impulses concerned with the action of the heart

S_1   the first heart sound, synchronous with the carotid pulse; systole

S_2   the second heart sound; diastole

semilunar valves   the aortic and pulmonary valves that separate the ventricles from the vena cava and aorta

sinus arrhythmia   a normal arrhythmia associated with respiration; the heartbeat becomes faster during inspiration and slower during expiration

splits   the double sound caused by the slightly asynchronous closing of two heart valves

sternoclavicular area   one of the classic areas for auscultation of the heart, lying directly over and to both sides of the sternoclavicular junction

systole   the S_1 of the cardiac cycle; the "lub" of the "lub-dub"; caused by the contraction of the ventricles

tachycardia   a rapid pulse

thrill   a palpable murmur

venous hum   a continuous low-pitched sound heard in normal children throughout the cardiac cycle, most clearly at the supraclavicular fossae or in the second and third interspaces on both sides of the sternum

Inspection of the Cardiovascular System*

Skin color	Yes	No	Not appli-cable	Describe (where appropriate)	Significance
1. Cyanosis					Any of these color changes may indicate cardiac, respiratory, or neurological problems.
2. Pallor					
3. Ruddiness					
4. Other					
Dyspnea					
1. Tachypnea					Any of these are signs of cardiac or respiratory problems which are fairly severe; they should be referred to a physician immediately.
2. Retractions					
3. Nasal flaring					
4. Other					
Visible vascular pulsations					
1. Neck					The only pulse which may be normally visible is the carotid; any excessive pulsation of the carotid or any visible pulsations elsewhere probably indicates a heart which is overworked; it should be referred to a physician.
2. Other pulses					

*These charts are meant to be used by beginning students as they perform their first physical assessments. Each item should be examined on the child and then checked off on the checklist. The significance of the items follows in the right-hand column.

201

Inspection of the Cardiovasular System (*Continued*)

Visible cardiac pulsations	Yes	No	Not appli-cable	Describe (where appropriate)	Significance
1. Aortic area					A thrill radiating from the aortic area to the right side of the neck may indicate aortic stenosis; vibrations of aortic closure may indicate hypertension; some pulsations may occur here with patent ductus arteriosus.
2. Sternoclavicular area					A very slight pulsation may normally be visible at this area.
3. Pulmonic area					A thrill radiating to the left side of the neck may indicate pulmonic stenosis; a slight brief pulsation may be normal, particularly if the child has a thin chest, but it may also indicate fever, hyperthyroidism, pregnancy, anemia, or other causes of increased cardiac output; a stronger pulsation may occur in hypertension or mitral stenosis.
4. Left lower sternal border (LLSB)					A thrill here may indicate ventricular septal defect; a pulsation may exist with any situation causing increased pressure in the right ventricle such as mitral stenosis, pulmonary stenosis, pulmonary hypertension, atrial septal defect, or ventricular septal defect; slight retractions in this area are normal, particularly in small children. Outward pulsa-tions may occur in any condition which increases cardiac output such as anemia, fever, pregnancy, or hyperthyroidism.
5. Apical area					A systolic thrill may be visible in mitral regurgitation; a diastolic thrill may occur with mitral stenosis. A displacement of the normally seen and felt point of maximal impulse (PMI) may indicate cardiac enlargement.
6. Epigastric area					Visible pulsations here can be normal, particularly in small children, but can also be indications of minor or major problems such as fever, tricuspid stenosis, tricuspid regurgitation, or thyrotoxicosis.
7. Ectopic area					All visible pulsations in ectopic areas should be considered abnormal and referred to a physician.

Palpation of the Cardiovascular System

Peripheral pulses	Yes	No	Not applicable	Describe (where appropriate)	Significance
1. Radial normal strength					All pulses should be symmetrical and of normal strength; weak, thready pulses or very strong bounding pulses can both be signs of cardiac malfunction; popliteal pulses are occasionally very difficult to feel and the pedis dorsalis and posterior tibial pulses are occasionally congenitally absent—all this is within the range of normal; femoral pulses should beat synchronously with radial pulses—if they do not, consider the possibility of coarctation of the aorta.
2. Brachial normal strength					
3. Carotid normal strength					
4. Femoral normal strength					
5. Femoral synchronous with radial					
6. Popliteal normal strength					
7. Dorsalis pedis normal strength					
8. Posterior tibial normal strength					

Cardiac pulsations					
1. Aortic area					Same significance as under inspection.
2. Sternoclavicular area					
3. Pulmonic area					
4. LLSB					
5. Epigastric area					
6. Apex					
7. PMI					

Percussion of the Cardiovascular System

Heart	Yes	No	Not appli-cable	Describe (where appropriate)	Significance
1. Normal cardiac borders					Usually judged by the position of the apex which should be at the fifth intercostal space in children 8 years and older in the midclavicular line; in younger children it is usually higher and more medial; in pregnancy, higher and more lateral.

Auscultation of the Cardiovascular System

B/P	Yes	No	Not appli-cable	Describe (where appropriate)	Significance
1. Normal in (R) arm					See chart on normal blood pressures below.
2. Normal in (L) arm					Systolic thigh pressures in infants under 1 year are similar to those of the arm; after that they may be 10 to 40 mm higher; diastolic should always be the same.
3. Normal in (R) leg					
4. Normal in (L) leg					
Respiratory noises					
1. Respiratory grunt					In an infant, this may indicate cardiac trouble.
Heart (sitting)					
A. Aortic area 1. S_1 of normal intensity					Normal.

	Comments
2. S_2 of normal intensity	Normal.
3. Split S_1	Should not be split in this area.
4. Split S_2	
a. increases with inspiration and decreases with expiration	Should not be split in this area.
b. increases paradoxically	
c. Does not change with respiration	
5. Murmur	Should be referred to a physician for further investigation.
B. Sternoclavicular area	
1. S_1 of normal intensity	Normal.
2. S_2 of normal intensity	Normal.
3. Split S_1	Should not be split in this area.
4. Split S_2	
a. increases with inspiration and decreases with expiration	Should not be split in this area.
b. increases paradoxically	
c. does not change with respiration	
5. Murmur	

205

Auscultation of the Cardiovascular System (*Continued*)

Heart	Yes	No	Not appli- cable	Describe (where appropriate)	Significance
C. Pulmonic					
1. S_1 of normal intensity					Normal.
2. S_2 of normal intensity					Normal.
3. Split S_1					Should not be heard at this area.
4. Split S_2					
a. increases with inspiration decreases or becomes single with expiration					This is the expected change.
b. decreases with inspiration and increases with expiration					Called "paradoxical splitting"; is abnormal and should be referred for further investigation.
c. does not change with respiration					Called "fixed splitting"; is abnormal and should be referred for further investigation.
5. Murmur					
D. Left lower sternal Border					
1. S_1 of normal intensity					In this area S_1 should be softer than S_2.
2. S_2 of normal intensity					See above.
3. Split S_1					A split of S_1 is normal in this area; it does not change with respiration.

4. Split S_2	
a. increases with inspiration and decreases or becomes single with expiration	
b. decreases with inspiration; increases with expiration	S_2 should not split in this area.
c. does not change with respiration	
5. Murmur	Needs referral.
E. Epigastric area	
1. S_1 of normal intensity	Normal.
2. S_2 of normal intensity	Normal.
3. Split S_1	Should not be split in this area.
4. Split S_2	
a. increases with inspiration and decreases with expiration	
b. increases paradoxically	Should not be split in this area.
c. does not change with respiration	
5. Murmur	Needs referral.

207

Auscultation of the Cardiovascular System (*Continued*)

Heart	Yes	No	Not applicable	Describe (where appropriate)	Significance
F. Apex					
1. S_1 of normal intensity					In this area S_1 is expected to be louder than S_2.
2. S_2 of normal intensity					See above.
3. Split S_1					S_1 should not be split at this area.
4. Split S_2					
a. increases with inspiration and decreases or becomes single with expiration					
b. decreases with inspiration and increases with expiration					S_2 should not be split in this area.
c. does not change with respiration					
5. Murmur					Needs referral.
With child leaning forward					This position is assumed only if questions arise during the other positions.
A. Aortic area					
1. S_1 of normal intensity					Normal.
2. S_2 of normal intensity					Normal.
3. Split S_1					Should not be split in this area.

4. Split S_2
   a. increases with inspiration and decreases with expiration | | | Should not be split in this area.
   b. increases para-doxically
   c. does not change with respiration

5. Murmur | Should be referred to a physician for further investigation.

In supine position

A. Aortic area
1. S_1 of normal intensity | Normal.
2. S_2 of normal intensity | Normal.
3. Split S_1 | Should not be split in this area.
4. Split S_2
   a. increases with inspiration and decreases with expiration | | | Should not be split in this area.
   b. increases para-doxically
   c. does not change with respiration

5. Murmur | Should be referred to a physician for further investigation.

Auscultation of the Cardiovascular System (*Continued*)

Heart	Yes	No	Not appli-cable	Describe (where appropriate)	Significance
B. Sternoclavicular area					
1. S_1 of normal intensity					Normal.
2. S_2 of normal intensity					Normal.
3. Split S_1					Should not be split in this area.
4. Split S_2					
a. increases with inspiration and decreases with expiration					
b. increases para-doxically					Should not be split in this area.
c. does not change with respiration					
5. Murmur					Should be referred to a physician for further investigation.
C. Pulmonic area					
1. S_1 of normal intensity					Normal.
2. S_2 of normal intensity					Normal.
3. Split S_1					Should not be heard at this area.

4. Split S_2	
a. increases with inspiration and decreases or becomes single with expiration	This is the expected change.
b. decreases with inspiration and increases with expiration	Called "paradoxical splitting"; is abnormal and should be referred for further investigation.
c. does not change with respiration	Called "fixed splitting"; is abnormal and should be referred for further investigation.
5. Murmur	Should be referred to a physician.
D. Left lower sternal border	
1. S_1 of normal intensity	In this area S_1 should be softer than S_2.
2. S_2 of normal intensity	See above.
3. Split S_1	A split of S_1 is normal in this area; it does not change with respiration.
4. Split S_2	
a. increases with inspiration and decreases or becomes single with expiration	
b. decreases with inspiration and increases with expiration	S_2 should not be split in this area.
c. does not change with respiration	

Auscultation of the Cardiovascular System (Continued)

Heart	Yes	No	Not appli-cable	Describe (where appropriate)	Significance
5. Murmur					
E. Epigastric area					
1. S_1 of normal intensity					Normal.
2. S_2 of normal intensity					Normal.
3. Split S_1					Should not be split in this area.
4. Split S_2					
a. increases with inspiration and decreases with expiration					Should not be split in this area.
b. increases para-doxically					Should not be split in this area.
c. does not change with respiration					
5. Murmur					Needs referral.
F. Apex					
1. S_1 of normal intensity					In this area S_1 is expected to be louder than S_2.
2. S_2 of normal intensity					See above.
3. Split S_1					S_1 should not be split in this area.
4. Split S_2					
a. increases with inspiration and decreases or becomes single with expiration					S_2 should not be split in this area.

212

b. decreases with inspiration and increases with expiration			S_2 should not be split in this area.
c. does not change with respiration			S_2 should not be split in this area.
5. Murmur			
G. General			
1. Regular rhythm			Normal.
2. Regular irregularity			These may be normal, but can be abnormal and should always be referred to a physician; the one exception is a sinus arrhythmia—this is an irregularity which changes with respiration; ask the child to hold his or her breath and if the arrhythmia disappears, you know it is sinus arrhythmia which is normal and does not have to be referred.
3. Irregular irregularity			Again these may be normal but are usually abnormal and always need to be referred to a physician for evaluation.
4. Normal rate			*Age* *Pulse rates* *Age* *Pulse rates* Newborn 70–170 6 years 75–115 11 months 80–160 8 years 70–110 2 years 80–130 10 years 70–110 4 years 80–120 Rate must be age appropriate; see above chart for specifics for various ages.
5. Tachycardia			
6. Bradycardia			

*If findings are questionable here, this area is also listened to with the child rolled onto his or her side.

Source: These checklists are printed with permission from Blue Hill Videotape Incorporated and are part of a more complete programmed learning approach to the physical examination, which includes a workbook and series of videotapes. The materials can be purchased from Blue Hill Educational Systems, Inc., 52 South Main Street, Spring Valley, New York 10977.

213

Chapter 12

The Abdomen

WHY THE CHILD IS EXAMINED

Careful examination of the abdomen can reveal many clues to the health or illness of a child. The abdomen contains many of the vital organs of the body, and careful examination of them is imperative. *Organomegaly,* tenderness, or masses are all important signs that should be sought for in the examination.

WHAT TO EXAMINE: ANATOMY OF THE AREA

In discussing the anatomy of the abdomen, the skin, fasciae, muscles, nerves, blood supply, and various organs must all be considered. Immediately beneath the skin there are several layers of fascia covering the abdomen. The superficial subcutaneous fascia is soft and movable and may contain some adipose tissue; in obese persons, this layer may be several centimeters thick. The deep subcutaneous fascia contains yellow elastic fibers and very little adipose tissue; it overlies the obliquus externus abdominis muscle.

The abdominal muscles are divided into two groups: the anterolateral muscles and the posterior muscles. The anterolateral muscles include the obliquus externus abdominis, the obliquus internus abdominis, the transversus abdominis, the rectus abdominis, and the pyramidalis. The *obliquus externus abdominis* is a large flat, irregular muscle covering the lateral portions of the abdomen. It aids in urination, defecation, vomiting, and parturition. Covering the entire ventral surface of the abdomen is the aponeurosis of the obliquus externus abdominis, a sheet of muscles which meets at the midline to form the *linea alba* (a line from the infrasternal notch to the pubic symphysis, intersected by the umbilicus). The thick, inferior edge of the aponeurosis of the obliquus externus abdominis forms the inguinal ligament. Superior and lateral to the pubis is an opening in the aponeurosis of the obliquus externus abdominis which is called the *superficial inguinal ring*. The spermatic cord passes through this opening.

The *obliquus internus abdominis* is a thin, small layer of muscle lying beneath the obliquus externus, which functions similarly to the obliquus externus. The *cremasteric muscle* is attached to the obliquus internus, inguinal ligament, and the rectus abdominis; it helps raise the testis into the inguinal ring. The *transversus abdominis* lies beneath the obliquus internus and has fibers running transversely across the abdomen towards the midline; it aids the other muscles in voiding, defecating, vomiting, and parturition. The *rectus abdominis* is a broad, thin muscle running parallel to the linea alba; it helps flex the vertebral column. The *pyramidalis* is a tiny, thin muscle running beside the lower rectus muscle; it helps tense the linea alba. Between the anterolateral muscles and the posterior muscles lie several additional layers of fascia. The four posterior muscles are the psoas major, psoas minor, iliacus, and quandratus lumborum. The *psoas major* is a long, thin muscle attached to all the lumbar vertebrae; its insertion is at the lesser trochanter of the femur. With contraction it flexes both the thigh and lumbar vertebral column. The *psoas minor* is a thin, long muscle running parallel to the psoas major; it is frequently congenitally absent. The *iliacus* is a thin, flat, broad muscle filling the fossa of the iliac; it is used in flexing the thigh. The *quadratus lumborum* is a broad, irregularly shaped muscle beginning at the iliac crest and inserting on the inferior border of the last rib. It aids in flexion of the rib cage and the lumbar vertebral column.

The abdomen has no bones, but is bordered by bony landmarks. The lower edge of the ribs forms the upper border of the abdomen while the bones of the pelvis form its lower border. The protruding tubercle on the iliac crest can be palpated, and the anterior superior iliac spine can often be felt at the outside end of the inguinal ligament.

Each layer of abdominal muscles is innervated by a specific group of nerves; in general, the spinal nerves involved are the seventh through the twelfth intercostals, the lower thoracic, lumbar iliohypogastric, and ilioinguinal.

Blood is supplied to the abdomen through the descending aorta which divides into the thoracic and abdominal aorta. The aorta contains three main subdivisions: the visceral aorta with 7 smaller branches; the parietal aorta with 3 smaller branches; and the terminal aorta with 1 branch. Blood returns from the abdominal cavity via the inferior vena cava and its tributaries.

It is important that the nurse-practitioner be familiar with the organs within the abdomen.

The stomach is located below the diaphragm between the spleen and the liver; its shape and position vary according to its contents, the digestive process going on, the gastric musculature, and the contents of the intestines. It has two openings: the cardiac and the pyloric orifices. The *cardiac valve* connects the esophagus and the stomach, and the *pyloric valve* joins the stomach to the duodenum. The stomach has two curvatures: the lesser and the greater. The lesser curvature forms the concave border of the stomach, while the greater curvature forms the ventral, longer curve. The stomach wall is composed of four layers: mucous, submucous, muscular, and serous. The mucous and submucous layers lie in deep, curving folds called *rugae.* These layers produce two types of muscular activity within the stomach: peristalsis and pressure. Peristalsis moves the food through the stomach into the intestine; pressure forces the food into contact with the stomach wall and gastric juices.

The small intestine is a 7-m-long tube extending from the pyloric orifice of the stomach to the ileocecal valve. It is divided into three parts: the duodenum, the jejunum, and the ileum. The *duodenum* is the beginning of the short intestine; it is the shortest and most immobile portion of the small intestine. The *jejunum* is found in the umbilical and left iliac portions of the abdomen; it is the most vascular portion of the small intestine and is liberally supplied with large villa for maximal nutrient absorption. The *ileum* is narrow, slightly vascular, and contains lymph nodules; its distal end lies within the pelvis and opens into the large intestine. Both the jejunum and ileum are connected to the abdominal wall by the mesentery (a large fold of peritoneum).

The large intestine or large colon is a 1.5-m tube extending from the ileum to the anus; it is composed of the cecum, appendix, colon proper, rectum, and anus; it lies in a large arch around the small intestine. The cecum begins below the ileocecal valve and runs in an upward direction 6.25 cm toward the right colic flexure. At its apex is a 5- to 10-mm projection called the *appendix.*

The colon proper has four portions: ascending, transverse, descending, and sigmoid. The ascending colon begins at the cecum and runs upward toward the right lobe of the liver. It turns then to the left to form the right colic (hepatic) flexure which can sometimes be palpated in the right upper quadrant of the abdomen. The transverse colon runs transversely across the epigastric areas where it bends downward to form the left splenic flexure (colic). The descending colon runs downward past the kidney, turns medially toward the psoas muscle, and then descends again to end in the sigmoid colon. The *sigmoid colon* is an S-shaped loop within the pelvis which ends with the rectum.

The liver is the largest and heaviest gland in the body; it lies beneath the diaphragm and fills most of the right upper quadrant. It weighs from 80 to 1800 g and is soft and highly vascular. It is divided into four lobes: the right lobe which is large, the left lobe which is smaller, and the caudate and quadrate lobes which are both quite small. The main functions of the liver are the production of bile for fat digestion, metabolism of proteins and carbohydrates, and the production of certain substances to aid in the development of red blood cells. The bile ducts, the hepatic artery, and the portal vein lie between the quadrate and caudate lobes on the undersurface of the liver. The two bile ducts join to form the common hepatic duct which meets the cystic duct from the gallbladder; all three then form the common bile duct which empties into the duodenum.

The gallbladder with the hepatic duct, cystic duct, and common bile duct form the excretory structures of the liver. It is a small, pear-shaped sac located under the right lobe of the liver, whose function is to store bile.

The pancreas is an exocrine and endocrine gland lying transversely on the posterior abdominal wall. It weighs between 70 and 106 g and is between 12 and 15 cm long. The exocrine portion secretes pancreatic juice into the duodenum for the digestion of proteins, carbohydrates, and fats, while the endocrine portion of the gland (the *island of Langerhans*) secretes insulin for the metabolism of sugars.

The spleen is a soft, highly vascular organ which lies between the stomach and the diaphragm. It grows from 17 g at birth to 170 g by 20 years of age and decreases to around 122 g by 75 years. Its function also seems to change throughout life. During the first year of life it helps with the production of red blood cells; thereafter it aids in the destruction of red blood cells and the formation of hemoglobin (see Fig. 12-1).

Also in the abdomen are organs of the genitourinary system. The ovaries and the fallopian tubes are in the lower quadrants of the abdomen; the ovaries can be palpated in a vaginal-abdominal examination. The uterus is midline and can also be palpated in this way. In the male the vas deferens and seminal vesicles are found low in the lower quadrants. The kidneys are two small (125 to 170 g, 11 by 7 cm) bean-shaped organs of the urinary system; the right kidney is normally 1 cm lower than the left. Both kidneys are attached to the posterior surface of the abdomen; they can occasionally be felt with deep palpation in the upper quadrants.

The urinary bladder is a muscular, membranous sac located at the midline of the lower quadrants. The size and exact position will vary according to the amount of urine being stored in the bladder, the size of the

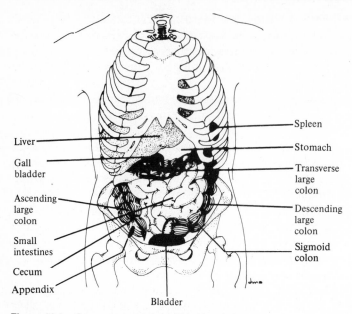

Figure 12-1   Organs contained within the abdomen.

person, and whether the person is male or female. In a child the urinary bladder lies between the symphysis pubis and the umbilicus. It descends lower into the abdomen in the adult, although a distended bladder holding as much as 500 ml of urine will rise into the abdomen even in an adult.

HOW TO EXAMINE

All four methods of physical examination are important in assessing the abdomen. Inspection, palpation, percussion, and auscultation are all utilized, but the order is slightly different from that used on other parts of the body, with auscultation rather than percussion following immediately after inspection. This is because percussion and palpation may disturb the normal sounds heard on auscultation.

WHERE TO EXAMINE

The entire abdomen must be carefully examined. There are two accepted methods of subdividing this region. The first is the traditional method and is less popular today. This method divides the abdomen into the nine sections shown in Figure 12-2. The current method of division is simpler and consists of only four divisions; it is also illustrated in Figure 12-2.

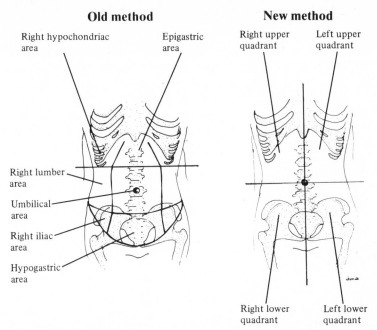

Old method

Right hypochondriac area

Epigastric area

Right lumber area

Umbilical area

Right iliac area

Hypogastric area

New method

Right upper quadrant

Left upper quadrant

Right lower quadrant

Left lower quadrant

Figure 12-2 The two accepted methods of subdividing the abdomen.

WHAT TO EXAMINE WITH

There is no specialized equipment for examining the abdomen except the stethoscope which is used for auscultation. This instrument was discussed more fully in the chapter "The Heart."

WHAT TO EXAMINE FOR

In this section, each method of examination will be considered separately and will specify what the examiner should be looking for in relation to the method discussed. Inspection is the first method of examination utilized when assessing the abdomen. First, the abdomen is observed for movement; normally there should be only respiratory and vascular movements visible. As discussed in the chapter "The Chest and Lungs," the child under about 6 or 7 years of age will usually breathe primarily with the abdominal muscles. A child over this age who is using the abdominal muscles for breathing should be examined carefully for the possibility of thoracic problems. Certain children (particularly those who are athletic or who sing), however, will usually use abdominal breathing. Greatly restricted abdominal movement in a child under 6 years old may indicate peritoneal irritation.

Peristalsis is not seen on a normal child. Visible peristaltic waves usually indicate an obstruction at some point along the gastrointestinal tract. Peristaltic waves which move from left to right are the classic sign of pyloric stenosis, but can also occur with malrotation of the bowel, duodenal ulcer, urinary tract infection, gastrointestinal allergy, or duodenal stenosis.

The contour of the abdomen should also be assessed. The abdomen normally bulges slightly at the beginning of inspiration; with certain central nervous system diseases such as chorea, it may retract rather than bulge; this is called *Czerny's sign* (paradoxical respiration).

Any localized fullness should be noted. Such a fullness found in the right lower quadrant, for instance, may be an appendicular abscess. In other areas it might indicate organomegaly or a tumor.

A mild potbelly is normal in young children, but should be carefully investigated, for it may conceal organomegaly, ascites, neoplasm, cysts, or defects in the abdominal wall.

Bulging of the flanks may indicate *ascites,* while a generalized scaphoid abdomen (an abdominal wall with a concave, depressed contour) in which the abdominal organs are unusually palpable may indicate extreme malnutrition.

Abdominal distention should be investigated for the possibility of pregnancy in older children, for feces (in the case of *megacolon* palpation will reveal a plastic feel to the mass), organomegaly, or ovarian cysts.

The superficial vessels of the abdomen should also be observed. It is sometimes possible to see a pulsating aorta over the epigastric area in normal children, but excess pulsation in this area may indicate an aortic aneurysm.

Many easily visible superficial veins are normally present in infancy, but in later childhood their presence may be a sign of abdominal distention or obstruction. Venous return in the abdomen should be checked if there is any question of vascular obstruction. Above the umbilicus the refilling of veins should take place from the bottom up; below the umbilicus the flow should be from the top down. This can be checked by occluding the vessel with two fingers and then "stripping" the vessel by spreading the fingers apart while continuing to maintain pressure. This should result in an empty vessel. One finger is then lifted to see if the vein refills from that side. If not, the other finger is lifted and filling should then be visible.

The skin of the abdomen should be inspected as skin anywhere else is on the body. For details the reader is referred to the chapter "The Skin." There are, however, a few specifics referring primarily to abdominal skin rather than skin elsewhere on the body. Abdominal skin should be carefully observed for scars, and an explanatory history should be obtained for each scar. Recent scars will appear pink or blue; older ones take on a silvery hue. In certain adrenal problems purple scars associated with fragile, easily broken skin may be seen. Scars may darken or lighten during pregnancy. *Striae* should also be noted on the abdomen as well as on the shoulders, thighs, and breasts; these may be the result of weight loss or previous pregnancies.

Glistening, thick skin may be a sign of underlying edema or ascites.

Spider nevi may appear with liver disease. These are spider-shaped reddened areas with a central arteriole and several extending rays. Pressure on the central arteriole will cause the entire marking to blanch.

Hair distribution on the abdomen is important. Excess hairiness may be a sign of adrenocortical problems. In older children, the nurse should expect to find a triangular distribution of hair in the pubic area in girls and a diamond-shaped distribution in boys. Alterations of the appropriate hair distribution for each of the sexes may indicate endocrine or liver disorders.

Grey Turner's sign is another possible finding on the abdominal skin. This consists of a massive ecchymosis with no history of trauma. It is usually reddish blue, bluish purple, or greenish brown, and is found primarily on the flanks and lower abdomen. It indicates extravasation of blood from some place in the abdomen.

The umbilicus is an important region of the abdomen and should be inspected thoroughly. A bluish umbilicus (*Cullen's sign*) may occur with intra-abdominal hemorrhage, while a nodular umbilicus (*Sister Joseph's nodule*) may be a sign of abdominal cancer. A recently everted umbilicus, if it occurs without hernia, may be the result of some kind of increased intra-abdominal pressure, although many normal children have everted umbiliculuses from birth.

The nurse should check carefully for umbilical fistulas. Drainage from the umbilicus may be urine in a case such as patent urachus, a small amount of feces, if a fistula to the colon exists, or pus, if a *urachal cyst* or abscess exists.

Sometimes an umbilical calculus will be found; it is not a true stone, but rather a hard mass of debris resulting from poor hygiene.

If serous or serosanguineous discharge continues after the cord has separated, a granuloma may be suspected. This consists of a small red solid button deep in the umbilicus. Most clinicians cauterize such granulomas with silver nitrate sticks, although some prefer borax powder.

Particularly in newborn infants, the umbilicus should be carefully inspected for any signs of infection. Foul-smelling discharge, periumbilical redness and induration, or skin warmth should alert the nurse to this possibility. This condition can be quite dangerous in a young infant, since the infection can travel up the open arteries into the peritoneum, causing a sepsis which is frequently fatal.

Omphaloceles are unusual defects of the umbilical area. In an omphalocele, the peritoneal contents bulge through a muscular defect in the umbilical area; these contents are covered only by a thick transparent membrane. One-third to one-half the number of children with this condition have associated defects, such as malrotation of the bowel, *Meckel's diverticulum,* cardiovascular problems, or patent vitelline ducts.

Umbilical *hernias* are a common finding. Their size should always be judged by palpating the actual opening, not by measuring the contents which protrude through the opening. They should be expected to attain their maximum size by about 1 month of age or sometimes later and will generally close by 1 year of age. There is great disagreement as to their treatment. Some clinicians operate on openings of more than 5 cm in early infancy. If the hernia is between 2 and 5 cm, they tape it and operate if its size has not decreased by age 6 to 8 months (Schaeffer, 1977, p. 395). Not all physicians will operate this early, and many will not tape an umbilical hernia at all, feeling that this procedure is useless. Whether taping is useful or not remains moot, and the practitioner may decide to follow this practice or not. The one practice that should definitely not be followed, however, is that of taping a coin into the umbilical ring; this can interfere with its closure.

Double or multiple herniations can occur in the region of the umbilicus and above; operations on these are usually not performed unless they are very small, but are usually taped for a year (Schaeffer, 1977, p. 395).

Finally, the umbilicus should be checked for a single umbilical artery. Realistically this can only be done in the delivery room because within a very short time, the cord is too dried out to discern the vessels clearly. If only a single artery is seen, the clinician must be alerted to search for other abnormalities, particularly abnormalities of the kidneys.

Other muscular defects of the abdominal wall can also occur. *Diastasis recti abdominis* is the condition in which the two recti muscles do not approximate each other. This is a rather common condition, particularly in black babies, and should be considered normal as long as no hernia is associated with it. Incisional hernias are a not infrequent occurrence, and any child with an operational scar should be observed while doing a sit-up. An incisional hernia will present as a protuberance adjacent to the scar.

Epigastric hernias are encountered occasionally. Usually, they are accompanied by pain resembling a chronic peptic ulcer. When the child stands, the examiner should run his or her finger down the midline of the abdomen. A small nodule protruding outward between the fibers of the linea alba will be felt if an epigastric hernia is present.

Inguinal hernias will be discovered in some children. The inguinal ligament runs from the anterior superior iliac spine to the pubic tubercle; the inguinal canal parallels this ligament and is about 3.5 cm long. The internal ring of this canal is located at the midpoint of this line but is not palpable; the external ring lies just lateral to the pubis and can be palpated in male through the scrotum. A *direct inguinal hernia* bulges through the posterior wall of this canal in an area called *Hesselbach's triangle,* directly behind the external ring. It seldom causes pain. It is never congenital, but always acquired. It is much more frequent in males than females. An indirect hernia does not bulge through the wall of the canal but actually enters it from the abdomen through the internal ring. It may protrude into the testes in a male (see Fig. 12-3). Direct hernias are very rare in children but indirect hernias are quite common.

The final type of hernia to be discussed here is the femoral hernia. This hernia will present as a small bulge adjacent and medial to the femoral artery by about two fingerbreadths. It is more common in females than males.

As explained before, auscultation should take place immediately after inspection, since percussion and palpation may disturb the bowel sounds.

The first sound the nurse should assess when auscultating the abdomen is peristalsis. The most important point is simply to ascertain that peristalsis exists. The clinician should be careful in concluding that it does not exist, however. Before concluding this, the examiner must listen at least 5 minutes, timed by the clock, since peristaltic sounds can be very irregular. *Paralytic ileus* is unusual in ambulatory children, and when it exists it is most often due to diffuse peritoneal irritation. Hyperperistalsis occurs with diarrhea or, more severely, with early obstruction in the intestine or pyloris. It presents as a frequent high-pitched tinkling sound accompanied by pain.

The nurse must also listen for vascular sounds. Venous hums similar to those which can occur in the neck may be found in cases of congenital ab-

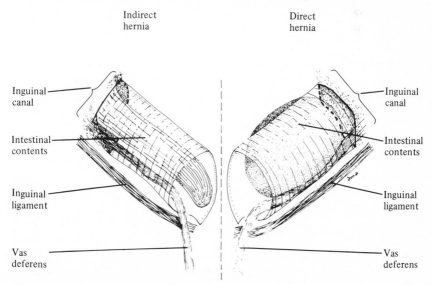

Figure 12-3 The direct and indirect hernia.

normalities of the umbilical vein, vascular problems located in the portal system, or hemangiomas of the liver.

A murmur heard near the umbilical area may indicate a renal artery defect. Occasionally similar defects can be heard over the femoral arteries.

Friction rubs can sometimes be heard in the abdomen. They may originate in an inflamed spleen or a liver with a tumor or with generalized peritoneal obstruction. These rubs are often quite soft and can be mistaken for breath sounds.

A bruit is important only if heard consistently with change of position and even with the stethoscope held very lightly against the abdominal wall. In such cases it may be a sign of some kind of vascular problem. A bruit may indicate a dilated, tortuous, or constricted vessel. If heard over the aorta, it may be a sign of aneurysm; if heard in other places, it may be a sign of congenital bands of tissue that constrict other branches of the vascular system.

Stomach contents may also be heard. To do this, the stethoscope should be held over the upper part of the stomach while the child's body is rocked back and forth. A splash will be heard if the stomach contains the normal amount of fluid. This maneuver is not routinely done.

After auscultation, percussion is performed. The examiner stands at the patient's right side and begins with the thorax, first going down the left midaxillary line. In this line, the nurse may encounter a tympanic note over the stomach bubble, just below the left diaphragm. Dullness above the ninth interspace in the left midaxillary line may originate with the spleen. Occasionally, a kidney or the left lobe of the liver or even consolidation of the left lower lung will produce the same note in this area. The lower edge of the spleen lies at about the eleventh interspace in the midaxillary line.

This procedure should then be repeated on the patient's right side. Liver dullness is expected at the sixth rib or interspace anteriorly and at the ninth rib posteriorly. Relative dullness may occur one or two interspaces above this. The lower border of the liver should be encountered at the costal margin or 2 to 3 cm lower. The liver moves with respiration, so that if it is percussed with held inspiration and expiration, its position should move about two fingerbreadths. Sounds in the rest of the abdomen should be tympanic or dull. This tympany may be more pronounced in children who swallow air extensively or in those with any obstructive lesions in the gastrointestinal tract. Dullness usually indicates feces, but should be further investigated to make sure it does not indicate a tumor.

Shifting dullness may indicate ascites. In this condition, dullness will be heard in the midabdomen when the child is standing, but will shift to the flank areas when the child is lying on his back. If the child is rolled from side to side, the area of dullness will shift to the dependent portion. A significant amount of fluid must be present for this type of percussion to be useful.

The final method of examination employed in assessing the abdomen is palpation. In general, a light touch should be employed. The examiner's hands should be warm; cold fingers usually cause muscular contraction to such an extent that the examiner's ability to palpate is severely impaired. Flexion of the knees and a pillow beneath the head may take strain off the abdominal muscles and result in less resistance to palpation. It is sometimes helpful to use the child's own hand to palpate, particularly if he or she is apprehensive. This, however, is a much less sensitive way to palpate. Distracting a child's attention is frequently a vital part of this examination, especially if the child is ticklish. The nurse should begin with superficial palpation, gradually increasing the pressure. Certain types of masses, such as various cysts and hematomas of the rectus muscles of the abdomen, may be felt in this manner. Rebound tenderness, or *Blumberg's sign,* may also be encountered in superficial palpation.

The nurse may also wish to test for cutaneous hyperesthesia. This may be done by gently stroking skin in parallel lines with a pin or by pulling the skin gently away from the abdomen. These maneuvers will be painful if hyperesthesia is present. Sometimes only a localized area of hyperesthesia will be found. This may be the case, for instance, in an inflamed appendix, where a small area of skin overlying it may manifest hyperesthesia.

Subcutaneous crepitus may also be discovered on palpation. The examiner will feel freely movable nontender bubbles directly under the skin. These may indicate subcutaneous emphysema or gas gangrene.

Muscle tone can also be evaluated through palpation. Involuntary muscle rigidity—sometimes unilateral, sometimes bilateral—may be an important sign of peritoneal irritation. Boardlike rigidity or spasm may occur in peritonitis, although in very young infants, peritonitis may not have any effect on the muscle tone at all.

Tissue turgor should also be tested in the adominal area by pinching a small piece of skin and then releasing it. Normally, the skin will quickly revert to its original position, but in dehydration, a peak of skin may remain standing out from the body, and return only very slowly.

After the entire abdomen has been superficially palpated, deep palpation should be performed over the same area. Deep palpation is important for discovering masses, tenderness, deep vessels, and palpable organs. All masses should be evaluated for size, consistency, tenderness, mobility, position, shape, pulsatility, and surface characteristics. If there is any suspicion of a neoplasm, palpation should be limited, since excess manipulation may spread it.

Fecal masses may sometimes be felt on palpation in children with constipation; if this seems excessive, the nurse should check for megacolon.

Wilms' tumor may sometimes be felt by deep palpation; this tumor is usually adjacent to the vertebral column and does not extend across the midline.

A pyloric tumor is palpable in about 95 to 98 percent of infants with pyloric stenosis. This is easiest to palpate immediately after vomiting, since the abdominal muscles are soft at this time. The examiner should stand at the child's left side and palpate with the middle finger held at a flexed right angle. The tumor is usually found deep between the edges of the rectus muscle and the costal margin on the right side; it is about the size and shape of an olive.

Tenderness in the abdominal area is very difficult to assess in a child. It is often very difficult for a child to be able to verbalize location and character of pain. Frequently, if a child is asked if something hurts, he will automatically say yes, thinking that the normal pressure he feels when the examiner palpates his abdomen should be interpreted as pain. It is probably best to avoid direct questions of this nature and rely more on such nonverbal clues as wincing. Distraction is extremely important because many children will complain of ticklishness. It is best not to reinforce this response by paying too much attention to it, since if a child is encouraged to continue this response, it will be almost impossible to examine him. Firm rather than light pressure may help avoid this response.

It is normal to complain of pain or wince during deep palpation of the midepigastrium, since this is the area of the aorta. Other areas of pain should be carefully noted. Many types of pain in the abdomen are referred to other locations. It is sometimes helpful to be aware of these referral pathways. For example, pain originating in the common bile duct may be referred to the midline in the upper abdomen; pain may be referred to the midline anterior wall of the abdomen from the stomach, liver, gallbladder, pancreas, and intestinal tract; pain in the kidneys, ovaries, fallopian tubes, or ureters may be experienced in the ipsilateral flank; and splenic pain may be referred to the left shoulder.

Rebound pain occurs only if the peritoneum is involved; this occurs even when pressure is exerted far from the diseased area and may occur merely from coughing or straining. In general, visceral pain is dull and difficult to characterize and localize; muscular pain is sharp and well localized. Some types of pain, like that originating in the appendix, will start out poorly localized and then gradually become more well defined, as in the case of appendicitis, to the right lower quadrant. Pain caused by inflammation is generally constant or increases when pressure is applied; visceral pain caused by distention or contraction of an organ decreases when constant pressure is applied.

Some vessels may also be encountered with deep palpation. Femoral pulses may have been felt with superficial palpation or may be felt better with deep palpation. The aorta can often be palpated and it should be carefully investigated to make sure there is no area where it seems to balloon out in width, indicating the possibility of an aneurysm. In this case the pulsations would be felt on the lateral sides of the aorta in addition to the anterior part where they are usually felt.

Palpable organs must be examined carefully. In order to palpate the spleen, the examiner should stand at the patient's right side with the left hand behind the child's left costovertebral area and push gently up from behind. Simultaneously the examiner should feel gently under the left anterior costal margin with the right hand. The child is then asked to take a deep breath; inspiration will push down on the spleen, causing the tip to strike the examiner's fingers (see Fig. 12-4).

Some clinicians prefer to palpate the spleen by *ballottement*. In this case, the nurse's left hand pushes gently in an anterior direction from behind the costovertebral angle, while the right hand pushes the abdominal wall directly below the costal margin in toward the backbone in short, ballottement movements. If the spleen is present, it will be felt bouncing back against the fingers. The spleen may be palpated more easily if the child rolls over onto his or her right side. Being able to feel the tip of the spleen is normal; it is more frequently felt in premature infants and thin children, but nothing more than the tip should normally be felt. In certain conditions such as erythroblastosis or infectious mononucleosis, in which spleen inflammation is likely, great care should be taken in palpating because it is possible to rupture an inflamed spleen.

Palpation of the liver should always be attempted, although in many normal children, it will not extend below the costal margin and consequently will not be felt. It is also normal, however, if the liver extends 1 to 3 cm below the costal margin in young children. If the examiner palpates with the flat of her fingers, starting at the lower abdomen and working gradually upward, the liver edge will be felt if it does extend below the costal margin. If

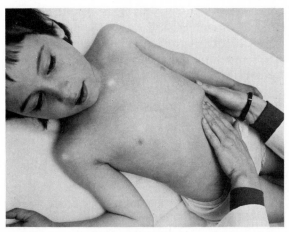

Figure 12-4 Palpation of the spleen.

the liver extends further than 3 cm or so below the costal margin, it should be considered enlarged, and the child should be referred to a physician. In rare instances of a congenital anomaly called *Riedel's lobe,* the liver will extend downward on the left side. At times systolic pulsations may be felt in the liver of a child with certain cardiac problems. Masses on the liver can also be palpated in certain conditions.

Liver tenderness may occur in children suffering from infectious hepatitis, infectious mononucleosis, liver abscesses, or certain other problems.

The nurse-examiner should attempt to palpate the kidneys. Although very few clinicians believe they can routinely feel a normal child's kidneys, the nurse-examiner might try to develop the ability to do so. The nurse-examiner should always attempt palpation of the kidneys, however, since this may reveal enlargement. Kidneys are retroperitoneal organs and very deep palpation is necessary to feel them. They lie immediately adjacent to the vertebral column and will descend slightly with inspiration. At most, the lower pole will be felt, particularly of the right kidney which is lower. The kidneys are easier to feel in premature infants and neonates, although even in infants it is very difficult, except immediately after birth.

Hydronephrosis may cause a constant or intermittent cystic enlargement that may be felt as will congenital polycystic disease of the kidneys, Wilms' tumor, or a perinephritic abscess.

The urinary bladder may be palpated, particularly during early infancy and early childhood. It should be checked for distention such as that which can occur with certain types of central nervous system defects or urethral obstruction.

Parts of the intestine can at times be palpated. The cecum will present as a soft, gas-filled object in the right lower quadrant. The sigmoid may be rolled over the pelvic brim in the left lower quadrant; it feels like a freely movable, sausage-shaped mass which may normally be tender. In chronic ulcerative colitis the ascending, descending, and sigmoid colons may be palpable and tender. At times it is possible to palpate bowel duplication as an extra movable, nontender, smooth, round mass. The newborn with meconium ileus may have palpable rubbery or hard masses. In intussusception a sausage-shaped tumor is present 85 percent of the time in either the right or left upper quadrant.

BIBLIOGRAPHY

Alexander, M., and M. Brown: "Examining the Abdomen," *Nursing '76,* vol. 6, no. 1, pp. 65–70, January 1976.

Mansell, Ellen, et al.: "Patient Assessment: Examination of the Abdomen," *American Journal of Nursing,* vol. 74, no. 9, pp. 1–24, September 1974.

Willacker, Jean: "Bowel Sounds," *American Journal of Nursing,* vol. 73, no. 12, pp. 2100–3101, December 1973.

Schaeffer and Avery: *Diseases of the Newborn,* Saunders, Philadelphia, 1977.

GLOSSARY

ascites an accumulation of serous fluid in the abdomen

ballottement a maneuver for palpating organs such as the spleen by placing one hand behind the organ and one in front of it, and literally bouncing it between the hands

cardiac valve the sphincter of the stomach through which food passes from the esophagus

cremasteric muscle the muscle attached to the obliquus internus, inguinal ligament, and rectus abdominis which helps to raise the testes into the inguinal ring

Cullen's sign a bluish umbilicus resulting from intra-abdominal hemorrhage

Czerny's sign (paradoxical respiration) a sign of certain nervous system diseases such as chorea in which the abdomen retracts rather than bulges at the beginning of inspiration

diastasis recti abdominis the condition in which the two rectus muscles separate, leaving the central area of the abdomen with fascia, but no muscular covering

direct inguinal hernia a herniation through the posterior wall of the inguinal canal directly behind the external ring at Hesselbach's triangle

duodenum the shortest, most immobile portion of the small intestine

Grey Turner's sign a assive ecchymosis, usually on the flanks and lower abdomen, without a history of trauma, indicating extravasation of blood from within the abdomen

hernia a muscular defect which allows internal organs to protrude

Hesselbach's triangle a triangular shape formed by inguinal ligament, the epigastric artery, and the rectus abdominis muscle, located in an area in the posterior wall of the inguinal canal

iliacus a thin, flat, broad muscle which fills the fossa of the iliac and functions in flexing the thigh

Meckel's diverticulum a blind pouch sometimes found in the lower ileum, at times forming a cord continuous with the umbilicus evident by a fistulous opening through the umbilicus

megacolon a very dilated, hypotonic colon usually with very little peristalsis

obliquus externus abdominis a large, flat, irregular muscle covering the lateral portions of the abdomen, which aids in urination, defecation, vomiting, and parturition

obliquus internus abdominis a thin small layer of muscle lying beneath the obliquus externus which functions in conjunction with it

omphalocele a muscular defect in the umbilical area which allows peritoneal contents covered only by a thin, transparent membrane to protrude externally

organomegaly enlarged palpable organs

paralytic ileus lack of peristalsis

psoas major   a long, thin muscle attached to all the lumbar vertebra which inserts on the lesser trochanter of the femur, flexing both the thigh and lumbar vertebral column

psoas minor   a thin, long muscle which runs parallel to the psoas major, flexing the thigh and lumbar vertebral column

pyloric valve   the sphincter of the stomach through which food passes as it leaves the stomach to enter the small intestine

pyramidalis   a tiny, thin muscle which runs beside the lower rectus muscle and aids in tensing the linea alba

quadratus lumborum   a broad, irregularly shaped muscle arising at the iliac crest and inserting on the inferior border of the last rib, functioning in flexion of the rib cage and lumbar vertebral column

rectus abdominis   a broad, thin muscle running parallel to the linea alba which helps to flex the vertebral column

Sister Joseph's nodule   a nodular umbilicus which may indicate abdominal cancer

spider nevi   spider-shaped, reddened areas with a central arteriole and several extending rays, pressure on it causing the entire mark to blanch; sometimes a sign of liver disease

splenic flexure   the junction of the transverse and descending colon located near the spleen

striae   bands of tissue differing from the surrounding tissue in color and/or elevation; "stretch marks"

subcutaneous crepitus   palpable, movable nontender bubbles directly beneath the skin

transversus abdominis   an abdominal muscle lying beneath the obliquus internus whose fibers run parallel to the linea alba

urachal cyst   a cyst formed in the tract between the umbilicus and the urinary bladder

Inspection of the Abdomen*

Skin	Yes	No	Not appli-cable	Describe (where appropriate)	Significance
1. Rashes					Usually the same significance as elsewhere on the skin; spider nevi may indicate liver disease.
2. Lesions					Same significance as elsewhere.
3. Striae					Usually indicate previous stretching of skin; may be due to weight loss, pregnancy.
4. Scars					Obtain a history of previous surgery or trauma. Purple scars associated with fragile, easily broken skin may be seen as certain adrenal problems.
5. Glistening, thin skin					May indicate underlying pressure—often from ascites, but sometimes from a tumor or other source of pressure; often seen in normal pre-mature infants.
6. Edema					Generalized ascites due to a variety of serious causes or local edema due to trauma.
7. Hair					Normal hair distribution.
8. Color a. jaundice					May be a sign of liver disease in the older child; in the infant can be a sign of blood group incompatibility, normal bilirubin production, sepsis, or a variety of other problems; the severity can be judged by how far down the body the jaundice extends—If it extends to the abdomen it is at least moderate; if it extends further (to the legs), it is severe.

*These charts are meant to be used by beginning students as they perform their first physical assessments. Each item should be examined on the child and then checked off on the checklist. The significance of the items follows in the right-hand column.

231

Inspection of the Abdomen (*Continued*)

Skin	Yes	No	Not appli-cable	Describe (where appropriate)	Significance
b. bluish discoloration of the umbilicus					Cullen's sign—indicative of intra-abdominal hemorrhage.
c. bluish discoloration of the flanks					Grey Turner's sign—indicative of extravasation of the blood from some-place in the abdomen.
9. Other					
Shape					
1. Symmetrically flat					Normal.
2. Symmetrically protruberant					May occur in ascites, indicative of a variety of problems including mal-nutrition; may also indicate feces, gas, obesity, tumor, or pregnancy.
3. Asymmetrically protruberant					May also indicate feces, gas, or tumor; might be indicative of a hernia or spinal deformity, organomegaly, defects in the abdominal wall.
4. Symmetrically scaphoid					In infancy may indicate absence of abdominal contents; may also be caused by a diaphragmatic hernia.
5. Lower abdominal fullness					May indicate pregnancy, feces, gas, tumor, or fluid.
6. Bulging flanks					Usually indicates fluid; will shift toward gravity if patient changes position.
7. Asymmetrical bulges					Same as 5.
8. Other					
Umbilicus					
1. Umbilicus deeply inverted					If symmetrical, probably a normal variant; if asymmetrical may indi-cate adhesion beneath it.

2. Umbilicus flat		Normal variant.
3. Umbilicus everted		Normal variant, but look carefully for underlying hernia.
4. Omphalocoele		Abnormal bulging of abdominal contents through abdominal wall.
5. Centrally located		Normal.
6. Drainage		Check the type of drainage: pus indicates infection; urine indicates a fistula to the bladder; feces indicates a fistula to the colon.
7. Granuloma		Presence on a newborn indicates need for cauterization.
8. Umbilical calculus		Not a true stone, but debris resulting from lack of hygiene.

Movement

1. Visible peristaltic waves		Occasionally normal, but may indicate bowel obstruction, or if in the classic left to right direction a pyloric stenosis.
2. Visible respiratory movement		Some is normally expected; the child under 6 breathes primarily with the abdomen; an older child who is breathing primarily with the abdomen may have chest pathology; the younger child who is not using abdominal breathing may have abdominal pathology.
3. Visible aortic pulsations		Normally visible, particularly in a young child in the epigastric area but, if increased, may indicate aortic aneurysm.
4. Fetal movements		A possibility in the adolescent.

Muscles

1. Diastasis recti		A normal variant, particularly in the black child.
2. Muscle atrophy		Can be a sign of muscle-wasting disease.
3. Muscle hypertrophy		Can also be a sign of muscle disease such as early muscular dystrophy.

233

Inspection of the Abdomen (*Continued*)

Muscles	Yes	No	Not applicable	Describe (where appropriate)	Significance
4. Herniations of muscle wall a. umbilical area					These are generally not corrected unless they fail to resolve by 1 year; more common in black children; don't judge the size by the visible protrusion; common in children's hypothyroidism.
b. periumbilical hernias					Hernias in the region of the umbilicus and above; these necessitate referral.
c. femoral bulges					May indicate hernias which need correction.
d. inguinal bulges					May indicate hernias which need repair.
e. epigastric bulges along the linea alba					May indicate epigastric hernias which need repair.
Vessels					
1. Distended abdominal veins					Normal in a newborn; after that, it may indicate vascular obstruction.
2. Spider nevi					May indicate liver problems.
3. Single umbilical artery					There are normally 2; only 1 may indicate renal problems—this can only be evaluated in the delivery room or soon after.
Hair distribution					
1. Pubic hair in the shape of a triangle with the base above the pubis					Normal distribution for a girl; if found in a boy, may indicate hormonal problems.
2. Pubic hair configuration is diamond shaped					Normal hair distribution for a boy; if found in a girl may indicate hormonal or liver problems.

234

	Significance
3. Hirsutism	May indicate adrenal problems.
4. Curly pubic hair	Is thought to indicate mature sperm formation in the boy.
5. Straight pubic hair	Is thought to indicate immaturity of sperm formation in the boy.
6. Pubic lice	Need for treatment.

Auscultation of the Abdomen

Peristaltic sounds	Yes	No	Not applicable	Describe (where appropriate)	Significance
1. Present					Normally peristaltic sounds will be present; absence is not assumed until you have listened for 5 min; total absence indicates paralytic ileus.
2. Absent					
3. Increased					Increased sounds may occur with diarrhea or intestinal obstruction.
4. Decreased					May herald a beginning paralytic ileus.
5. High-pitched, tinkling					Same as 3.
6. Gurgling, rushing sounds					May indicate obstruction.
7. Other					
Vascular sounds					
1. Venous hum					May indicate abnormalities of the umbilical vein, vascular problems in the portal system, or hemangioma of the liver or cirrhosis.
2. Bruits					May indicate aneurysm.
3. Other					

235

Auscultation of the Abdomen (*Continued*)

Subcutaneous crepitus	Yes	No	Not appli- cable	Describe (where appropriate)	Significance
					May indicate gas gangrene or escape of air into tissue.
Friction rub					
1. Liver					Inflammation of the liver peritoneum.
2. Spleen					Inflammation of the spleen peritoneum.
Succussion splash					
					Sound of fluid in the stomach.

Percussion of the Abdomen

Liver	Yes	No	Not appli- cable	Describe (where appropriate)	Significance
1. Upper limit of liver dull- ness in the midaxillary line from fifth to seventh interspace					Height changes with respiration; higher limit may indicate liver enlargement.
2. Liver height 4–8 cm in midsternal line					Greater height may indicate enlargement.
3. Liver height 6–12 cm in right midclavicular line					Same as above.

236

4. Liver edge not more than 6–7 cm below costal margin		Lower edge may indicate enlargement.
Stomach		
1. Tympany in area of left lower anterior rib cage		Indicates normal stomach bubble; absence does not indicate pathology.
Spleen		
1. Dullness near left 10th rib slightly posterior to mid-axillary line		If dullness extends down to the lowest rib even when child takes a deep breath this may indicate enlargement.
Bladder		
1. Dullness above the pubis		Dullness indicates distention of the bladder; the bladder cannot usually be percussed.
Tympanic areas over entire abdomen		Tympany is expected over any bowel containing gas.
Other		
1. Dull areas in abdomen		May indicate masses or feces; further examination is needed.
2. Shifting dullness		Dullness which shifts toward gravity when the child changes position indicates fluid.

Palpation of the Abdomen

Skin	Yes	No	Not appli-cable	Describe (where appropriate)	Significance
1. Normal turgor					Dehydration may be indicated by lack of normal turgor.
2. Subcutaneous crepitus					Gas gangrene; air escaping into tissues.
Muscle					
1. Hernias					
a. epigastric					
b. periumbilical					
c. umbilical					Same significance as under inspection.
d. femoral (right)					
e. femoral (left)					
f. inguinal (right)					
g. inguinal (left)					
2. Tone					
a. normal					
b. increased					May be increased in muscle guarding from peritonitis or general hypertonicity.
c. decreased					Poor muscle tone from neurological or muscular problems.

Vessels

1. Palpable aorta	Usually normal.
2. Aorta with lateral expansion	Pulsations of the aorta are transmitted forward, not laterally; a lateral expansion may indicate an aneurysm.

Organs

1. Palpable liver	May normally be palpable 5–7 cm below costal margin.
2. Enlarged liver	Liver extending downward more than 5–7 cm below costal margin should be considered enlarged.
3. Enlarged spleen	Palpable spleen should be considered enlarged; can be a sign of a multitude of diseases; a small tip may be normally palpated.
4. Enlarged right kidney	Any kidney large enough to be palpated after the newborn period should be considered enlarged; it may be a sign of Wilm's tumor or other kidney problems.
5. Enlarged left kidney	Same as above.
6. Palpable uterus	May indicate pregnancy or uterine pathology such as fibroids.
7. Palpable bladder	Probably indicates distention due to a variety of causes.
8. Palpable feces	May be normal or due to constipation, aganglionic colon, or other pathologies but can be normal.
9. Palpable cecum with flatus	Usually normal but may indicate aganglionic colon.

Masses

	May indicate benign or cancerous tumors or feces.

239

Palpation of the Abdomen (*Continued*)

Tenderness	Yes	No	Not appli-cable	Describe (where appropriate)	Significance
					Rebound tenderness indicates peritoneal inflammation.
					Pain from the gallbladder is often referred to the right shoulder.
					Pain from the spleen to the left shoulder.
					Pain from the stomach, liver, gallbladder, pancreas, and intestine is usually referred to the midline anterior wall.
					Pain from the kidneys, ovaries, fallopian tubes, and ureters is usually referred to the flank on the same side.
					Pain from the common bile duct is usually referred to the midline in the upper abdomen.
					Pain from the appendix usually starts as diffuse, localizes to umbilicus and then to right lower quadrant.
					Visceral pain is dull, difficult to characterize and localize.
					Somatic pain is usually sharp and well localized.
					Pain from inflammation is constant or increases when pressure is applied.
					Pain emanating from distention or contraction of an organ decreases with constant pressure applied.

Source: These checklists are printed with permission from Blue Hill Videotape Incorporated and are part of a more complete programmed learning approach to the physical examination, which includes a workbook and series of videotapes. The materials can be purchased from Blue Hill Educational Systems, Inc., 52 South Main Street, Spring Valley, New York 10977.

Chapter 13

The Male Genitalia

WHY THE CHILD IS EXAMINED

Every complete examination should include a thorough evaluation of the boy's genitalia. It may seem easier to skip this part of the examination for some boys because they are so upset by it; however, this is not wise. The procedures should be done as quickly and matter-of-factly as possible, but it is important that the examiner is certain that no abnormalities exist. This is particularly true in cases of undescended testicles which may be a problem and should definitely be diagnosed before the prepubertal period. Other conditions, such as hermaphroditism, should be diagnosed even earlier, in fact, during the neonatal period.

Another reason that this part of the examination is so important is because so many parents and children (particularly adolescents) are concerned with the genitalia and yet do not feel free to voice these concerns.

Because our culture puts great emphasis on the genital area and because many parental and child anxieties are concerned with this area, the physical examination of the genitalia must be done with great care and tact.

Many parents and children will hesitate to ask questions concerning this part of the examination, and for that reason, it is important that the examiner verbalize his or her findings. This is particularly true with the adolescent patient. If the findings are normal, this should be plainly stated. If there are findings which, although normal, may be a possible cause of concern to the parent or child, the nurse should be alert to this and reassure the parent, without waiting for specific questions. By the time a child is 3 years old or even younger, he may well have incorporated many of his parents' feelings about his genitalia. If the child lives in a home where sexuality is a subject surrounded with an air of shamefulness, he will soon learn that his genitals may be regarded by some as shameful, and the child himself may begin to regard them in this way. If this is the case, a physical examination performed brusquely may indeed be traumatic, and the nurse-examiner must be extremely sensitive to the patient's feelings. Although reticence on the part of the child is no excuse for skipping this part of the examination, it is reason enough to proceed with it in the least possible traumatic manner. Usually a firm, matter-of-fact, and rapid but thorough examination is the best approach. Immediately after it is completed the child should be briefly reassured that the examination showed that all is normal, if such is the case, since many unmentioned fears may center around this area. Discussion of other less threatening topics might be useful at this time to reestablish rapport if this has been lost.

WHAT TO EXAMINE: ANATOMY OF THE AREA

For purposes of study, we can divide the male genitalia into two parts, the *penis* and *scrotum* (see Fig. 13-1). The penis consists of a shaft, a retroglandular sulcus meatus, prepuce, glans, and corona. The *penile shaft* is made up of three cylindrical structures: one, called the *corpus spongiosum* (sometimes called the *corpus cavernosum urethrae*) and the two structures called the *corpora cavernosa*. The corpus spongiosum is the medial cylinder of the penis and contains the urethra. The anterior end of the corpus spongiosum forms a rounded balloon called the *glans penis,* the border of which is called the *corona glandis.* The urethra is located within this structure. The *retroglandular sulcus* is the proximal end of the corona and forms the neck of the penis.

The two corpora cavernosa form the major portion of the shaft of the penis and are composed of strong erectile tissue and many fibrous columns. The skin covering the shaft is thin, darkly pigmented and loosely connected to deeper fascia. The *prepuce* (foreskin) is the fold of skin at the neck of the penis, while a secondary fold of skin from the meatus to the neck is termed the *frenulum.* The glans skin contains no hairs, but small papillae and glands which secrete an odoriferous sebaceous material that mixes with epithelial cells to form smegma.

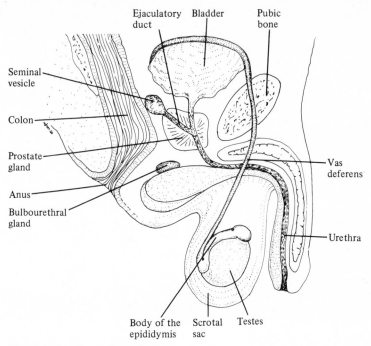

Figure 13-1 The male genitalia.

This penile shaft is supplied with strong ligaments, muscles, and blood vessels.

The scrotum contains the *testes,* the *epididymis,* and the tail of the *vas deferens.* The left and right side of the scrotum are divided by a raphe (ridge) and are covered by a layer of skin and by the dartos tunica.

The testes are the most palpable structures in the scrotum; they are two smooth olive-shaped masses which produce sperm. Prenatally, they develop in the abdominal cavity, but by birth they descend along the inguinal canal into the scrotum.

The *spermatic cord* extends from the testes to the deep inguinal ring. The right cord is shorter, causing the right testis to hang higher than the left. The epididymis can be felt as a long, thin mass along the lateral edge of the posterior border of the testes. It consists of three parts: head, body, and tail. The upper pole is called the head, or globus major; the body is an elongated cone down the posterior axis of the testes; and the tail, or globus minor, forms the tip of this cone. The vas deferens, or minor ductus deferans, is a whiplike cord continuous with the tail of the epididymis.

The *seminal vesicles* are pouches lying along the side of the vas deferens; they secrete a liquid into the semen as it passes from the testes. The opening of the seminal vesicles joins the vas deferens to make up the ejaculatory ducts which are 2 cm long, and extend from the prostate base to the borders of the *utricle* (the blind pouch between the prostate gland and pelvic connective tissue). The *prostate gland* is a small, round, firm mass, the size of a walnut, lying within the pelvic cavity. The urethra and ejaculatory ducts run through this gland. The *bulbourethral glands* (Cowper's glands) are two pea-sized masses lying along the urethra. Both the prostate and bulbourethral glands produce secretions that neutralize the acidity of the urethra and vagina, which might cause damage to the semen.

HOW TO EXAMINE

The primary methods for examining the male genitalia are inspection and palpation. Very rarely a clinician will choose to use auscultation to help ascertain whether the bowel has slipped through a hernia, by listening for bowel sounds in the scrotum. Percussion is of no use in this area. In general, the nurse-examiner should exercise great care and tact in this part of the physical examination. Many children are quite sensitive about their genitals by the time they are 4 or 5 years old. A kind, firm, and quick examination is best. It must be remembered that the *cremasteric reflex* in boys can be activated by cold, touch, or emotion, so that if he is frightened or embarrassed, his testes may ascend into the abdomen before the examiner has palpated the scrotum. It can be very difficult in this case to determine for sure whether the testes had ever descended. This will be discussed at greater length later, but is mentioned here only to remind the nurse that if at all possible, it is helpful to keep this part of the examination as untraumatic as possible, both for psychological well-being of the boy and for the accuracy of physical findings. Also, it is wise to begin by blocking the inguinal canals by applying pressure with the index finger before palpating the testes. If this is done at the beginning of this part of the examination, it will prevent the passage of the testes into the abdomen if the child should later become cold or upset.

WHERE TO EXAMINE

The entire genital and surrounding area must be carefully inspected and palpated. All parts of the penis and scrotum, as well as nearby lymphatic chains, should be included.

WHAT TO EXAMINE WITH

Elaborate equipment is not necessary for this examination. A good light and careful technique are essential. Sometimes an examiner will wish to use a stethoscope for auscultating bowel sounds, as mentioned before. A good penlight with a protruding neck is also necessary for transillumination.

WHAT TO EXAMINE FOR

There are two primary areas of examination, the penis and the scrotum with its contents. All parts of the penis must be carefully evaluated. In newborns and sometimes on older children, the foreskin may be an area of concern to the mother. In an uncircumcised child, the foreskin is normally quite tight for 2 to 3 months and does not retract easily. There is some disagreement on whether it should be forcibly retracted during the first few months. Some clinicians feel that it should not be retracted for cleaning or other purposes, since the thin membrane which connects it to the shaft of the penis may tear, causing adhesions and making retraction even more difficult later. This tightness gradually diminishes naturally, and by 4 or 5 years of age it should be completely retractable. If after this time the condition persists it should be considered to be *phimosis.* Starting at about 4 months, the foreskin should be gently retracted at monthly intervals until it retracts easily and without trauma. Other clinicians forcibly retract the foreskin from birth. Once this has been done it is important to continue to do it regularly since tiny scar tissues can replace the membrane once it is broken.

The question of circumcision is controversial. Basically it is important to remember that this decision belongs to the parents. The nurse-examiner, however, should be aware of the advantages and disadvantages of this procedure and should carefully explain them to the parents. The primary advantage of circumcision is the ease of cleanliness. It eliminates the necessity for cleaning between the foreskin and the penile shaft, an area where smegma can easily accumulate. It is easier not only for the mother to keep this area clean but also for the preschooler who is beginning to take care of himself. The second advantage is based on some experimental data that suggest that wives of uncircumcised males have a higher incidence of cervical cancer. These data are not totally conclusive, however. The disadvantage of circumcision seems to be the procedure itself. Not all circumcisions are performed well. There is always the possibility of excessive bleeding, but even more important, of infection. A few cases of gangrene have been reported following a bell clamp circumcision, and there has been a suspicion that some cases of sepsis may have originated with a local infection in this area. Some authors mention the possibility that because the *meatus* is more exposed to irritation from ammonia from urine breakdown in the diaper area the penis may be more likely to become ulcerated.

During the examination the foreskin must always be carefully retracted in any child over the age of 4 months, if it retracts easily. It must be inspected and palpated carefully. Small white cysts may normally be seen on the distal prepuce in neonates. In older children a condition called *paraphimosis* may be seen. In paraphimosis the foreskin is permanently retracted behind the corona of the glans and cannot be slipped forward; edema of the glans almost always accompanies this condition, since the free flow of blood is constricted by the band of foreskin. This should be brought to the attention of the physician immediately. *Balanoposthitis* is another condition which may be noticed. Balanoposthitis is the local infection of both prepuce and glans, characterized by redness and tenderness in that area and sometimes accompanied by discharge. *Preputial calculus* should also be checked for. Rarely these are renal calculi passed into the prepuce, but more often they are actually solidified dirt and smegma caught beneath a phimosis. *Preputial adhesions* may be another problem found in this area. Most often these are in young infants and are the result of circumcision. They can usually be gently separated and covered with petroleum jelly to keep them from readhering.

Next, the meatus is examined; it should be carefully checked for ulceration, a condition much more common in circumcised children than in uncircumcised ones of diaper age. The ulceration itself is usually not a major problem but may result in stricture which can, if it leads to a small pinpoint meatus, cause urinary obstructive symptoms and will significantly increase the possibility of acute pyelonephritis. The stricture may initially be manifested by frequency, dysuria, and possibly by enuresis. The meatus should also be palpated; a papilloma or benign tumor may at times be found immediately inside it. Urethritis of the meatus results in the edges being erythematous, swollen, and everted. Micturition and erection may be painful, and the nearby lymph nodes will be tender and swollen. If this condition is accompanied by conjunctivitis and arthritis, it forms a triad of symptoms called *Reiter's syndrome. Morgagni's folliculitis* is another condition of this area. These follicles are located just inside the meatal lips, and when infected, the openings will enlarge and a puslike drainage will be seen.

The position of the meatus is also important; normally the meatus is centered at the tip of the shaft (see Fig. 13-2). If the opening is found on the dorsal shaft, it is called *epispadias.* This is a rarer condition than hypospadias and is usually associated with extrophy of the urinary bladder. There are three types of epispadias, depending on the exact position of the meatus; when it is located on the glans, it is called *balanic epispadias*; when on the shaft, it is called *penile epispadias*; and if it is not on the penis at all, but directly below the symphysis, it is called a *penopubic epispadias.* All types should be referred to a physician.

Hypospadias refers to the location of the meatal opening on the ventral surface of the penis. It is often associated with fibrotic chordee which restrict the penis on erection, causing a downward curvature. Again, there are three types. *Balanic hypospadias* or glandular type is located at the base of the glans. It is usually asymptomatic and no treatment is necessary unless the opening is too narrow, in which case a meatotomy is indicated. In *penile hypospadias* the meatus is found somewhere between the glans and the scrotum. As in epispadias, this type is often associated with chordee, as well as a flattened glans and an absent ventral foreskin. Surgical correction is

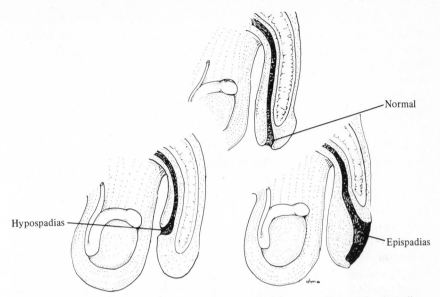

Normal

Hypospadias

Epispadias

Figure 13-2 Three types of meatal openings: normal, hypospadias, and epispadias.

usually begun at about 4 years of age. A child with this condition should definitely not be circumcised, since the foreskin will be needed in the later operation. The final type is called *penoscrotal* (perineal) *hypospadias.* In this type the meatus is located at the penoscrotal junction and often associated with a bifid scrotum. The penis is usually small and the meatus large; the testes are often undescended in such situations. A thorough investigation into the possibility of hermaphroditism is indicated. The incidence of hypospadias is 1 in 500.

A thorough inspection of the meatus should also include an evaluation of its size. The difficulty of a pinpoint meatus has been discussed previously. Usually this is due to stricture, but it can be congenital. Actual meatal atresia is usually due to an obstruction caused by a thin membrane. Deeper obstructions may also cause failure to void. All nurses working with newborns are aware of the importance of observing the neonate for first voiding.

Next in the examination of the genitalia is the glans. Venereal warts (*condyloma acuminatum*) are a possible finding in this area. They appear as pointed projections, either singly or in groups, often extending to the anus. These are frequently a site of secondary infection. *Condyloma latum* is a symptom of secondary syphilis and appears flat and wartlike. *Erosive balanitis* is an infection sometimes found on the glans in which the superficial skin appears eroded where small ulcers form and coalesce. The etiology of this infection is unknown.

The shaft of the penis must also be examined. Acute urethritis may cause palpable, long cords extending the length of the penis; a cord palpable only at one point in the shaft may indicate stricture. Visible swelling associated with a soft midline mass in the penoscrotal juncture may indicate an underlying diverticulum. A *periurethral abscess* is another condition of the penile shaft. In this situation, pus will accumulate in the middle of the shaft in Littre's follicle and will be palpable. Inflammation of the glans, which spreads and results in a palpable cord about 1 mm in diameter in the midline area of the shaft, may be an indication of dorsal vein thrombosis. The shaft should also be inspected for varicosities as well as for cavernositis (a palpable hard irregular mass in the lateral or ventral shaft). This condition can be from thrombosis, leukemia, septicemia, trauma, or infection. It is accompanied by inflammation and often by priapism and edema. Drainage may appear through the skin or urethra. *Priapism* is another possible abnormality of the shaft, although again, it is very rarely found in this age group. This is the condition of continuous erection without sexual desire. It is quite painful and may have either a local or central nervous system etiology. If of central nervous system in origin, the cause is usually lesions in the spinal cord or cerebrum. Local causes include neoplasms, inflammation, hemorrhage, and thrombosis. It is often associated with leukemia and sickle-cell anemia. This must not be confused with the transitory erections of infancy, which are completely normal. The size of the penile shaft must also be evaluated. Penile hypoplasia (*microphallus*) is a possibility. The nonerect length of the infantile penis is about 2 to 3 cm at birth. A penis smaller than this should not be worrisome unless there is a possibility that it is actually an enlarged clitoris rather than a small penis. In any situation of such ambiguity, the possibility of hermaphroditism must be thoroughly explored. A penis which remains infantile in size at adolescence may be an indication of hormonal abnormalities.

Penile hyperplasia (*megalopenis*) usually does not appear until 1 year of age. Possible causes of this condition are a tumor of the pineal body, a tumor of the hypothalamus, or a tumor of the adrenal glands.

The scrotum and its contents are the second major area of examination. The scrotal wall must be carefully checked for edema such as occurs in nephrosis, local inflammation, or portal vein obstruction and for purpura such as occurs in Schoenlein's disease. Sebaceous cysts will frequently be found in this area and are considered normal. Gangrene is a possibility, particularly when acute urethritis may have resulted in extravasation of urine. This is also a possible site for neoplasms. The color is important. Red, shiny skin may indicate an underlying orchitis. A very dark scrotum, particularly in a child of light-skinned race, may indicate adrenal hyperplasia. It is also important to note rugae. Well-formed rugae usually indicate that the testes have descended at some time even though they may not be palpable at the time of the examination. The normal scrotal contour in the neonate is quite variable. Scrotal skin may be tight and small or loose and hanging. During infancy, the proximal end is widest; the opposite is true after the hormonal influence of adolescence.

Most important of the scrotal contents are the testes. Except in premature infants, the testes should be descended by birth. As previously mentioned, it is wise to palpate for the testes at the very beginning of the genital examination; this lessens the chance of activating the cremasteric reflex by exposing the infant to cold or the older child to embarrassment. Before palpating for them, the inguinal canals should be blocked by the examiner's index finger (see Fig. 13-3). It is extremely important to palpate the testes at each visit. This is even more important if there is a question of undescended testes. The term *undescended* refers only to testes which have never descended. Once you are assured that they have been felt at any time in the boy's life, there will no longer be a need to consider surgery. Accurate recording is extremely important because of this. If there is a question of undescended testes, the examiner should attempt to palpate them with the child in a supine and standing position. If neither of these positions is helpful, the child should be asked to sit in a chair with knees flexed against the chest and feet placed on the seat of the chair. This usually forces the testes down. Heat also influences their descent, and an examination in a warm tub of water may be necessary. Because there is disagreement as to when surgical intervention is indicated, the nurse must find out at what age the physicians in the community would like boys referred for undescended

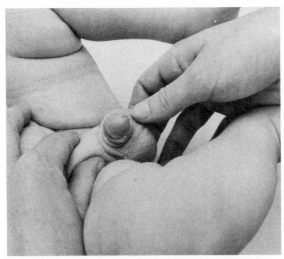

Figure 13-3 Procedure for blocking the inguinal canal when examining the scrotal contents.

testes. If they are not palpable in the scrotum, the examiner should palpate the femoral, inguinal, perineal, and abdominal areas to see if they are palpable in these areas. About one-half of the cases of undescended testes at birth will descend by the end of the first month, and one-fourth by the end of the first year.[1] The normal length of the testes at birth is 1.5 to 2.0 cm. The size remains constant until about 11 years of age. Between the ages of 11 and 18, the size increases to about 3.5 to 5.0 cm. Abnormal enlargement may occur in certain boys with neurogenic or idiopathic sexual precocity; it can also occur from a testicular tumor, but in such cases only one testes will enlarge. Testes will be small in *Klinefelter's syndrome,* in *hypopituitarism,* or in *adrenal hyperplasia.* If both are undescended, the examiner should consider the possibility of *intersex.*

Another important structure in the scrotum is the epididymis. This can be palpated as a vertical ridge of soft nodular tissue extending from the superior testicular pole to the inferior testicular pole, usually behind the testis, but in front of them in 7 percent of boys (a normal condition known as anteversion of the epididymis). The examiner must compare both for size and consistency. A mass may be palpated in some epididymides; this may indicate a *spermatocele* or *retention cyst.* In such a case the mass can be transilluminated. A mass may also fail to transilluminate and appear opaque; the possibility of neoplasm should always be considered in this situation. Nodularity of the epididymis may be a result of syphilis and is palpable though not painful. Hard nodules adherent to the scotum also may be a result of tuberculosis. Another possible finding is acute *epididymitis,* usually resulting from trauma or an adjacent infection. This condition is painful and tender and is associated with fever and an increase in the number of white blood cells.

The spermatic cord should be palpated in the scrotal sac. Both sides should be felt simultaneously and compared. The vas deferens should be felt as a hard distinct cord, while the more ambiguous cords are nerves, arteries, and fibers of the cremasteric muscle. These cords should be traced with the fingers to their origin in the testes. A thickening of the vas deferens may be due to inflammation. This may be from syphilis or tuberculosis or may be an extension of any nearby infection. If the inflammation is chronic, nodular formations may be felt. *Hydrocele* of the cord will be palpable as a sausage-shaped, smooth bulge above the testes which can be transilluminated. *Hematoma* of the cord, on the other hand, is opaque and feels like a boggy mass in the same area. Usually it is associated with a history of trauma and often other signs of trauma of the scrotal skin. *Gumma* or *granuloma* is a tertiary sign of syphilis. It also appears as an opaque mass when transilluminated. It is nontender, and if it extends to the testes, they will lose their sensitivity to pain. These are very rare in the pediatric age

[1] C.B. Scorer, "A Treatment of Undescended Testicles in Infancy," *Archives of Diseases of Childhood,* vol. 32, p. 520, 1957.

group. Neoplasms are indistinguishable from gumma and can be either benign or malignant. Torsion of the cord is a painful emergency occasionally encountered in children. This is the condition in which the spermatic cord becomes twisted, resulting in edema and congestion and a tender, irregular, swollen mass. At times the examiner will actually be able to feel the twist of the cord and will notice that the testis on the affected side is a great deal higher than the other side. The leg on the involved side is usually flexed to alleviate the pain. A similar condition is epididymitis which is less of an emergency. Palpation will determine an enlarged epididymis posterior to the testis; it is thickened or nodular and elevation of the scrotum for an hour or so usually relieves it.

Generalized masses in the scrotal sac will also be encountered occasionally. One such mass may be a *scrotal hydrocele.* In a scrotal hydrocele, transillumination will show the testes and epididymis as shadows behind the transilluminated mass. The external inguinal ring should be examined. A very large ring associated with a communicating hydrocele (one that continues from the testes into the abdomen) is reason for referral. If it is communicating, it will be slightly larger at night after the child has been on his feet all day, and frequently a hernia will be associated with it. Treatment is usually indicated only if a communicating hydrocele contains a hernia or if a noncommunicating one is extremely large and lasts for many months.

Hematoceles are very similar to hydroceles, except that they are filled with blood rather than with clear fluid, and for this reason, do not transilluminate. They are usually associated with a history of trauma and are often accompanied by other signs of trauma. *Chylocele* is a mass very similar to hydrocele, except that the fluid that fills the sac is lymph. Like a hydrocele it will transilluminate. This condition is unusual in this country and is usually a result of filariasis.

A *varicocele* is a scrotal sac filled not with fluid but with multiple varicose veins. Palpation reveals a sensation often said to be similar to a bag of worms. Most often this condition is more prominent on the left side and felt only when the patient is standing up. Such a condition should lead the examiner to suspect an obstruction above the scrotal sac. Surgeons will operate on these to prevent any chance of bowel herniation.

A malignant condition located in the scrotum may also appear as a mass; in this situation the mass will appear hard, opaque, and usually nontender. More often this type of malignant mass does not appear until after puberty.

Orchitis is another problem found in this area; usually, it is a sequela of mumps, but sometimes it is a result of other infections. In orchitis there is an acute, tender, painful hydrocele and erythematous scrotal skin.

Hernias are an important finding and can be abdominal or inguinal. For purposes of clarity both types are considered in the chapter, "The Abdomen."

Regional lymph nodes may be an important manifestation of disease of the genitalia. Both femoral and inguinal nodes must be palpated. Many individuals, however, have chronic, painless nodes in these areas which are usually insignificant, and are a residual of previous infections such as diaper rash.

BIBLIOGRAPHY

Alexander, Mary M., and Marie S. Brown: "Physical Examination: Male Genitalia," *Nursing '76,* vol. 6, no. 2, pp. 39–43, February 1976.

Gott, Laurence J.: "Common Scrotal Pathology," *American Family Physician,* vol. 15, no. 5, pp. 165–173, May 1977.

GLOSSARY

balanic epispadias the condition in which the urinary meatus is malpositioned dorsally on the glans penis

balanic hypospadias the condition in which the urinary meatus is malpositioned ventrally at the base of the glans penis

balanoposthitis a condition of local infection of the penis

bulbourethral glands (Cowper's glands) the two pea-sized masses lying along the urethra which produce secretions to neutralize the acidity of the urethra and vagina, which might damage semen

corona glandis the border of the glans penis

corpora cavernosa the two cylindrical masses that form the major portion of the shaft of the penis and which are composed of strong erectile tissue and many fibrous columns

corpus spongiosum the medial cylinder of the penis which contains the urethra

cremasteric reflex a reflexive withdrawal of the testes into the abdomen when the individual is stimulated by cold, emotion, or stroking of the inner thighs

epididymis a long, thin mass along the lateral edge of the posterior border of the testes which constitutes the first part of the excretory duct of each testis

frenulum a fold of skin extending from the meatus to the neck of the penis

glans penis the anterior end of the corpus spongiosum, which forms a rounded balloon-shaped structure

hematocele a generalized scrotal mass consisting of blood

meatus the opening in the corpus spongiosum to allow excretion of urine

megalopenis hyperplasia of the penis

microphallus hypoplasia of the penis

Morgagni's folliculitis the condition in which the follicles located just inside the meatal lips are infected

paraphimosis the condition in which the foreskin is permanently retracted behind the corona of the glans and cannot be slipped forward

penile epispadias the condition in which the meatus is malpositioned dorsally on the penile shaft

penile hypospadias the condition in which the urinary meatus is malpositioned ventrally between the glans and the scrotum

penile shaft the main body of the penis, composed of one corpus spongiosum and two corpora cavernosa

penopubic epispadias a condition in which the urinary meatus is malpositioned dorsally directly below the symphysis

penoscrotal (perineal) hypospadias the condition in which the urinary meatus is malpositioned ventrally at the perineum

phimosis a narrowing of the tip of the foreskin in such a way that it can no longer be slipped back over the shaft of the penis

prepuce (foreskin) the fold of skin at the neck of the penis

preputial calculus hard gritty material found in the prepuce, sometimes passed from the bladder, but more often formed by an accumulation of solidified dirt and smegma caught beneath a phimosis

priapism a condition of continuous erection without sexual desire

Reiter's syndrome a triad of conjunctivitis, arthritis, and urethritis

retroglandular sulcus the proximal end of the corona glandis which forms the neck of the penis

scrotal hydrocele a generalized scrotal mass consisting of clear fluid

scrotum the pendulous sac containing the testes and their excretory apparatus

spermatic cord the cord extending from the testes to the deep inguinal ring

testes the two smooth olive-shaped masses that produce sperm and are located in the scrotal sac

variocele a generalized scrotal mass filled not with fluid but with multiple varicose veins

Inspection of the Male Genitalia*

Hair	Yes	No	Not appli-cable	Describe (where appropriate)	Significance
1. Stage I[†]					May indicate delayed puberty if inappropriate for age.
2. Stage II					May indicate delayed or premature puberty if inappropriate for age.
3. Stage III					Same as above.
4. Stage IV					Same as above.
5. Straight					Thought to indicate lack of mature sperm production.
6. Curly					Thought to indicate onset of mature sperm production.
7. Diamond shape distribution					Normal male distribution; if replaced by the female diamond it may indicate hormonal problems; if generalized hirsutism, it may indicate adrenal problems.
Penis					
A. Skin 1. Normal color					Color expected to darken with puberty; if darker than normal, may indicate adrenal problems.
2. Lesions					Same significance as elsewhere, but more likely to be from venereal disease.
3. Other					
B. Foreskin 1. Present					Present if circumcision not done or poorly done.

254

2. Retractable			If it is forcibly retracted, it may be retractable from birth; if allowed to retract normally, may not be totally retractable until 4–5 years; can grow adherent without good hygiene.
3. Lesions			Same significance as elsewhere.
4. Color a. normal			Expected to darken with puberty; otherwise may indicate adrenal problems.
b. darkened			Darker in Mexican-American and black children.
c. erythematous			Irritation often secondary to infection.
5. Rash			Same significance as elsewhere.
6. Other			
C. Glands 1. Lesions			Same significance as elsewhere, but more likely to be venereal in origin.
2. Normal color			Same significance as color of penile shaft.
3. Other			
D. Corona 1. Lesions			Same significance as elsewhere, more likely to be veneral in origin.
2. Normal color			Same significance as penile shaft.

*These charts are meant to be used by beginning students as they perform their first physical assessments. Each item should be examined on the child and then checked off on the checklist. The significance of the items follows in the right-hand column.

†Stage I   No change is seen in the penis, testes, or scrotal area, and pubic hair is not present
Stage II   Light colored, soft pubic hair appears at the penile base, and the penis and testes become enlarged
Stage III Dark, coarse pubic hair begins to replace the soft, childish hairs, and the penis lengthens
Stage IV Coarse, pigmented pubic hair resembles the adult pubic hair but covers a smaller area, and the testes and penis increase in size
Stage V   Pubic hair, testes, and penis resemble the adult genitalia in size, shape, and texture

255

Inspection of the Male Genitalia (*Continued*)

Penis	Yes	No	Not applicable	Describe (where appropriate)	Significance
E. Urinary meatus					
1. Position					
a. hypospadias					If it extends beyond the glans, will need surgical correction; make sure child is not circumcized since this skin will be needed in surgical correction.
b. epispadias					Will need surgical correction; often associated with extrophy of the bladder.
c. midline					Normal.
2. Discharge					Infection.
3. Erythema					Irritation, often secondary to infection.
4. Inflammation					Infection.
F. Penile shaft					
1. Enlarged					May be secondary to a tumor of the pineal body, a tumor of the hypothalamus, or a tumor of the adrenals.
2. Size normal for age					
3. Size small for age					If this continues through adolescence, it may reflect hormonal problems; if during infancy, investigate to make sure that it is not an enlarged clitoris rather than a small penis.
4. Erections					Normal unless continuous and painful (priapism).
5. Other					

256

G. Scrotum

					Significance
1. Skin color					
a. normal					
b. erythematous					Irritated, sometimes from infection, sometimes in infants from diaper rash.
c. darkened					May indicate adrenal problems.
d. other					
2. Lesions					Same significance as elsewhere.
3. Rugae present					Usually indicates that testes have at some time been in the scrotum; helpful in ruling out undescended testes.
4. Visible bulging					May indicate tumor, hydrocele, hematocele, spermatocele, or varicocele.

Palpation of the Male Genitalia

Hair	Yes	No	Not appli-cable	Describe (where appropriate)	Significance
A. Normal texture					Same significance as elsewhere.
B. Other					
Penis					
A. Normal texture					
B. Palpable nodules, cysts, or other masses					Same significance as elsewhere.
C. Other					

Palpation of the Male Genitalia (*Continued*)

Scrotum and contents	Yes	No	Not appli-cable	Describe (where appropriate)	Significance
A. Scrotum					
1. Normal texture					Same significance as elsewhere.
2. Palpable nodules, cysts, or other masses					
3. Other					
B. Testes					
1. Present bilaterally					If undescended during examination, ascertain if they have ever been descended; if so, there is no concern; if neither has descended by 1 year, a consultation is necessary. If neither descend, they must be brought down before puberty. Opinion differs on the best time or method. If one is descended, fertility is assured, but the undescended testis is at high risk for cancer.
2. Size normal for age					Testes will be small in Klinefelter's syndrome, hypopituitarism, or adrenal hyperplasia; may be large in neurogenic or idiopathic sexual precocity.
3. Normal shape					Same significance as penile shaft.
4. Normal consistency					Abnormal fluctuant consistency may indicate hydrocele or hematocele; bag of worms feeling may indicate varicocele.
5. Tenderness					May occur with trauma or infection.
6. Right testis higher than left					Normally expected.
7. Other					

C. Palpable intrascrotol masses		
1. Hydrocele		Common in newborns; usually resolves by itself.
2. Hematocele		Same as above.
3. Chylocele		Unusual in this country; usually indicates filiarisis.
4. Varicocele		Multiple varicose veins; leads to high index of suspicion of some vascular obstruction proximal to the scrotum.
5. Solid mass		May be benign or malignant.
D. Epididymis		
1. Bilaterally posterior to testes		Usually posterior, but 7 percent of normal boys have anteversion, that is, the epididymis is in front—a normal variant.
2. Spermatocele		Accumulation of sperm within the epididymis.
3. Other masses		May be nodular and indicative of syphilis, or hard and indicative of benign or malignant growth.
4. Tender		May indicate epididymitis from trauma or infection.
5. Other		
E. Spermatic cord		
1. Palpable vas deferens (normal consistency)		Vas is expected to be palpable but may be enlarged due to infection.
2. Palpable nerves, vessels, etc.		Should normally be palpable but less distinct than the vas.
3. Hydrocele		Same significance as in scrotum.
4. Hematoma		Same significance as in scrotum.
5. Other mass		Possibility of malignancy should be considered.
6. Tenderness		May indicate trauma or infection.
7. Twisted cord		An acute emergency, very painful.

Palpation of the Male Genitalia (*Continued*)

Scrotum and contents	Yes	No	Not applicable	Describe (where appropriate)	Significance
F. Inguinal canal 1. Size a. enlarged					Usually a normal variant, but may be accompanied by hydrocele and hernia.
b. normal					
c. bulges					May indicate direct or indirect hernia; check to see if it is reducible.
d. other					

Source: These checklists are printed with permission from Blue Hill Videotape Incorporated and are part of a more complete programmed learning approach to the physical examination, which includes a workbook and series of videotapes. The materials can be purchased from Blue Hill Educational Systems, Inc., 52 South Main Street, Spring Valley, New York 10977.

Chapter 14

The Female Genitalia

WHY THE CHILD IS EXAMINED

The genitalia are an important part of the physical examination of girls as well as of boys. In the infant, it is most important that the genitalia be judged to be unambiguous; any question in this regard should be fully investigated before the child is any older. In the toddler or preschool girl, this part of the examination remains an important one, not only in checking for abnormalities, but in providing an excellent opportunity for discussing questions of bodily acceptance and sexuality both for the parents and the child. In the adolescent girl, especially, this part of the examination can be a chance for important counseling in the areas of human sexuality and body image. It is also important baseline data for contraceptive counseling.

WHAT TO EXAMINE: ANATOMY OF THE AREA

For purposes of study the female genitalia can be divided into the internal and external structures. The internal structures include the ovaries, uterine

261

tube, uterus, and vagina, all of which are contained within the pelvis (see Fig. 14-1); the external structures are the mons pubis, labia majora, labia minora, clitoris, bulbus vestibuli, and Bartholin's and Skene's glands (see Fig. 14-2). These are more easily inspected, since they are superficial urogenital structures. In young girls the examiner is concerned mostly with these external structures and the vagina. For a more detailed description of the anatomy of the internal structures the reader is referred to a good text book on obstetrics.

The external genital structures are sometimes referred to as the *vulva* or pudendum. The first of these, the *mons pubis,* is a pad of adipose tissue anteriorly surmounting the *symphysis pubis.* At *puberty,* the mons becomes covered with hair, the distribution of which forms an inverted triangle in the normal female. If it is diamond-shaped as in males, the examiner should be concerned about possible hormonal abnormalities. The base of this triangle is called *female escutcheon.*

The *labia majora* are two fatty folds running from the mons pubis posteriorly, containing fat, nerves, and blood vessels. The outer surface is pigmented and covered with thick, curly hairs while the inner surface is smooth, with many sebaceous follicles.

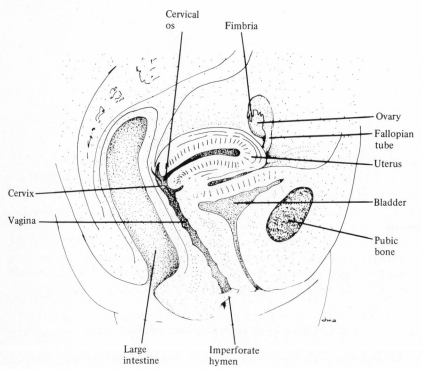

Figure 14-1 Internal female organs.

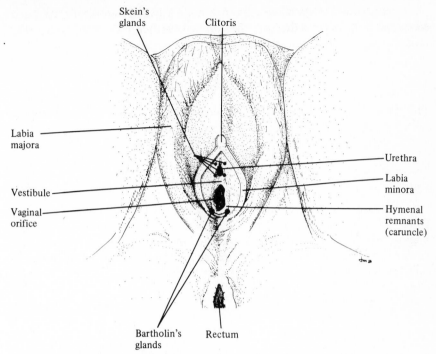

Figure 14-2 External female genitalia structures.

The *labia minora* are two smaller folds of tissue running parallel to the labia majora; their tissue ends about 4 cm from the vagina, and in the virgin the two labia minora are joined by a fold of skin called the *frenulum* (fourchette). The surface of the labia minora contains many sebaceous follicles.

The *clitoris* is an organ composed of erectile tissue and joins the labia minora anteriorly. Dense fibrous tissue covers the two corpora cavernosa which are surrounded by folds of the labia minora. These corpora cavernosa are the preputium clitoridis and the frenulum of the clitoris. The clitoris is an erectile homologue of the penis.

The *vestibule* is the cleft between the labia minora which contains the urethral and vaginal orifices. The urethral meatus is 2.5 cm posterior of the clitoris, and contains *Skene's glands,* which are homologues of the male prostatic gland. The vaginal orifice is immediately posterior to the meatus.

The *hymen* is a thin membrane covering part of the vaginal orifice. Although it is usually a perforated ring with the widest opening posteriorly, sometimes it is cribiform, fringed, or even imperforate. After rupture, only caruncles (small rounded bumps) remain.

The bulb of the vestibule is a 2.5-cm mass of erectile tissue located along both sides of the vaginal orifice.

The greater vestibular glands (*Bartholin's glands*) are small, rounded elevations on both sides of the vaginal orifice. They resemble the bulbourethral glands of the male.

HOW TO EXAMINE

The methods of examination for evaluating the female genitalia are inspection and palpation. Neither auscultation nor percussion has any usefulness in this area.

WHERE TO EXAMINE

The genitalia examination in the young girl should almost always be confined solely to the external genitalia. Seldom is an examination of the vagina, cervix, uterus, or adnexa indicated in prepubertal girls. In the case of the adolescent girl desiring contraceptives or a confirmation of pregnancy, an examination of the internal reproductive organs is obviously indicated.

WHAT TO EXAMINE WITH

For an examination of the external genitalia of infants and very young girls, no special equipment is required. If for some reason an examination of the internal genitalia is indicated, pediatric speculums and other specialized equipment are useful. In most instances, it will not be the nurse who does this kind of examination of a very young child. Because of the possibility of venereal disease, gloves are suggested.

WHAT TO EXAMINE FOR

All parts of the external genitalia are carefully inspected and palpated. The examination is begun with the mons pubis which in the very young child is inspected for any skin discolorations or abnormalities and palpated for any masses; in the older child, the appearance of hair and its distribution will be used as indicators of adequate hormonal functioning. At this point also, the possibility of pubic lice or crabs must be considered.

Proceeding posteriorly the labia majora are evaluated next. Again the skin is inspected, particularly for its integrity. At times ulcerations will be found. Usually these will be of nonspecific origin, but they should always be cultured. They can be a result of venereal disease, although this finding is more common in older children. *Chancres, chancroids, granuloma inguinales, lymphogranuloma venereum* and *herpes progenitalis* are all possible findings. These are discussed more completely in a good book on gynecology.

Vulvitis, another possible finding, is a condition in which the skin will be warm, erythematous, and swollen. The usual cause is an extension of some type of vaginitis with an accompanying irritating discharge. This may result from a trichomonal or gonorrheal infection or, less frequently, from a monilial or nonspecific infection. Vaginitis resulting from a foreign body should also be considered, particularly in preschool-age children.

The vulva should also be palpated and inspected for any masses. *Condyloma acuminatum* and *condyloma latum* may be present just as in males. Neoplasms should also be considered.

Swelling of the vulva may be a symptom of *lymphedema* resulting from an obstruction of the lymphatic system anywhere above the vulva, or, if large, painful, and bluish, may be a hematoma. Usually this will appear within a few hours after trauma. It should always be documented, particularly, of course, if there is any question of sexual molestation. A more localized swelling may result from a *labioinguinal hernia,* the homologue of a scrotal hernia in the male. Careful palpation will reveal whether this swelling communicates with the abdomen.

The vulva should be further examined for any areas of *cellulitis* or any suggestion of *varicosities.* Varicosities in a young child usually suggest a blockage of the circulatory system in any area above the varicosities. Possible causes of such blockage are tumors or enlarged organs which may be obstructing venous return.

Lichen sclerosus et atrophicus is a condition of the vulva in which the skin is white, thin, atrophied, wrinkled, and excoriated. It is usually accompanied by some pruritis. This is quite rare in premenarchal or young adolescent girls, however.

Next Bartholin's glands are inspected and palpated. Normally they are neither visible nor palpable. If they are palpable, enlargement exists and is almost always due to infection, usually gonorrhea.

Skene's glands are likewise not normally seen or felt. Again, Skene's glands which are large enough to be visible or palpable are abnormally enlarged, most often from acute or chronic gonorrhea, although sometimes from other infections.

The labia minora are the next structures to examine. They are normally quite large in the newborn and will frequently be seen protruding from the labia majora. This is even more obvious in premature infants. The edges may show a rather darkly pigmented border; this is to be considered normal in the young infant.

Adhesions are one of the most common difficulties in the infant and young child. Sometimes they are actually present from birth and appear as a transparent membrane which partially or totally occludes the vaginal orifice. Usually there are no symptoms although occasionally complaints of frequency and dysuria will be heard. Adhesions may also follow vulvovaginitis. This must be carefully distinguished from a thick sticky collection of smegma due to lack of hygiene. This frequently appears not because mothers are remiss in caring for their child, but because their own sexual inhibitions prevent them from handling the baby's genitals to any great extent.

Hypertrophy of the labia minor is fairly common and usually has no clinical significance. Some authors feel that it may at times be an indication of excessive masturbation, but this is not usually thought to be the case.

The clitoris also must be inspected closely, although, because of its sensitivity, it is not palpated unless there is definite indication to do so. The clitoris is normally large in newborns, but the examiner must evaluate its size carefully, since hypertrophy of the clitoris is its most common abnormality. When such hypertrophy exists, the clitoris should be thoroughly investigated. This is even more a possibility if there is an anterior displacement of the urethral meatus associated with the clitoral hypertrophy. Inflammation is uncommon but may present as cellulitis or abscess.

Hypoplasia of the clitoris, on the other hand, is exceedingly rare and has very little clinical significance although some authors have indicated the possibility that this may result later in an individual who has difficulty with sexual arousal. There is some question about this.

The vestibule should be examined next. Although it is the most common site of cancer in the elderly and is a fairly common site of granulomatous and ulcerative venereal lesions in older girls, there are generally very few physical findings in children of this age in this area.

The meatus is a very important area for examination in little girls. Any urethritis, indicated by inflammation, erythema, and discharge, should be cultured. Prolapse of the mucosa should also be sought for, and if found, the mother should be carefully questioned concerning a history of *hematuria, dysuria,* or other urinary symptoms. Position of the urethra is important in little girls, as well as in little boys. If epispadias is found, accompanied by a complete or partial midline division of mons and clitoris, the possibility of hermaphroditism must be fully investigated. Palpation is also important. *Urethral caruncles* may appear and be palpated as small red masses, visible just inside the meatus. They are tender and painful on urination and are a complication of urethritis. It is quite unusual to find them in this age group, however.

The final structures to be examined are the vaginal opening and hymen. Congenital absence of a vagina is a possible finding as is an imperforate hymen. In a small infant or young girl, this will not usually be apparent unless there is some type of fluid retained by the hymen. If the fluid is a collection of vaginal secretions, the condition is called *hydrocolpos* and may appear as a small midline lower abdominal mass or a small cystic movable mass between the labia. This condition may clear spontaneously or surgery may be needed. If the fluid retained by the hymen is blood, the condition is called *hematocolpos* and the mass will usually be suprapubic. The hymen may be bluish and bulging, and there may be associated lower abdominal pain. This condition may occur either in the newborn who has absorbed enough hormones from her mother to set up a small pseudomenstruation or in the adolescent who is actually menstruating. In the newborn, the blood will gradually be reabsorbed if the pressure does not rupture the membrane. In the adolescent, the condition is more serious, mostly because the amount of blood is greater. A back pressure is generated, resulting eventually in cervical dilation. The blood then backs up to the uterus and tubes, making the girl strongly susceptible to infection. Bladder pressure, dysuria, frequency, urinary retention, *amenorrhea,* and lower abdominal pain are accompanying symptoms in the adolescent. If not corrected, the condition may lead to sterility.

Sarcoma botryoides is another unusual but possible finding in the vaginal area. This growth is a grapelike, fleshy group of tissue masses originating beneath the vaginal epithelium. It is extremely malignant and any suspicion of it requires immediate referral.

Vaginal discharge is the final subject to be discussed in the physical examination of the vagina of little girls. A small amount of bloody discharge is normal, though uncommon, in newborns up to 1 month of age. It results from the absorption of hormones from the mother during pregnancy. Newborns may also exhibit mucoid discharge which is generally also normal. Foul discharge in older children can be due to a foreign body in the vagina, tight pants, pinworms, masturbation, or infection. It should be fully investigated.

In the adolescent girl seeking oral or intrauterine contraceptive devices, a speculum or bimanual examination of the internal genitalia is also necessary. This examination can be very traumatic for a young girl, and a good explanation and gentle procedures are essential. The girl should fully understand the procedure before the examination is begun, and detailed explanations of what sensations she should expect should be given at each stage of the process. The girl is first helped to put her feet into the stirrups of the gynecological table. (A few examiners are comfortable in doing this exam with the girl's feet flat on the table flush against her buttocks. This is a more comfortable position for the girl, but requires greater skill on the part of the examiner.) She is then asked to slide down until her buttocks are extending about 1 in over the edge of the table. The examiner then warns her that she will be feeling two fingers inserted into her vagina—this creates the sensation of pressure, but not pain. The lower vaginal wall is then pushed downward in such a way that the vaginal opening is enlarged for the speculum insertion. The fingers at this time are inserted as far as the cervix and remain in place, if possible, while the speculum is inserted above them. They serve to cushion the speculum insertion. Enlarging it in this way prior to insertion of the speculum avoids much of the pain and tissue trauma often associated with this insertion. After telling the girl the speculum is to be inserted, the insertion is begun at an oblique angle (inserting the speculum horizontally is unnecessarily painful and inserting it vertically can traumatize the urethra). After it is inserted a few centimeters, it is gently turned to a horizontal position and pushed back (still in the closed position) until it is at the level of the cervix. At this time the girl is told that she will feel some more pressure and it is gently opened so that the cervix is visible. The cervix should appear pink and smooth without erythema or nodules. The os of the nullipara should be small and smooth. A bluish tint to the cervix may indicate an early pregnancy; an os which is surrounded by *eversion* (i.e., the mucous membrane from inside the os is everted resulting in a darker color red surrounding the os) may be present, particularly if the girl has been pregnant previously. *Erosion* (i.e., where the cervical epithelium is debrided from some kind of friction, occasionally by frequent intercourse or frequent vaginal infections) may be present although it is more common in older women. *Nabothian cysts* (slightly bluish tinged cystic protrusions) may be present, although again they are more common in older women. Any discharge must be carefully evaluated. Normal discharge should be creamy white; the consistency varies somewhat with the part of the menstrual cycle. Thick, curdlike white discharge accompanied by severe pruritis and plaques on the cervix of the vaginal wall usually indicates monilia (or candida) infection. (The same organism causes oral thrush and the plaques look very similar to oral thrush.) Greenish, foul-smelling discharge accompanied by erythematous mucosa, sometimes with bright red pinpoints usually indicates a trichomonas infection. Greyish discharge may indicate a nonspecific infection or a haemophilus infection. Thick yellow discharge, particularly accompanied by severe pain on examination may indicate a gonococcal infection. All suspicions of infection processes should be confirmed by culture.

After a thorough inspection of the cervix and cervical os, the speculum is withdrawn slowly while the examiner inspects the vaginal wall. Again it should be smooth and pink.

Palpation is the next part of the examination of the internal genitalia. It is begun by inserting the index and middle finger of the right hand gently into the vagina, feeling carefully for any irregularities to the vaginal walls. These fingers then palpate the cervix and cervical os, again noting any palpable hardness or irregularities. These two fingers are then left in place but the hand is turned palm upward while the left hand is used to palpate the uterus and annexa abdominally. While the right hand balances the uterus, the left hand palpates it for position, mobility, size, consistency, and lesions. All surfaces should be carefully felt. Most uteruses are anteverted and anteflexed (i.e., they bend forward at the cervix toward the abdominal wall and flex downward at the junction of the cervix and the uterine body). However, retroverted and retroflexed uteruses are also normal. They may be more difficult to palpate until the rectal exam is performed, however.

The normal uterus should be freely movable. Any restriction of movement should make the examiner suspicious of adhesions and should be carefully investigated.

Sizing of a uterus is extremely important, particularly if contraceptives are to be prescribed. To prescribe contraceptives to a girl who is already pregnant could cause serious harm to the fetus. Any questions of a beginning pregnancy should be thoroughly investigated. A pregnancy test and good menstrual history are also necessary before contraceptive prescriptions.

The consistency of the normal uterus should be quite firm. Any bogginess, particularly with a history of abortion, is worrisome and should be investigated. Lesions or irregularities in surface contour are never normal and demand a further workup.

Next, each ovary and fallopian tube is palpated. Tubes are not usually palpable, and if one is felt, abnormality is suspected. Ovaries are sometimes, but not always palpable. The absence of a palpable ovary is not worrisome, but the nurse must become skillful enough to recognize an enlarged one. They should be no larger than an olive. Palpation of these organs may involve some transient pain and the girl should be warned of this ahead of time. This palpation requires that the vaginal fingers be placed lateral to the cervix and pushed in an upward direction while the abdominal hand is pushed inward and downward in a sweeping movement so that the ovary, if palpable, will be caught between the fingers of the two hands. This is done bilaterally. Ovaries should be palpated for possible enlargement. Their surfaces should be smooth and any irregularities require further workup.

The vaginal fingers are then removed and the index figure is reinserted into the vagina at the same time that the middle finger is inserted into the anus. For many girls, this is the most uncomfortable part of the exam and they should be warned beforehand that it will involve a sensation of pressure and many will feel that they are having an involuntary bowel movement. Often this embarrassment is the worst part of the exam. Once the fingers are inserted, the posterior vaginal wall should be between them; this makes very thorough bimanual palpation possible. Any irregularities here should be considered abnormal until proven otherwise. Finally, the finger in the vagina is removed and palpation by the finger in the anus is continued first by palpating all walls of the anus for any lesions or irregularities and then by palpating the posterior wall of the uterus. This can often (particularly in the case of the retroverted or retroflexed uterus) be done more thoroughly through the rectal wall than in the previous vaginal-abdominal palpation. Again, the uterus is checked for position, mobility, size, consistency, and lesions.

BIBLIOGRAPHY

Brown, Marie S., and Mary M. Alexander: "Physical Examination: Female Genitalia," *Nursing '76,* vol. 6, no. 3, pp. 39–41, March 1976.

GLOSSARY

amenorrhea   absence of menstruation

Bartholin's glands   the two small mucous glands situated on either side of the posterior wall of the vaginal opening

chancre   an ulcer of primary syphilis appearing on mucous membrane, usually in the genital area

chancroid   a highly infectious nonsyphilitic genital ulcer

clitoris   an organ composed of erectile tissue which joins the labia minora anteriorly; considered the erectile homologue of the male penis

condyloma acuminatum   a pointed wartlike nonsyphilitic projection of the genital area

condyloma latum   a flat, wartlike syphilitic lesion of the genital area

dysuria   difficulty or pain on urination

escutcheon   the base of the triangular hair formation on the female pubic area

hematocolpos   the condition in which blood is retained by an imperforate hymen, resulting in distention of the internal genitalia

hematuria   blood in the urine

herpes progenitalis   a herpetic disease of the genital region

hydocolpos   a condition in which vaginal secretions are retained by an imperforate hymen, resulting in distention of the internal genitalia

hymen   a thin membrane covering part of the vaginal orifice

labia majora   two fatty ridges running from the mons pubis posteriorly

labia minora   the two small folds of tissue running parallel to the labia majora, extending about 4 cm into the vagina

labioinguinal hernia   a herniation of the abdominal contents into the labioinguinal area, the female homologue of the scrotal hernia

lymphogranuloma venereum   a viral venereal disease

puberty   period of development when the individual becomes capable of reproduction

sarcoma botryoides   a grapelike fleshy group of tissue masses originating beneath the vaginal epithelium

Skene's glands   tiny glands whose openings are just inside the urinary meatus in the female

urethral caruncles small red masses visible just inside the meatus

vestibule the cleft between the labia minora which contains the urethral and vaginal openings

vulvitis inflammation of the vulva

Inspection of the Female Genitalia*

Hair	Yes	No	Not appli-cable	Describe (where appropriate)	Significance
1. Straight					Straight hair may indicate lack of mature egg formation (this is not fully proven).
2. Curly					Curly hair may indicate onset of mature egg formation.
3. Diamond distribution					Normal male distribution; in a female may indicate endocrine or liver pathology.
4. Triangle distribution					Normal female distribution.
5. Stage I*					If inappropriate for age, may indicate delayed puberty.
6. Stage II					If inappropriate for age, may indicate delayed or early puberty.
7. Stage III					Same as above.
8. Stage IV					Same as above.
9. Pubic lice					Need treatment and education.
10. Other					
Labia majora					
1. Color a. normal					
b. erythematous					May indicate local infection or irritation from vaginal infection.
c. darkened					May indicate adrenocortical pathology.
2. Lesions					Same significance as elsewhere, may also have lesions of venereal disease, chancres, etc.
3. Rash					

272

4. Swelling			May be from trauma, lymphedema, labio inguinal hernia.
5. Masses			May be from venereal disease or benign or malignant problems.
6. Other			

Labia minora

1. Color a. normal			
b. erythematous			May be from local infection or irritation from drainage.
c. darkened			May indicate adrenocortical problems.
d. other			
2. Lesions			Same as with labia majora.
3. Rash			Same as with labia majora.
4. Swelling			Same as with labia majora.
5. Other			

Clitoris

1. Present			
2. Enlarged			Probably a variant of normal; occasionally is said to result from excessive masturbation, but this is controversial.
3. Extremely small			Probably a variant of normal; some feel it may contribute to sexual dysfunction in the adolescent or adult but this is highly controversial.

*These charts are meant to be used by beginning students as they perform their first physical assessments. Each item should be examined on the child and then checked off on the checklist. The significance of the items follows in the right-hand column.

273

Inspection of the Female Genitalia (*Continued*)

Vestibule	Yes	No	Not appli-cable	Describe (where appropriate)	Significance
1. Lesions					Same significance as on the other parts of the genitalia.
2. Rash					Same significance as on the other parts of the genitalia.
3. Other					
Skene's glands					
1. Visible					Visibility indicates enlargement usually due to infection.
2. Discharge					Infection.
3. Other					
Urinary meatus					
1. Erythematous					Irritation, possibly due to infection, trauma, or frequent rubbing such as may occur with excessive masturbation.
2. Discharge					Infection.
3. Other					
Urinary stream					
1. Straight					Normal.
2. Strong					Normal; dribbling may indicate obstruction or a small meatus.
3. Normal color					Very light colored urine may indicate lack of concentration due to diabetes insipidus, granular kidney, nervous conditions, or a high fluid intake. Very dark urine may indicate dehydration or febrile disease.

| | | | Milky urine may be present in chyluria or purulent infection. Orange urine may occur with such drugs as pydridine, santonin, or chrysophanic acid. Brown or black urine may indicate methehemoglobin uria with bile pigments excreted. Green-blue may occur with methylene blue medication or cholera or typhus. |
| 4. Normal odor | | | Musty odor may indicate phenylketonuria. Maple sugar smell occurs with maple sugar disease. Sweaty feet odor occurs with butyric/hexanoic acidemia or isovaleric acidemia. An odor of stale fish occurs with trimethylaminuria. A rancid butter smell accompanies hypermethioninemia. A brewery smell accompanies methionine malabsorption and oasthouse disease. |

Bartholin's glands

1. Visible			Visibility indicates enlargement and probably infection.
2. Erythematous			Infection, often gonnorhea.
3. Other			

Vaginal orifice

1. Patent			Cannot always be ascertained without a speculum exam.
2. Discharge			Postpuberty midcycle clear discharge is normal; otherwise, may indicate a variety of infections or foreign body.
3. Erythematous			Irritation, often secondary to infection or discharge.
4. Lesions			Same significance as elsewhere; likely to be venereal disease lesions.
5. Other			

Inspection of the Female Genitalia (Continued)

Hymenal ring	Yes	No	Not applicable	Describe (where appropriate)	Significance
1. Visible					Usually visible.
2. Perforate					Cannot always be ascertained without a speculum exam; if imperforate, may be cribiform or completely closed. If completely closed, may appear as a bluish painful bulge with first period; needs immediate referral to prevent damaging the reproductive tract because of back pressure.

Rectum	Yes	No	Not applicable	Describe (where appropriate)	Significance
1. Rash					Same significance as elsewhere; venereal lesions may occur with anal intercourse.
2. Lesions					Same as above.
3. Fissures					Must spread buttocks to see fissures; may be caused by hard stools; will often cause painful defecation and secondary constipation.

Palpation of the Female Genitalia

Hair	Yes	No	Not applicable	Describe (where appropriate)	Significance
1. Normal texture					Same significance as the hair on the head.
2. Other					

Labia majora

1. Skin and mucous membrane of normal texture			Same significance as elsewhere.
2. Palpable nodules, cysts, or masses			Same significance as elsewhere.
3. Other			

Labia minora

1. Mucous membrane of normal texture			Same significance as elsewhere.
2. Palpable nodules, cysts, or other masses			Same significance as elsewhere.
3. Other			

Clitoris (not palpated unless there is a specific indication)

1. Mucous membrane of normal texture			Same significance as elsewhere.
2. Palpable nodules, cysts, or other masses			Same significance as elsewhere.
3. Other			

Palpation of the Female Genitalia

Vestibule	Yes	No	Not appli- cable	Describe (where appropriate)	Significance
1. Normal texture					Same significance as elsewhere.
2. Palpable nodules, cysts, or other masses					Same significance as elsewhere.
3. Other					
Skene's glands					
1. Palpable					If palpable, they are enlarged, usually secondary to infection, often gonorrhea.
2. Normal texture					Same significance as elsewhere.
Urinary meatus					
1. Normal texture					Same significance as elsewhere.
2. Palpable nodes, cysts, or other masses.					Same significance as elsewhere.
Bartholin's glands					
1. Normal texture					Same significance as elsewhere.
2. Palpable					If palpable, they are enlarged, usually secondary to infection, most often to gonorrhea.

278

Vaginal orifice

1. Normal texture		Same significance as elsewhere.
2. Palpable nodes, cysts, or other masses		Same significance as elsewhere.

Hymenal ring

1. Normal texture		Same significance as elsewhere.
2. Palpable nodes, cysts, or other masses		Same significance as elsewhere.

Rectum

1. Normal texture		Same significance as elsewhere.
2. Palpable nodes, cysts, or other masses		Same significance as elsewhere.
3. Tight sphincter		Some feel this is a possible cause of painful defecations in infants, but this is controversial.

*Stage I Pubic area is covered with the same soft, fine hair as the rest of the body, and only the papilla of the breast shows slight elevation.

Stage II The area around the labia develops several long, pigmented hairs, and the breast papilla becomes slightly erect with some of the surrounding tissue becoming fuller.

Stage III There is development of additional long, pigmented, coarser hairs from the labia to the mons, and the breast areola and surrounding tissue show continued expansion.

Stage IV The pubic hair becomes darker, coarser, more curled and covers the labia and mons, while the subareolar and papilla area of the breat becomes distinct from the surrounding breast tissue.

Stage V The pubic hair becomes more adult-like in appearance and covers the general adult triangular pattern over the pubic area, and the breast shows the projecting papilla with areola and surrounding tissue rounded in contour.

Source: These checklists are printed with permission from Blue Hill Videotape Incorporated and are part of a more complete programmed learning approach to the physical examination, which includes a workbook and series of videotapes. The materials can be purchased from Blue Hill Educational Systems, Inc., 52 South Main Street, Spring Valley, New York 10977.

279

Chapter 15

The Rectum

WHY THE CHILD IS EXAMINED

The American culture places a good deal of emphasis on good health in the rectal area. Parents frequently worry about their child's bowel habits, if the child's hands are massaging the area, rectal itching, and any skin rashes or redness. Careful examination of this area is an important part of the physical examination.

WHAT TO EXAMINE: ANATOMY OF THE AREA

The rectum and anus are the terminal ends of the digestive system. The *rectum* comprises the last 10 to 14 cm of the sigmoid colon. The last 2 to 4 cm of the rectum (the part which leads to the outer surface) is called the *anal canal*; it terminates in the *anus* (opening). The canal is surrounded by layers of voluntary external muscles and internal involuntary muscles. The canal slants obliquely downward and backward.

280

The outer surfaces of the anus should be covered with smooth, folded skin, which may be slightly darker in pigment than the surrounding genital area.

HOW TO EXAMINE

This area is examined by inspection and palpation of the external surfaces. Internal palpation is not done routinely on children, but is done if the history and symptoms indicate its usefulness.

WHERE TO EXAMINE

The examination of the rectal area is generally included when doing the examination of the genital area. This is less embarrassing for the child and more efficient for the examiner.

WHAT TO EXAMINE WITH

No special equipment is necessary for this part of the examination. If an internal examination is needed, then a rubber glove (or finger cot) and lubrication must be used.

The child may be positioned on his back with the knees flexed and spread, on his side with his knees drawn toward his chest or standing with his back to the examiner and the torso bent forward. The examiner must be gentle but firm in the palpation. The *buttocks* should be pulled away from the midline for better visualization of the area.

WHAT TO EXAMINE FOR

The anus is inspected for any redness or signs of inflammation and irritation. The skin should be smooth with no scratch marks or rashes. As the buttocks are parted, anal *fissures* (small, slitlike cuts with raw edges) may become apparent. They are often accompanied by bleeding, a history of constipation, pain on bowel movements, and blood on diapers or panties.

Any protrusions from the anus should be inspected. The rectal mucosa, flat skin tags (*condylomas*), tiny mucosal tags, *polyps* (bright red protrusions), or rectal veins (*hemorrhoids*) may emerge through the anal opening.

The anus is palpated for sinuses, fistulas, abscesses, and strictures. Tone can be checked by lightly touching the anus and observing for anal contraction. Lack of this reaction may indicate lack of muscle tone due to low spinal cord injury (such as a myelomeningocele). Constipation or painful bowel movements may be caused by stenosis or tight sphincter tone.

If internal palpation is performed, a small finger should be gloved, lubricated and inserted through the anal opening and past the *rectoanal ring*. Palpation may reveal fistulas, strictures, masses, tenderness, any fecal matter and, in older children, some organs. The pubertal boy may have a small, palpable prostate and the pubertal girl can have a uterus and ovaries palpable to touch.

GLOSSARY

anal canal last 2 to 4 cm of rectum
anus terminal opening of anal canal
buttocks firm, rounded protruberance of the gluteal muscles
condylomas flat skin tags protruding from the rectum through the anus
fissures small, slitlike cuts with raw, and sometimes bloody, edges
hemorrhoids rectal veins protruding through the anus
polyps bright red protrusions through the anus
rectoanal ring firm, muscular layers at the rectal-anal junction
rectum lower, last 10 to 14 cm of the sigmoid colon

Chapter 16

The Skeletal System: Spine and Extremities

WHY THE CHILD IS EXAMINED

Because of its central function in giving structure to the soft tissues of the body, the health of the skeletal system is extremely important in maintaining the health of the individual. For this reason, a thorough examination of the skeletal system and its functioning is an important part of the examination of every child. Another reason is the fact that the skeletal system is frequently an area of many parental concerns, especially because there are several normal developmental conditions of the skeletal system (for instance, the slight bow-leggedness of the newborn or the knock-knees of the preschooler) which closely resemble pathologic conditions, and parents often worry about them. A third reason for this part of the examination is that there are many minor orthopedic abnormalities (for instance, subluxation of the hip in the newborn) which can be remedied rather easily in the newborn, but which will become major problems if not discovered early.

WHAT TO EXAMINE: ANATOMY OF THE AREA

The skeletal system is a bony structure held together by *ligaments,* attached to muscles by *tendons,* and cushioned by cartilage. In this section we will be primarily concerned with the bones themselves. There are 206 bones in the body, and they can be divided roughly into three categories. The first is the axial skeleton which comprises the vertebral column, the skull, the hyoid bone, the ribs, and the sternum—a total of 74 bones. The second major category is the appendicular skeleton which is made up of the 64 bones of the upper limbs and the 62 bones of the lower limbs. (The auditory ossicles total 6 bones and are usually considered separately.) This section will be primarily concerned with the appendicular skeleton, as well as the vertebral column. In discussing the anatomy, the upper extremities, lower extremities, and spine will be considered. In each of these areas the bones, muscles, and blood and nerve supply will be described. First, however, a general introduction to the joint system will be given.

Joints

Joints are classified as immovable, slightly movable, or freely movable. Immovable joints are found in the skull at the suture lines. Slightly movable joints and freely movable joints include most of the joints in the body and are classified by the kind of motion permitted. *Hinge joints* permit motion in one plane only; an example is the movement of the humerus and the ulna. *Pivot joints* allow rotation only; examples of pivot joints are the radioulnar articulations and the juncture of the atlas and axis vertebrae. *Condyloid joints* allow flexion, extension, adduction, abduction, and circumduction, but not axial rotation; the wrist is a joint of this type. *Saddle joints* are very similar to condyloid joints except that the adjacent surfaces form a concavoconvex fit; the carpometacarpal joint of the thumb is of this type. *Ball-and-socket joints* have a rounded head fitted into a deep concave cavity which allows motion around many different axes; the hip and shoulder joints are ball-and-socket joints. Finally, the *gliding joints* allow a gliding motion between two flat surfaces; the vertebral and carpal joints are gliding joints. Types of motion which can be produced by these joints are basically of only four types, but in combination, these movements produce a variety of actions (see Fig. 16-1).

Gliding movements, in which two surfaces slide past each other, are the simplest and most common. Angular movements increase or decrease the angle of the two bones. *Flexion* describes a decrease in the joint's angle; *extension* increases the joint's angle; *hyperextension* increases the angle beyond the usual arc. *Abduction* is movement away from the medial line of the body; *adduction* is movement towards the medial line of the body. *Circumduction* movement is a rotation of one bone around a stationary disk.

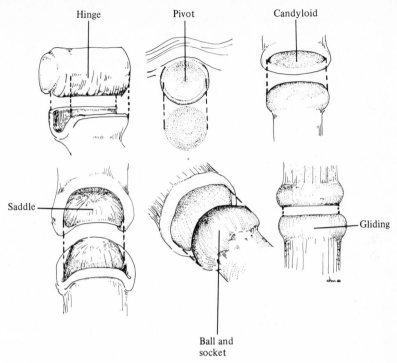

Figure 16-1 Types of skeletal joints.

Rotation movement is motion around a central axis, such as that seen when the radius rotates around the ulna during pronation.

Terms

It is also important for the nurse-examiner to know certain terms used in describing different positions of the extremities. *Supination* refers to the position of the hand in which the palmar surface faces upward, while *pronation* describes the position in which the palmar surface faces downward (see Fig. 16-2). *Inverted* refers to a "turning in" position, such as that seen in the feet of pigeon-toed children. *Eversion* is a term used to describe a situation in which an extremity, or part of an extremity such as the foot, turns outward.

The Upper Extremities

Discussion of the anatomy of the sections of the skeleton will begin with a description of the important bones, muscles, blood and nerve supply of the upper extremity (see Fig. 16-3). The bones of the upper extremities form the shoulder girdle and the arm. The shoulder girdle includes two bones, the

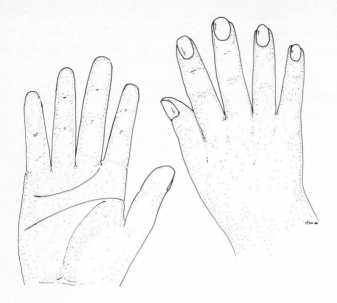

Supination   Pronation

Figure 16-2 Supination and pronation.

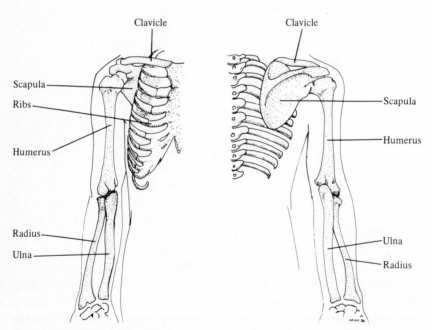

Figure 16-3 The upper extremity.

clavicle and scapula. The clavicle is a long slender bone curved like a shallow S. It is at a horizontal plane directly above the first rib and extends from the sternum to the superior surface of the scapula. The scapula is a large, flat triangular bone forming the posterior portion of the upper extremity. It contains two surfaces, three borders, and three angles, with the superior, lateral angle containing the articulating capsule for the humerus. Attached to the scapula is the humerus, the first of the arm bones. The humerus is a shaft divided into a head, body, and condyle. The rounded head articulates with the scapula; directly below this head is an indentation called the *anatomical neck* which is not to be confused with the surgical neck at the upper end of the shaft. The body ends at the broad, flattened condyle with its two articulating surfaces. This area is divided into the medial *epicondyle* and the lateral epicondyle. The ulna is a slender bone on the medial, or little-finger, side of the arm. Its thick, broad proximal end attaches at the articulating surfaces of the humerus; the outer rounded distal surface of the ulna, called the olecranon, forms a major portion of the elbow. The distal end is small and articulates with the wrist bones. Along the lateral, or thumb, side of the arm is the radius, the proximal end of which attaches to the humerus at the elbow, while the small distal end forms a large portion of the wrist. The hand contains 14 small bones, 8 carpal bones, 5 metacarpal bones, and 14 phalanges. The carpal bones are arranged in two rows and comprise the wrist; the first row includes the scaphoid, lunate, triangular, and pisiform bones, while the distal row includes the trapezium, trapezoid, capitate, and hamate. At birth many of the carpal bones are cartilaginous. An x-ray of a child's hand at $2\frac{1}{2}$ years of age will show only the capitate and hamate bones ossified, but by the 11th year ossification has occurred in all the carpal bones except the pisiform, which develops during the 12th year. The metacarpals are slender bones with the distal ends forming the knuckles of the hand. These articulate with 3 phalanges on each finger and 2 on the thumb (see Fig. 16-4).

The upper extremity is held in place by large muscles: the pectoralis major, pectoralis minor, subclavius and serratus anterior. These attach at different spots and angles along the vertebral column and are woven into the superior muscles of the upper arm. The shoulder itself contains six big muscles: the deltoid, subscapular, supraspinatus, infraspinatus, teres minor, and teres major; while the upper arm contains four muscles: the coracobrachialis, biceps brachii, brachialis, and triceps brachii. The muscles of the lower arm are smaller and more numerous, allowing for increased dexterity. A good anatomy book will be more descriptive of the muscles in this area.

Blood is supplied to the upper extremities through the subclavian artery. Although this is one vessel, it has different names at different points; for instance, it is called the axillary artery at the axilla, the brachial artery

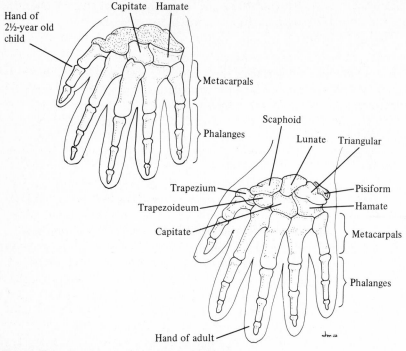

Figure 16-4 The bones of the hand of a child.

coming through the branchial muscles and the radial and ulnar arteries along the radial and ulnar bones. Blood drains from the upper extremities through both a deep and a superficial set of veins.

The nerve supply for the upper extremities comes from the cervical and thoracic nerves of the spinal nerves in the vertebral column. These nerves form the brachial plexus which supplies the entire shoulder, arm, and fingers.

The Lower Extremities

The lower extremities are attached to the body at the pelvic girdle. The pelvic girdle is a large, rigid, heavy structure made up of four bones: two hip bones placed anteriorally and laterally and the *sacrum* and *coccyx* -placed posteriorly. The pelvis is divided into the *false pelvis* (greater pelvis) and the *true pelvis* (lesser pelvis). The borders of the greater pelvis are formed by the *ilium* and the base of the sacrum. The lesser pelvis forms a cavity bounded posteriorly by the sacrum and coccyx and anterolaterally by the *pubis,* the *ischium,* and a small part of the ilium. It should be remembered that the pelvis of a child is different from an adult's, a man's is different from a woman's; there are also differences of pelvic structure in different races. A more detailed description of the pelvis can be found in a good anatomy or obstetric textbook.

The hipbone contains three distinct parts in childhood, which are fused in adulthood. The ilium is the superior, broad, flat surface of the hipbone; the ischium is the strongest portion of the hipbone and contains a portion of the acetabulum and an opening called the *obturator foramen* which carries nerves, muscles, and ligaments; the pubis contains the medial portion of the acetabulum and joins at midline with the opposite pubis to complete the pelvic girdle.

Attached to the hipbone at the acetabulum is the *femur,* which is the longest and strongest bone of the body. The femur begins ossification during the seventh week of fetal life but does not become completely ossified until the fourteenth year of life. The head of the femur becomes completely ossified sometime during the first year of life. During infancy a major portion of the ends of the long bones are cartilage which gradually ossifies during early and late childhood. Growth in length of the bone will continue as long as this epiphyseal cartilage continues to grow, and bone tissue will gradually replace the cartilage. Epiphyseal cartilage disappears in girls about three years before it disappears in boys. A dense, fibrous tissue called *periosteum* covers the bone shaft and produces layers of bone to widen the shaft. It also produces new bone cells when a fracture occurs. The femur contains five parts: a head (which articulates with the *acetabulum*), a neck, the greater trochanter (a curved projection), a shaft, and two *condyles* at the distal end. The *patella* (kneecap) is a small, triangular bone over the junction between the femur and the tibia. The lower leg contains two bones: the larger is the *tibia,* and the smaller is the *fibula.* The tibia consists of a shaft with two enlarged ends; the proximal end articulates with the condyle of the femur, while the distal end forms the medial malleolus at the ankle, which articulates with the tarsal bones. The fibula is smaller and lateral to the tibia. It consists of a shaft with the proximal head resting against the tibia and the distal end spreading to form the lateral malleolus of the ankle (see Fig. 16-5).

The foot contains 7 tarsal bones, 5 metatarsal bones, and 14 phalanges. They include the talus, calcaneus, cuboid, navicular, and 3 cuneiforms. The calcaneus ossifies at the sixth month of fetal life; the talus is formed by the seventh month of life; the cuboid appears by the ninth month; and the lateral cuneiform is formed during the first year. During the third year the medial cuneiform develops, and by the fourth year the intermediate cuneiform and navicular are formed. The phalanges continue their ossification process until the tenth to eighteenth years (see Fig. 16-6).

Four areas of muscles are involved in the lower extremities: muscles of the iliac region, the thigh, the leg, and the foot. The iliac region contains the psoas minor and major and the iliacus which work together to flex the lum-

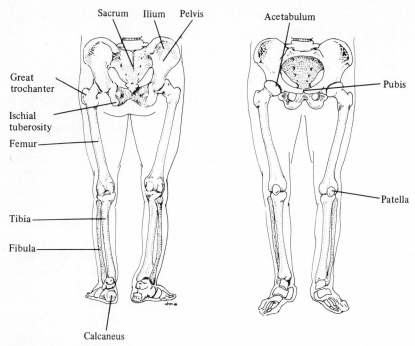

Figure 16-5 The pelvis and the lower extremity.

bar vertebrae, pelvis, and thigh. There are four large groups of muscles that move the thigh. They are six anterior femoral muscles, including the sartorius, rectus femoris, vastus lateralis, vastus medialis, and vastus intermedius. The five medial femoral muscles include the gracilis, pectineus, adductor longus, adductor brevis, and adductor magnus. There are 10 muscles from the gluteal region, including the gluteus maximus, gluteus medius, and gluteus minimus. The three posterior femoral muscles are the biceps femoris, semitendinosus, and the semimembranosus. Movement of the leg is produced by 13 muscles divided into three groups: the 4 anterior crural muscles, 7 posterior crural muscles, and 2 lateral crural muscles. The foot contains four layers of highly coordinated small muscles.

The lower extremities are supplied blood from the iliac branches of the aorta. This is a single artery with different names applied as it passes different parts of the leg. The proximal end is called the external iliac artery; the medial portion is the femoral artery; and the distal portion is the popliteal artery. Blood is drained from the lower extremity by the great saphenous vein and its branches. This is the longest vein in the body, starting at the dorsum of the foot and ending at the femoral vein in the pelvic region.

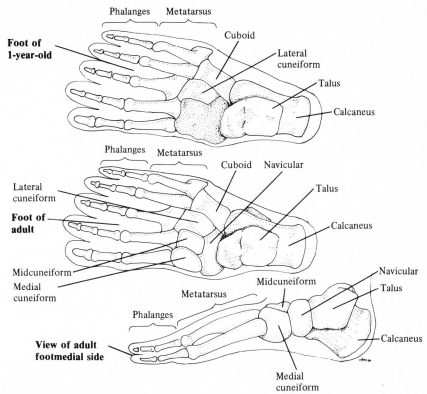

Figure 16-6 Bone changes in the foot—1-year-old and adult.

The nerve supply of the lower extremities follows much the same route as the blood supply. The leg is innervated primarily by the tibial and peroneal nerves and their branches.

The Spinal Column

The vertebral column is a series of 33 connecting bones which support the trunk and protect the spinal cord. These bones are divided into five groups: 7 cervical, 12 thoracic, 5 lumbar, 5 sacral, and 3 to 4 coccygeal, which form four curves. The cervical curve is a *ventral,* convex line, while the thoracic curve is concave. This is followed by the lumbar curve which is ventrally convex and more pronounced in the female. Finally, the pelvic curve is concave, with a caudal and ventral direction. Only the thoracic and pelvic curves are present at birth, thus they are called the primary curves and give the infant a spinal curve shaped like a C rather than the double S of later life (see Fig. 16-7). The secondary (or compensatory) curves are the cervical and

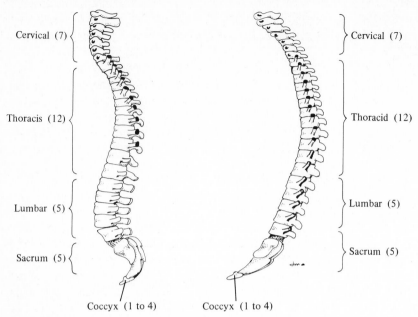

Cervical (7)

Thoracis (12)

Lumbar (5)

Sacrum (5)

Cervical (7)

Thoracid (12)

Lumbar (5)

Sacrum (5)

Coccyx (1 to 4)   Coccyx (1 to 4)

Figure 16-7 Spinal curves of the adult (left) and infant (right).

lumbar because they develop later in life. The cervical is apparent around 3 to 4 months of age when the child begins to hold up his head. The lumbar appears when the child begins to walk, around 12 to 18 months.

The structure of each vertebra is basically the same. The heavy, rough, cylindrical base of the bone is called the body. At the posterior of this body two roots (or pedicles) are formed; these roots surround an opening, meeting midline posteriorly to form a bridge called the lamina. This opening is the vertebral foramen through which the spinal cord passes. Posteriorly there is a palpable projection from the lamina called the spinous process.

The first two cervical vertebrae are known as the *atlas* and *axis* because of their direct support of the cranium and are slightly different in structure from the rest of the vertebrae. The first cervical vertebra (atlas) has no body, only a slight knob for a spinous process and the addition of two transverse processes and two large articulating surfaces to receive the occipital condyles from the skull. The second cervical vertebra (axis) serves as a pivot for the first vertebra and contains a body, 2 roots, 1 spinous process, and 2 articulating surfaces, plus an extra bony projection called the dens protruding from the anterior surface of the body. The seventh (and last) cervical vertebra is similar to the rest of the vertebrae, but has an especially long spinous process which can be useful as a landmark when palpating the vertebrae.

The thoracic vertebrae are structurally similar to those already described, but are slightly larger than cervical vertebrae. The lumbar vertebrae are again structurally similar and are the largest vertebrae in the spinal column. The final section of the spinal column is the sacrum which, at birth, is composed of five separate bones; by 18 to 20 years of age these fuse into one large bone. The sacrum is wider and shorter in women than in men, and it has greater curvature and wider angles to increase the pelvic size for childbearing. The coccyx (or tail bone) consists of three to five small rudiments of vertebrae which begin ossification between the 1st and 4th years of life and become fused into one bone by age 25.

To help the spinal column move and to protect against harmful movement each vertebrae is separated from the rest by intervertebral disks. These disks are composed of soft, elastic, fibrous tissue and comprise one-fourth the length of the entire vertebral column.

The vertebrae contain three kinds of joints: synovial, fibrous, and cartilaginous. The synovial joints allow for gliding movements of the joints and for flexion, extension, lateral bending, and rotation; the fibrous joints connect the arches and allow flexion and extension to some degree; and the cartilaginous joints combine with the intervertebral disks to give support as well as some flexion and extension.

The muscles of the spine are difficult to describe because they are usually discussed in connection to other portions of the body. The deep muscles of the back are divided into two groups: the superficial iliocostalis group and the deeper transversospinal group which crosses medially. The iliocostalis group contains three muscles: the splenius capitis, splenius cervicis, and erector spinae; the transversospinal group contains five muscles: semispinalis, multifidus, rotatores, interspinales, and intertransverse. The superficial muscles of the back are also used to connect the upper extremities to the trunk. There are five of these muscles: the trapezius, latissimus dorsi, rhomboideus major, rhomboideus minor, and levator scapulae.

The blood supply to the spinal column originates with the descending aorta. This branches into two posterior intercostal arteries and finally becomes the spinal branch. Blood is drained from the area through the vertebral vein. The spinal column is a primary innervation source for the entire body. Well protected within the vertebral foramen of each vertebra lies the spinal cord. This cord is protected both by the bony framework of the vertebrae and by several layers of protective covering. The first of these layers is a thin membrane called the pia mater. Between the pia mater and the next layer, the arachnoid layer, are loose spaces called the subarachnoid spaces. These allow cerebrospinal fluid to continually bathe the spinal cord. Above the arachnoid layer is the dura mater, the outer covering of the cord composed of tough connective tissue. Meninges and fatty connective tissue further cushion the cord from the bony foramen. The internal portion of the spinal cord is composed of ascending and descending tracts from which project 31 pairs of nerves innervating most of the body. The pairs of spinal nerves are divided into sections corresponding to the vertebrae from which they emerge: 8 cervical, 12 thoracic, 5 lumbar, 5 sacral and 1 coccygeal. A good anatomy book will give a more complete description of their locations and functions.

HOW TO EXAMINE

It is difficult to find a child who is motionless. Therefore, much of the musculoskeletal examination can be done while watching or playing with the child before the examination. Some of this examination will depend upon the age of the child. An older child will perform when asked to sit, stand, walk, pick up a ball, or reach. A young infant will have to be helped and supported to be observed for sitting or weight bearing, and much of his range of motion will have to be passive. Some parts of the skeletal examination are fun and an easy way to establish rapport with the child. The child should be fully undressed for the skeletal examination. Older children may be allowed to keep their underpants on, but babies should have their diapers removed. Much of the skeletal system is examined during other parts of the physical examination, but the nurse-examiner must remember to compile all this information at the end of the examination and to record the evaluation of the skeletal system as a whole. Inspection and palpation are the primary methods of examination used in evaluating the musculoskeletal system. Every inch of the body must be thoroughly observed and felt.

Inspection should proceed from the general to the specific. In other words, note how the child walks into the room, how he sits in a chair, etc., before looking at specifics like his legs and spine. This general observation will include symmetry inspection of the skeleton for movement as well as general alignment, position, deformities, shortenings, lengthenings, and unusual postures. Observe the soft tissues and muscles for symmetry, swelling, and muscle wasting. Inspect the skin for color, texture, redness, cyanosis, pigmentation, bruises, and scratches. Scars should be noted and described: linear scars are usually from surgery; irregular scars, from trauma; and puckered scars, from suppuration. Observations should also include the presence or absence of a part, such as *polydactyly* or *syndactyly*.

Palpation is the next important part of the examination. The examiner must run the hands over every inch of the spine and extremities to gather all the data needed to make a decision. The bones are palpated for general shape and outline. Any thickening, abnormal prominence, or indentations are noted. The skin is palpated for temperature, tenderness, and pain. Erythema, swelling, tenderness, and heat may indicate inflammation. In feeling for temperature it is best to compare sides; the examiner should place the hands on both joints for 30 seconds and then switch hands. Palpation may help to localize tenderness or pain. The examiner must also palpate the soft tissues and muscles for swellings, wastings, and contractures. All joints should be checked for a full range of motion, and this motion should be described in degrees of a circle (see Fig. 16-8).

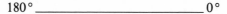

$180°$ _____ $0°$

Motion may be active or passive—active if the child will do it herself and passive when the examiner must help her. Unless there is paralysis or damaged muscles or tendons, active and passive motion should be the same. Motion should be checked for extension, flexion, and rotation such as supination and pronation of the palms. Strength and power must be checked. Strength of movement with gravity, against gravity, and against resistance should be tested, and symmetry of strength noted. Different muscle groups can be tested for strength. In testing the upper extremities, the child should be asked to raise both arms over the head, out to both sides, and out in front. The child should be able to hold her arms and hands in these positions while the examiner applies pressure to force the arms in the opposite direction. The examiner can also ask the child to squeeze her two index fingers to feel the symmetry of strength in both arms and fingers.

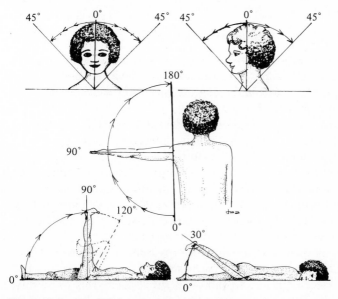

Figure 16-8 Degrees for the range of motion.

Joints that are functioning properly should not exhibit muscle spasms or sudden loss of control. Tests for function include watching the child walk, stand, sit, bend, jump, skip, and run. Most children will be able to do these with symmetry, smoothness, and ease.

WHERE TO EXAMINE

The examination of the skeletal system requires both a total examination of the child as a whole and many very specific evaluations of individual parts of the skeletal system, such as the upper extremities, and even smaller parts, such as each finger.

WHAT TO EXAMINE WITH

No specialized equipment is needed for the examination of the skeletal system, although a plastic tape measure will sometimes be useful in evaluating symmetry of parts.

WHAT TO EXAMINE FOR

Some specifics the nurse may encounter during the examination will be discussed under the portion of the skeleton where it is most likely to occur. As in the discussion of the anatomy, the upper extremities, lower extremities, and spinal column will all be considered.

The Upper Extremities

In the upper extremities, the clavicles must be palpated, and full range of motion of the arms must be observed to make sure clavicular fracture does not exist; this is particular true in the neonate, since a broken clavicle is one of the more common birth injuries.

The long bones of the arm must be examined to rule out *subluxation*. Subluxation of the radius is most common in children from 2 to 4 years old. The child may complain of pain either in the elbow or the wrist. Passive range of motion is possible in all directions except supination. Subluxation of the shoulder is another occasional finding in the preschool child. It is usually caused by an adult lifting the child off the ground by holding him by the hands or wrists; this puts undue strain on the shoulder. It may be heralded by swelling, pain, and refusal to use that arm.

The elbow should also be inspected for increased carrying angle. This is frequently associated with gonadal dysgenesis, and is a danger signal that should alert the nurse-examiner to thoroughly investigate this possibility. This can be done by asking the child to hold his arms straight out at right angles to his body, palms facing forward. In this position the upper and lower arms should form a relatively smooth continuous line. If the lower arm angles upward toward the ceiling forming an angle less than 180° with the lower arm the child is considered to have an increased carrying angle (see Fig. 16-9).

The nurse then examines one hand at a time carefully. Each should be checked for number of fingers, noting any polydactyly or syndactyly. (Polydactyly is frequently associated with Ellis–van Crevel syndrome and syndactyly with premature closure of the sutures.) The length of the fingers—long, narrow, short, stubby, or clubbed—is important. A short, broad, clawlike hand may indicate Hurler's syndrome; a trident hand (short, broad hands with the index, middle, and fourth fingers about equal length and a space between the thumb and first finger and between the second and third fingers) is often associated with chondrodystrophy; short fingers, an incurved little finger, a low-set thumb and a simian crease should make the nurse investigate the possibility of Down's syndrome; digits may be unusually short in children with myositis ossificans or pseudohypoparathyroidism; macrodactyly or an enlarged digit may be normal or may be a sign of neurofibromatosis; an overlapping of the second and third fingers should make one think of trisomy 18 syndrome.

The creases of the palms are inspected. Although a simian crease is often associated with Down's syndrome, it is often found in normal individuals. There is an entire field of investigation called *dermatoglyphics*

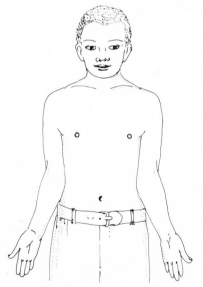

Figure 16-9   Child with increased carrying angle.

that is finding correlations between certain congenital anomalies and palmar crease patterns. The nurse should stay informed of the current findings from these studies.

The nurse then feels across the knuckles to ascertain the presence of four knuckles and gently runs his or her fingers up the length of the arm feeling and looking for radial pulses, widening of the wrist bones as seen in rickets, dryness, roughness or scaliness of the skin, skin color, as well as any bruises, scratches or bites, muscle wasting, swelling or lumps, and enlargement of epitrochlear lymph nodes at the elbow and axillary nodes at the axilla. The examiner then repeats this process with the other hand and checks both arms and hands for symmetry of length, width, and color.

The Lower Extremities

In examining the lower extremities, the nurse observes the shape of the legs, noting the presence of *genu varum* (bowleggedness) or *tibial torsion. Genu valgum* (knock-knees) is present if the medial malleoli are more than 1 in apart when the knees are touching. Genu valgum may be normal in children between 2 and $3\frac{1}{2}$ years of age. It may persist in mild form until age 6. Genu varum is present when the medial malleoli are touching and the knees are more than 1 in apart. Infants are frequently bowlegged until they have been walking for a year. However, severe genu varum may be due to such nutritional deficiencies as rickets (see Fig. 16-10). Tibial torsion is a twisting of

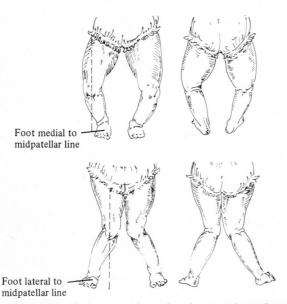

Foot medial to midpatellar line

Foot lateral to midpatellar line

Figure 16-10   Genu varum (upper) and genu valgum (lower).

the tibia which is sometimes initiated by an intrauterine position and aided by the child sitting in a TV squat (the buttocks on the floor with the knees and ankles flexed and flat against the floor to the side) (see Fig. 16-11).

Tibial torsion can be tested for in one of three ways. The first way is to have the child lie on his back with his knees facing upward. The forefoot and hindfoot should be in line with the knees. The examiner places the thumb and index fingers on the lateral and medial malleoli. In an infant the four malleoli should be parallel to the table. In older children the external malleoli may rotate up to 20° and still be normal. The second way is to have the child sit on the examining table while the examiner draws a circle over the patellar and external malleoli. With the patella facing forward only the anterior edge of the malleolar circle should be seen. If one-half to three-fourths of the malleolar circle is seen, tibial torsion is present and the child needs to be referred (see Fig. 16-12). The third test requires the child to stand while a plumb line is drawn from the great iliac crest downward. The line should intersect the toes between the second and third toe. If the medial malleoli are posterior and the lateral malleoli are anterior, the child needs to be referred to the physician.

The strength of the legs should be tested by having the child flex his legs while the examiner tries to straighten them. The nurse should check complete range of motion at the toes, ankles, knees, and hips. In infants it is especially important to check hip rotation to rule out congenital dislocation of the hip. Congenital dislocation of the hip is more common in girls than in

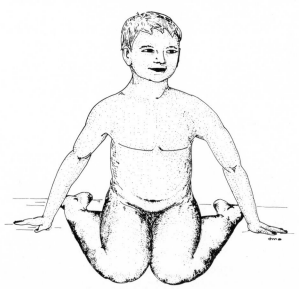

Figure 16-11 Child in the position called "TV squat."

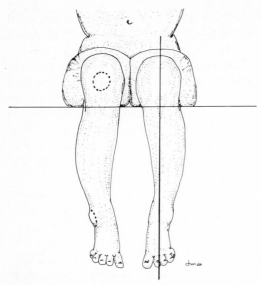

Figure 16-12   One test for tibial torsion.

boys and should be suspected if the mother complains of trouble in diapering the child due to the tight adductor muscles. A normal newborn should have bilateral hip rotation of almost 160 to 175°, which means the flexed hips are almost flat on the bed. There are several methods of checking for hip dislocation. One way is to check the leg length. If the femur rides upward above the acetabulum it shortens that leg and makes the opposite knee seem lower. When the feet are kept flat on the bed, with the knees flexed, and the examiner observes the height of the knees, it will be apparent if one knee is lower than the other. This is called the *Allis's sign* and indicates possible dislocation (see Fig. 16-13). The examiner should also check for unequal gluteal or leg folds. Although this is not a completely reliable sign of dislocated hip since most children have slightly asymmetrical folds, any significant asymmetry should be investigated thoroughly. *Ortolani's sign* is probably the most reliable test for a dislocated hip. The examiner flexes the knees and applies slight downward pressure (to dislocate the hip) and then abducts the hips up and out (the click is felt during inward movement). A dislocated hip may be present if there is resistance to having the leg rotate the 175° or if a click can be heard as the femur slips out of the acetabulum.

The lower extremities are also examined as the child stands. In this position the examiner can note foot arches. *Pes cavus* (a very high arch) may be normal or a symptom of Friedreich's ataxia. All children have a fat pad under their medial arches until they have walked for 1 to 2 years, giving the appearance of flat feet. Many parents are concerned about this in their young children, and the nurse-examiner should reassure them that flat feet are normal in a child of this age and that even if they are found in older

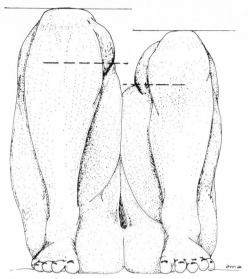

Figure 16-13 Allis's sign.

children, there is no reason for concern unless the problem is causing symptoms. An easy way to test arches is to wet the child's feet and have him stand on two paper towels and then examine the imprints left on the paper.

As the child stands, her feet should point straight ahead. *Pes valgus* (toeing out) may be causing or caused by *tibial torsion; pes varus* (toeing in, pigeon-toes) may be causing or be caused by an anteverted femur or tibial torsion. Pes valgus and pes varus refer to the entire foot turning, while *metatarsus varus* refers to the turning in of the forefoot alone. When the child with metatarsus varus is standing, the heel is straight and in line with the leg, but the front half of the foot toes inward (see Fig. 16-14). This conditions needs referral for treatment. In infancy many of these positions may be seen as a remnant of intrauterine life. If this is the case, passive manipulation will correct the deformity. If it cannot be corrected in this way, a referral is needed. When evaluating the feet of a child past the age of walking, it is also important to assess the straightness of the heel cords when standing behind the child. It is normal for these tendons to slant medially before the age of 5 or 6, but after that age this may be an indication of pronated feet.

Such conditions as tibial torsion, genu valgum, and genu varus are apparent as the child stands. Looking at the child's shoes and their pattern of wear (e.g., is only the inside of the heel worn down?) may also give clues to the position of feet and legs. Finally, the child should walk, run, and skip while the examiner watches. Gait, balance, and stance should be observed. The new walker (between 12 to 18 months) has a wide-based gait and very little balance, but the older child has a very narrow-based gait and enough

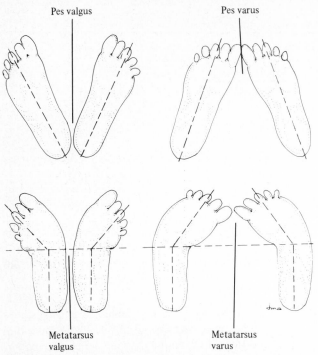

Pes valgus

Pes varus

Metatarsus
valgus

Metatarsus
varus

Figure 16-14 Child with pes valgus and pes varus, metatarsus valgus and metatarsus varus.

balance to stand on one leg for varying periods of time. Most children learn to skip fairly well by age 5 or 6. Evaluation of gait in the older child is also important. In general, the examiner should watch for smoothness of movement and position of arms, legs, and toes. The opposite arm and leg should move forward at the same time. Toes should always be pointed straight ahead. There are two phases to the gait: the stance phase and the swing phase. Each of these consists of three stages. The stance phase begins when the heel strikes the ground; this is called "heel strike"; next is the "midstance," and finally the "push-off" stage. The second phase, the swing phase, also consists of three stages: The acceleration stage, the "swing-through" stage, and the deceleration stage. Any abnormality noted should be described specifically in relation to the appropriate phase and stage.

Also important in evaluating the lower extremities of children who complain of pain is the rotation and telescoping of the joint for possible Legg-Perthes and rotation and telescoping of the knee joint for possible Osgood-Schlatter's disease. These maneuvers will result in pain if the joint is involved. Observe the child's spine and palpate when the child is in the standing position. Watch the infant on his back and then turned over and observe for alignment and symmetry of movements, as well as for skin manifestations such as dimples, cysts, and tufts of hair and discoloration of the coccygeal area. Run the fingers down the spine to feel the lack or presence of the spinous processes. In older children the spine is also inspected in the upright position for masses, tenderness, stiffness, mobility, and posture. Posture is observed from the front, side, and back and when flexed. Normally the spine curves forward and backward but should have no side curves.

Criteria for good posture include the following:

1 The head should be centered on the spine in such a way that if a plumb-line were dropped from the occiput it would fall directly in the midline of the sacrum.

2 The level of the shoulders should be equal (within about $\frac{1}{2}$ in); this level will be significantly different in scoliosis if the legs are of unequal length. The shoulders should be neither unequally elevated nor rounded.

3 The scapulae should be symmetrical with a distance of 3 to 5 in between them. Poor muscle tone in the deltoid or pectoralis will result in inequality.

4 The spine should be straight in flexion and extension.

5 Each of the four curves should be smooth and balanced.

If the forward and backward curves are exaggerated, they are considered pathologic. *Kyphosis* is the term given to an exaggerated concave curve in the lumbar region. *Scoliosis* is a lateral curvature of the spine and may be pathologic. Normally infants and small children with protuberant abdomens have a slight degree of lumbar *lordosis,* which is normal. This is more pronounced in black children. Some adolescents display rounded shoulders with slight kyphosis. Children displaying kyphosis usually have an interscapular distance of more than 5 to 6 in. Usually this reflects a habitual posture rather than a permanent skeletal deformity. Some children develop a functional scoliosis (see Fig. 16-15). The fact that it is functional can be proved by having the child bend forward toward his toes, as the examiner stands behind him and looks up the spine toward his head. The spine should be flexed approximately 60°. Functional scoliosis will disappear under these conditions. If the scoliosis is not functional but due to a pelvic tilt, decreased vital capacity, or muscle contractures, the bent-over position will not correct it; in such case, the child needs to be referred.

Another orthopedic condition sometimes encountered is overlapping toes. In older children this may come from shoes that are too narrow. In infancy this is usually a hereditary condition. Sometimes strapping the toe into the correct position with an adhesive bandage for 6 weeks will correct it.

In recent years, an area of health care called *sports medicine* has evolved which has required nurses working with school-age children to keep abreast of the developments in this area in relation both to physical ex-

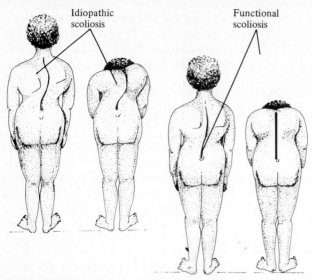

Figure 16-15 Child with functional scoliosis.

amination and to the prevention, recognition, and decision making about the types of injuries occurring in sports. There is currently a feeling among proponents of sports medicine that a physical examination of a school-aged child which reveals hyperextensibility of the joints may warrant counseling of the child away from contact sports and into other types of sports. The idea is that young children with this type of "loose joint" may be more vulnerable to dislocations of the joints and other serious injuries involved in heavy contact such as occurs in football. Although this is not yet proven, it would seem wise to keep this possibility in mind when doing physical examinations on children of this age group.

There are a variety of special maneuvers related to suspected problems of the skeletal system which are not done on a routine physical examination, but may be done if a special complaint occurs.

1 Tenderness in "tennis elbow" may be detected by palpation of the lateral epicondyle of the elbow.

2 A "bulge sign" is positive if, after milking in an upward direction along either side of the patella, the examiner can see a bulge of returning fluid medial to the patella when tapping on the lateral hollow next to the patella.

3 Another method for determining whether excess fluid exists under the patella is to push downward above the patella (thus pushing any fluid from that area beneath the patella) and then tapping the patella briskly against the femur. If an audible or palpable tap results, the sign is positive, indicating that fluid exists under the kneecap.

4 If after holding the child's wrists in full flexion for one or two minutes, he complains of numbness and tingling in the palm, thumb, index, middle, and part of the ring finger (the distribution of the median nerve), the *carpal tunnel sign* is positive. This indicates compression of the median nerve at the wrist.

5 A test for torn medial or collateral ligaments is important, particularly after sports injuries. This is done by extending the child's leg, holding the femur tightly in one hand and grasping the ankle with the other hand; the hand holding the ankle then attempts to adduct and abduct the leg at the knee. Neither adduction or abduction should be possible. If there is any movement, collateral ligament injury is suspected.

6 Another concern after sports injuries is damage to the anterior or posterior cruciate ligaments. To test for this, have the child lie down, flexing the knee to a 90° angle while stabilizing the lower leg by sitting on the foot. The examiner then holds the leg below the knee and exerts pressure both toward and away from the table. Neither maneuver should elicit any movement if the cruciate ligaments are stable.

7 *McMurray's test* is designed to detect a torn meniscus of the knee. The child is asked to lie flat on the back and the knee is then completely flexed so that the foot is flat on the table next to the buttocks and held in that position with one hand, using the thumb and index finger to stabilize the knee on either side of the joint space. The examiner's other hand holds the child's heel and rotates the foot and lower leg in a lateral direction. Maintaining the leg in this outward rotation, the knee is then extended to a 90° angle. A palpable or audible click in the knee may occur if a torn meniscus is present.

BIBLIOGRAPHY

Alexander, M., and M. Brown: "Physical Examination: The Musculoskeletal System," *Nursing '76*, vol. 6, no. 4, pp. 51–56, April 1976.

American Academy of Pediatrics: "American Academy of Pediatrics Policy Statement on Cardiac Evaluation for Participation in Sports," *New and Comments*, vol. 28, no. 4, pp. 1–2, April 1977.

Kadkhoda, Mohamad, et al.: "Congenital Dislocation of the Hip—Diagnostic Screening & Treatment," *Clinical Pediatrics*, vol. 15, no. 3, pp. 239–246, March 1976.

Sells, Clifford J., and Eleanor A. May: "Scoliosis Screening in Public Schools," *American Journal of Nursing*, vol. 74, no. 1, pp. 60–62, January 1974.

GLOSSARY

abduction movement away from the medial line
acetabulum the large, rounded cavity of the pelvis which holds the head of the femur
adduction movement toward the medial line

Allis's sign the unequal height of the knees with the feet flat and the knees flexed; a test for dislocation of the hip

ankylosis stabilization of a joint that should be movable

atlas the first cervical vertebra

axis the second cervical vertebra

ball-and-socket joint a rounded head of a bone fitted into a deep concave cavity, as seen in the hip joints

circumduction rotation of one bone around a stationary disk

condyle the rounded protuberance on the end of a bone

condyloid joint a joint, such as the wrist, which allows flexion, extension, adduction, abduction, and circumduction but not axial rotation

dermatoglyphics the study of the patterns of lines on the palms and fingers

dorsal posterior, as of a surface, organ, or other area

epicondyle a rounded protuberance above the condyle at the end of a bone

epiphysis the end of the long bones which is cartilage during early childhood and ossified during late childhood

eversion turning out and away from the midline of the body

false pelvis (greater pelvis) the border of the pelvic girdle formed by the ilium and base of the sacrum

flaccid flabby, weak, as an abnormal muscle

genu the knee

genu valgum knock-knees

genu varum bowleggedness

gliding joints a joint that allows a gliding motion between two flat surfaces, as in the carpal joints

ilium the upper portion of hipbone

inverted turning inward; toward the midline of the body

ischium the lower, posterior portion of the hipbone

kyphosis an exaggerated concave curve in the thoracic region of the spine

ligament the tough, fibrous tissue connecting two bones

lordosis an exaggerated convex curve in the lumbar region of the spine

pes cavus a very high arch of the foot

pes valgus toeing out

pes varus toeing in

polydactyly extra digits on the hands or feet

pronation the position of the hand in which the palmar surface faces downward

pubis the pubic bone

sacrum the final section of the spinal cord, containing five bones

scoliosis a lateral curvature of the spine

subluxation a dislocation which is incomplete

supination the position of the hand in which the palmar surface faces upward

syndactyly the fusion or webbing of 2 or more phalanges

tendon the fibrous connective tissue joining muscle to bone

tibial torsion twisting of the tibia

true pelvis (lesser pelvis) the pelvic cavity bounded posteriorly by the sacrum and coccyx and anterolaterally by the pubis, the ischium, and a small part of the ilium

ventral anterior, as of a surface, organ, or other area

Inspection of the Skeletal System*

Spine	Yes	No	Not appli-cable	Describe (where appropriate)	Significance
A. Curvature					
1. Scoliosis					If scoliosis persists when bending over, it is pathological.
2. Kyphosis					Need for referral.
3. Lordosis					A moderate amount may be a racial variant—particularly for blacks.
4. Cervical curve present					Expected by age 3–4 months.
5. Thoracic curve present					Expected at birth (at that time only the concave curves are present giving the back a "C" shape rather than an "S" shape).
6. Lumbar curve present					Expected to appear when the child begins to walk—about 13–18 months.
7. Other					
B. All spinous processes present					Absence may indicate underlying bony defect.
C. Pilonidal dimple					May also indicate underlying bony defect such as meningocele.
D. Hair tuft along spine					Same as lordosis.

*These charts are meant to be used by beginning students as they perform their first physical assessments. Each item should be examined on the child and then checked off on the checklist. The significance of the items follows in the right-hand column.

307

Inspection of the Skeletal System (Continued)

Spine	Yes	No	Not appli-cable	Describe (where appropriate)	Significance
E. Range of motion					
1. Bends 30° back					
2. Bends 75-90° forward					
3. Bends 35° laterally to right					
4. Bends 35° laterally to left					
5. Twists 30° with (R) side moving anteriorly					Any limitation needs further investigation.
6. Twists 30° with (L) side moving anteriorly					
7. Flexes chin on sternum					
8. Bends neck backward 55°					
Upper extremities					
A. Shoulder girdle					
1. Scapulae symmetrical					In newborn, particularly, asymmetricality may indicate fracture.
2. Clavicles symmetrical					
3. (R) shoulder higher than (L)					Asymmetricality may indicate scoliosis.
4. (L) shoulder higher than (R)					Asymmetricality may indicate scoliosis.

5. Range of motion
  a. raises straight arm
    upward 180°
						Limitation may indicate pathology; excessive motion may indicate hyperextensibility; some authorities feel that this is a contraindication to participation in certain sports for the school-age child since they feel that this kind of hyperextensibility is predisposed to injury in body contact sports such as football. This is controversial, however.

b. extends straight arm
    downward and back-
    ward 50°						

c. raises arm flexed at
    elbow 90° (external
    rotation)						

d. lowers arm flexed
    at elbow 90°
    (internal rotation)						

e. adduction 50°						
f. abduction 180°						
g. other						

B. Arms, wrists, and hands
  1. Visible deformities of
    (R) humerus						

2. Visible deformities of (L) humerus						Same significance as above
3. Visible deformities of (R) radius or ulna						

4. Visible deformities
    of (L) radius or
    ulna						

5. Visible deformities
    of (R) wrist and
    hand bones						

Inspection of the Skeletal System (*Continued*)

Upper extremities	Yes	No	Not appli-cable	Describe (where appropriate)	Significance
6. Visible deformities of (L) wrist and hand bones					
7. (R) elbow increased carrying angle					
8. (R) elbow flexion 160°					Same significance as above.
9. (R) elbow extension 180°					
10. (R) elbow supination 90°					
11. (R) elbow pronation 90°					
12. (L) elbow increased carrying angle					May indicate Turner's syndrome.
13. (L) elbow flexion 160°					
14. (L) elbow extension 180°					Same significance as above.
15. (L) elbow supination 90°					
16. (L) elbow pronation 90°					

17.	Abnormally wide wrist			May indicate rickets.
18.	(R) wrist radial deviation 20°			
19.	(R) wrist ulnar deviation 55°			
20.	(L) wrist radial deviation 20°			
21.	(L) wrist ulnar deviation 55°			
22.	(R) wrist flexion 90°			
23.	(R) wrist extension 70°			
24.	(L) wrist flexion 90°			Same significance as above.
25.	(L) wrist extension 70°			
26.	(R) finger joints all flex completely			
27.	(R) finger joints all extend completely			
28.	(L) finger joints all flex completely			
29.	(L) finger joints all extend completely			

Inspection of the Skeletal System (*Continued*)

Upper extremities	Yes	No	Not applicable	Describe (where appropriate)	Significance
30. (R) polydactyly					
31. (L) polydactyly					
32. (R) syndactyly					
33. (L) syndactyly					
34. (R) fingers a. clubbed					
b. short					
c. broad					
d. trident					
e. claw-like					Present in a variety of mental retardation syndromes and genetic abnormalities.
f. middle and 4th fingers equal length					
g. incurved 5th finger					
h. low set thumb					
i. overlapping fingers					
j. macrodactyly					
35. (L) fingers a. clubbed					
b. short					

312

c. broad				
d. trident				
e. claw-like				
f. middle and 4th fingers equal length				
g. incurved 5th finger				Present in a variety of mental retardation syndromes and genetic abnormalities.
h. low set thumb				
i. overlapping fingers				
j. macrodactyly				
36. Simian crease				
37. Abnormal dermatoglyphics				

Lower extremities

A. Pelvic girdle				
1. (R) straight leg hyperextension 15°				Same significance as above.
2. (R) straight leg flexion 90°				
3. (L) straight leg hyperextension 15°				
4. (L) straight leg flexion 90°				

313

Inspection of the Skeletal System (*Continued*)

Lower extremities	Yes	No	Not appli-cable	Describe (where appropriate)	Significance
5. (R) leg (flexed at knee) flexion 120°					
6. (L) leg (flexed at knee) flexion 120°					
7. (R) leg abduction 45° (straight leg)					
8. (R) leg adduction 30° (straight leg)					
9. (L) leg abduction 45° (straight leg)					
10. (L) leg adduction 30° (straight leg)					Same significance as above.
11. (R) leg external rotation (flexed at knee) 40°					
12. (R) leg internal rotation (flexed at knee) 45°					
13. (L) leg external rotation (flexed at knee) 40°					
14. (L) leg internal rotation (flexed at knee) 45°					

15. Ortolani's sign negative		Abnormality raises suspicion of dislocated hip.
16. Piston maneuver negative		Same as Ortolani's.
17. Allis maneuver negative		Same as Ortolani's.
B. Legs		
1. Equal length (within $\frac{1}{4}''$) (Measure from anterior iliac crest to medial malleoli)		Greater leg length discrepancy requires referral.
2. Visible abnormalities of upper or lower leg bones		
3. Genu varum		Considered true knock-knees if medial malleoli are more than two fingerbreaths apart with knees together.
4. Genu valgum		Considered true bow-legs only if knees are more than two fingerbreaths apart with medial malleoli touching.
5. (R) tibial torsion		May require correction.
6. (L) tibial torsion		May require correction.
7. (R) knee flexion 130°		
8. (L) knee flexion 130°		

315

Inspection of the Skeletal System (*Continued*)

Lower extremities	Yes	No	Not appli-cable	Describe (where appropriate)	Significance
9. (R) knee hyper-extension					
10. (L) knee hyper-extension					
11. (R) foot dorsiflex-ion 20°					Same significance as upper extremities.
12. (R) foot plantar-flexion 45°					
13. (L) foot dorsi-flexion 20°					
14. (L) foot plantar-flexion 45°					
15. (R) pes cavus					Flat feet only need treatment if symptomatic. Young children (under about 3 years) have fat pads under their arches, giving the false appear-ance of flat feet.
16. (L) pes cavus					Same as above.
17. (R) pes valgus					May be caused by deformities of the foot itself, but more often indi-cates tibial torsion.
18. (L) pes valgus					Same as above.
19. (R) pes varus					May be caused by deformities of the foot itself, but is more likely to indicate anteversion of the femur.
20. (L) pes varus					Same as above.
21. (R) metatarsus varus					Needs treatment.

	Yes	No	Not appli-cable	Describe (where appropriate)	Significance
22. (L) metatarsus varus					Same as above.
23. Overlapping toes					Common in certain mental retardation syndromes.

Palpation of the Skeletal System

Spine	Yes	No	Not appli-cable	Describe (where appropriate)	Significance
A. Spinous processes all present					Absent spinous process may indicate underlying bony defect.
B. Any palpable abnormalities					Require further investigation.
Upper extremities					
A. Shoulder girdle 1. Palpable crepitus in shoulder joint on movement					May be normal variant, but indicates referral if accompanied by pain or other symptoms.
2. Swelling in shoulder joints					May indicate arthritis, gout, trauma.
3. Bone irregularities (masses, fractures, etc.)					Require further investigation.
4. Bones normally shaped					
5. Other					

317

Palpation of the Skeletal System (*Continued*)

Upper extremities	Yes	No	Not applicable	Describe (where appropriate)	Significance
B. Arms					
1. Crepitus in elbow joint					Same as A1.
2. Swelling in elbow joint					Same as A2.
3. Crepitus in wrist joint					Same as A1.
4. Swelling in wrist joint					Same as A2.
5. Crepitus in finger joint					Same as A1.
6. Swelling in finger joint					Same as A2.
7. Bone irregularities (masses, fractures, etc.)					Same as A3.
8. Bones normally shaped					
9. Other					
Lower extremities					
A. Pelvic girdle					
1. Palpable crepitus on movement					May be normal variant or may indicate pathology if accompanied by pain.
2. Palpable swelling					Pathological.
3. Palpable bone irregularities					May indicate old healed fracture or current pathology.
4. Other					

B. Legs and feet		
1. Crepitus in knee		Same as A1.
2. Swelling in knee		Same as A2.
3. Crepitus in ankle		Same as A1.
4. Swelling in ankle		Same as A2.
5. Crepitus in toes		Same as A1.
6. Swelling in toes		Same as A2.
7. Any bone irregularities		Same as A3.
8. All bones normally shaped		
9. Other		

Source: These checklists are printed with permission from Blue Hill Videotape Incorporated and are part of a more complete programmed learning approach to the physical examination, which includes a workbook and series of videotapes. The materials can be purchased from Blue Hill Educational Systems, Inc., 52 South Main Street, Spring Valley, New York 10977.

Chapter 17

The Neurologic Examination

WHY THE CHILD IS EXAMINED

The evaluation of the central nervous system is one of the most important assessments made during a physical examination. So many of the functions which give life its human quality are closely related to a healthy nervous system. Not only is gross neurologic impairment, such as severe cerebral palsy or meningomyelocele, important to the child's future life, but the more subtle defects, such as hyperactivity or the controversial "minimal brain dysfunction," will make a large qualitative difference in his general health and happiness. This is an area where preventive health measures and early recognition of problems are of the utmost importance.

WHAT TO EXAMINE: ANATOMY OF THE AREA

The nervous system is complex and delicately balanced. It is composed of a _central nervous system_ and a _peripheral nervous system._ Each of these systems is composed of basic units, called *neurons,* and their protective coverings. Each neuron contains a nucleus, cell body, organelles, and inclusion bodies, as well as two types of processes: *dendrites* and *axons.* Dendrites are branches of the cell body cytoplasm, some of which are covered by myelin and some of which are not. Each neuron has one axon, but may have several dendrites. Impulses are received through the dendrites, travel into the cell body, and leave through the axon where they can be transmitted through a synapse to the dendrite of the next neuron. Axons may or may not be covered with a myelin sheath (a lipid material) and a neurilemma (sheath of Schwann) (see Fig. 17-1).

There are two kinds of peripheral nerves: myelinated and unmyelinated. *Myelinated* nerves make up the spinal and cranial nerves; the *unmyelinated* nerves form the autonomic nervous system. Groups of nerves found outside the central nervous system are called *ganglia;* these can be either sensory or autonomic.

The central nervous system contains the brain (*encephalon*) and spinal cord (*medulla spinalis*). The brain includes both the *cortex* (gray matter), and the white matter. The bones covering the brain form the cranial cavity. These include the 8 skull bones (1 parietal, 1 occipital, 2 frontal, 2 temporal, and 2 sphenoid) and many facial bones. The brain and spinal cord both are covered with three layers of membranes (*meninges*): the *dura mater,* the *arachnoid,* and the *pia mater* (see Fig. 17-2). The dura mater is composed of several layers of tough, fibrous connective tissue which lies directly beneath the periosteum of the bone. The arachnoid is a web-like, avascular membrane lying between the dura mater and the pia mater. It is separated from

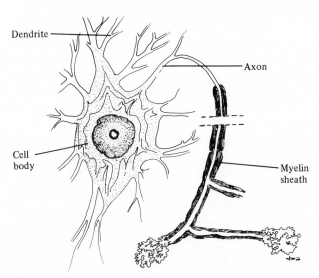

Figure 17-1 A neuron.

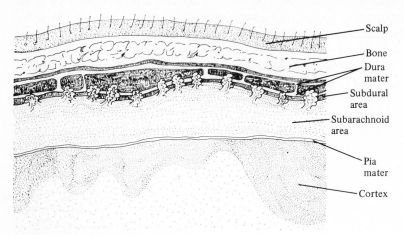

Scalp
Bone
Dura mater
Subdural area
Subarachnoid area
Pia mater
Cortex

Figure 17-2   The meningeal layers.

the dura mater by the subdural space and the pia mater by the cerebrospinal fluid in the subarachnoid space. A spinal puncture in the lumbar region enters the subarachnoid space between the third and fourth lumbar vertebrae. The deepest layer of the meninges is the pia mater, which is a delicate, highly vascular layer attaching directly to the gray matter of the brain.

The next layer, or cortex, is actually the surface of the brain itself. Each hemisphere of the brain has a convex superior surface, a convex lateral surface, a medial surface which is flat, and an inferior (or basal) surface which is irregular. The entire surface is covered with irregular, convoluted grooves and fissures called *sulci*. These surfaces, generally called the cortex, are further divided into 11 areas thought to control specific functions.

The *precentral cortex* (or motor area) includes the precentral gyrus, the posterior frontal gyri, and the giant pyramidal cells of Betz. This area is located on the superior surface of the hemisphere and controls voluntary muscle contraction. Removal of this area causes paralysis.

The *premotor areas* initiate head and eye movements, and the *suppressor areas* cancel motor activity innervated by the other areas. The *frontal area* exerts some control over circulation, respiration, and pupillary reaction. This is the area removed in the surgical procedure called lobotomy thought to improve severe psychotic problems.

The speech region (*Broca's area*) controls the ability to articulate speech. Motor aphasia can result from damage to this area.

The *postcentral area* receives stimulation from the spinal cord and controls the sensory areas of the body.

The visual sensory area (or *striate area*) integrates visual stimulation for size, form, motion, and color; the visual psychic, or *parastriate area* recognizes, integrates, and associates visual images with past experiences.

The *auditory sensory area* integrates sound stimulus into pitch, quality, and loudness; the *auditory psychic area* recognizes and integrates these sound stimuli with past experiences (see Fig. 17-3).

The *parietal area* integrates several types of stimuli from various sensory areas.

The innermost layer of the brain is called the *basal ganglia* and contains several layers which will not be described here.

The central white matter (or *centrum ovale*) is the layer beneath the cortex; it is composed of three types of fibers: *projection fibers, commissural fibers,* and *association fibers.* The projection fibers contain both afferent and efferent fibers that connect the cortex, brain, and spinal cord; the commissural fibers connect the two hemispheres through the corpus callosum, anterior commissure, hippocampal commissure, fornix commissure, and posterior commissure. The association fibers connect different portions of the cortex to each other.

The brain can also be divided by sections: the *cerebrum,* the *cerebellum,* the *pons,* and the *medulla oblongata* (see Fig. 17-4). An important part of the brain is its system of ventricles called *ventricles of the brain* which is located within several of these sections. The cerebrum occupies the greatest area within the *cranium* and is divided into two hemispheres joined by the *corpus callosum;* it contains three sections called the *telencephalon, diencephalon,* and *mesencephalon,* each of which contains important structures.

The telencephalon contains part of the walls of the third ventricle. The diencephalon contains the *thalamus, pineal body, hypothalamus,* and parts

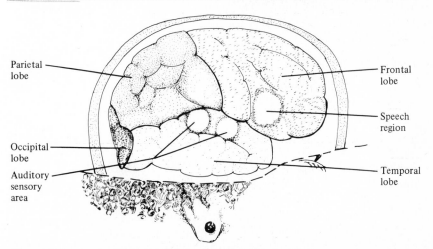

Figure 17-3 Areas of thought which control specific functions.

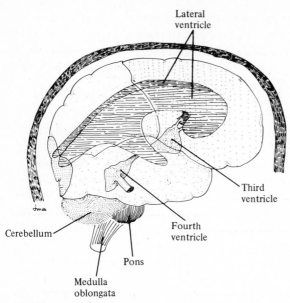

Lateral
ventricle

Third
ventricle

Fourth
ventricle

Cerebellum

Pons

Medulla
oblongata

Figure 17-4 Areas of the brain.

of the third ventricle. The thalamus is a large mass (about 4 cm) of gray matter, forming the lateral wall of the third ventricle which functions in the transmission of sensory impulses to the cortex. The pineal body lies posterior to the thalamus; its function is unclear but seems to be more active in childhood than in adult years. The hypothalamus is composed of gray matter and is located inferior to the thalamus. The *optic chiasm* is located in the hypothalamus, as are the mammillary bodies and a small bean-sized gland called the *hypophysis.* The hypothalamus has many functions, the most important of which are temperature control, water balance, and some visceral activities important in digestion.

The mesencephalon is a small constricted region joining the pons and cerebellum to the diencephalon.

The cerebellum is the next largest section of the brain. It is located between the occipital lobes of the cerebrum and the brainstem. The outer gray ridged cortex is divided into two lobes and covers a core of white matter. The cerebellum is important in the control of balance, movement, and posture.

The pons is a ventral protuberance of the brainstem. Several of the cranial nerves, such as the abducent, facial, trigeminal, and cochlear, arise in this area. Many descending and ascending nerve fibers come through the pons, and in general, it serves as a neural transmission center.

The medulla oblongata is a continuation of the spinal cord; it is tucked between the pons anteriorly and the cerebellum posteriorly. The rounded swelling on the anterior surface of the medulla contains the pyramid which holds many motor fibers. Some of these fibers cross the midline at the pyramidal decussation. The medulla performs many vital functions in addition to transmitting impulses along the spinal cord. It plays a major role in circulation and respiration; damage to this area often causes death. It also controls such activities as yawning, coughing, vomiting, and sneezing.

There are four ventricles of the brain: the two lateral ventricles, the third ventricle, and the fourth ventricle. A series of openings allow the cerebrospinal fluid to flow from ventricle to ventricle. The left and right lateral ventricles lie within the basal ganglia of the telencephalon. Fluid drains from these ventricles into the third ventricle via the *foramen of Monro*. The third ventricle lies midline between the right and left thalamus and communicates with the fourth ventricle via the *aqueduct of Sylvius*. The fourth ventricle lies in the cerebellum, pons, and superior portion of the medulla. The roof of the fourth ventricle contains three openings for spinal fluid to pass into the subarachnoid space. The brain and spinal cord are bathed in cerebrospinal fluid—a clear, watery liquid, which is formed in the ventricles, drains through the entire system of ventricles, and finally flows into the subarachnoid space.

The *spinal cord* is composed of a group of fibers running from the lumbar region to the medulla oblongata. Like the brain, it contains both gray and white matter. In the cord the gray matter forms two large lateral masses and one small midline strip that forms an H-shaped cross section. The areas are designated the *dorsal horn* (posterior column) and the *ventral horn* (anterior column). The dorsal horns receive and transmit impulses from the peripheral nerves to muscles. The lateral horns are composed of preganglionic fibers of the sympathetic nervous system along the thoracic and lumbar regions; in the sacral region, they comprise part of the sympathetic nervous system.

The white matter contains myelinated and unmyelinated fibers and, like the gray matter, is divided into sections (or fasciculi) according to location. The dorsal part consists of 2 large ascending fasciculi, 1 small descending fasciculus, and 1 intersegmental fasciculus. Its main functions are muscle, tendon, and joint *proprioception;* tactile sensation; and fine discriminatory sensation.

The ventral funiculus contains 2 ascending tracts and 5 descending tracts. They transmit impulses of touch and pressure, visual reflexes, eye and head movements, and muscle tonus and equilibrium. The lateral funiculus contains 10 tracts: 2 ascending and 8 descending. Proprioception, temperature, and pain impulses are transmitted via the lateral funiculus.

The peripheral nervous system consists of the cranial nerves, spinal nerves, and the autonomic nervous system. *Afferent (sensory) fibers* carry impulses from the organs to the central nervous system, while *efferent (motor) fibers* transmit impulses from the central nervous system to the organs.

There are 12 pairs of cranial nerves arising in the cranium.

1 Cranial nerve I: The *olfactory nerves* originate in the cranial cavity and emerge through the ethmoid bone into the nasal cavity. They terminate in a bundle of nerve fibers in the mucous membrane of the superior nasal tuberinates, and are needed for the sense of smell.

2 Cranial nerve II: Most of the *optic nerve* fibers originate near the thalamus, converge at the optic chiasm, cross and travel through the optic foramen into the retina. *hypothalmus*

3 Cranial nerves III: The *oculomotor nerves* arise near the floor of the third ventricle of the brain and innervate several of the muscles surrounding the eye. The control the movement of the eye within the socket.

4 Cranial nerves IV: The *trochlear nerves* are the smallest cranial nerves; they originate near the cerebral aqueduct; they innervate the obliquus superior oculi muscle of the eye and control ocular movement.

5 Cranial nerves V: The *trigeminal nerves* are the largest of the cranial nerves containing somatic sensory, special visceral, efferent, and proprioceptive fibers. They arise near the pons and middle cerebellar peduncle and innervate the sensory portions of the face, the mucous membranes, and internal structures of the head; they also supply the muscles of mastication.

6 Cranial nerves VI: The *abducent nerves* originate near the floor of the fourth ventricle and innervate the rectus lateralis bulbi muscle of the eye. Stimulation of these nerves causes the muscles to rotate the corneal surface of the eye laterally.

7 Cranial nerves VII: The *facial nerve* has two roots originating in the pons. The larger roots control facial expression while the smaller roots supply the front two-thirds of the tongue with the sensation of taste; they also innervate sections of the external acoustic meatus, soft palate, and pharnyx. From this root, parasympathetic fibers control secretions from the submandibular, sublingual, lacrimal, nasal, and palatine glands.

8 Cranial nerves VIII: The *acoustic nerves* are each composed of two fibers—the cochlear branch concerned with hearing and the vestibular branch concerned with sensory and equilibratory functions. The cochlear branch innervates the organ of Corti within the internal ear, and the vestibular branch innervates the internal acoustic meatus at its superior lateral end.

9 Cranial nerves IX: The *glossopharyngeal nerves* consist of sensory and motor fibers which innervate the tongue and pharnyx. They originate in the medulla oblongata.

10 Cranial nerve X: The *vagus nerves* are the longest of the cranial nerves; they originate in the medulla oblongata, wander through the neck and thorax, and terminate in the abdomen. Their somatic sensory fibers innervate the skin of the posterior surface of the external ear, and the external acoustic meatus, while the visceral afferent fibers control the mucous membrane of the pharynx, larynx, bronchi, lungs, heart, esophagus, stomach, kidneys, and intestines.

11 Cranial nerves XI: The *accessory nerves* originate in the medulla oblongata and each splits into the cranial section and the spinal section. The motor nerves of the cranial part innervate the pharynx, larynx, and esophagus. The motor nerves of the spinal section innervate the trapezius and sternocleidomastoid muscles.

12 Cranial nerves XII: The *hypoglossal nerves* originate in the medulla oblongata and supply the motor fibers of the tongue.

Leaving the spinal cord between the cervical area and coccygeal area are 31 pairs of spinal nerves. There are five main divisions each of which contains several subdivisions. The primary divisions are 8 cervical pairs, 12 thoracic pairs, 5 lumbar pairs, 5 sacral pairs, and 1 coccygeal pair. Each spinal nerve contains a dorsal (posterior) root and a ventral (anterior) root. The dorsal roots attach to the cord along the lateral surfaces and carry impulses up the spinal cord from the body. The ventral roots attach to the cord along the anterior surface and carry impulses from the cord to the muscles. There are four main types of fibers carried via the cord: somatic afferent, visceral afferent, somatic efferent, and visceral efferent. Somatic afferent fibers carry sensations for pain, temperature, touch, and sensations from the muscles and joints to the dorsal root of the spinal cord; visceral afferent fibers carry reflex impulses to the cord; somatic efferent fibers carry motor impulses from the ventral roots of the spinal cord to the voluntary skeletal muscles; and visceral efferent fibers carry motor impulses from the ventral roots of the spinal cord to the involuntary muscles of the viscera, secretory glands, and blood vessels.

The peripheral part of the autonomic nervous system is divided into the *sympathetic* (thoracolumbar) nervous system and the *parasympathetic* (craniosacral) nervous system. The two systems are frequently found in the same areas but are physiologically antagonistic toward each other. Generally, the sympathetic nervous system activates increased energy for bursts of activity, while the parasympathetic restores stability for quieter activity. The autonomic nervous system contains two types of fibers: visceral afferent and visceral efferent. The visceral afferent fibers carry impulses from the organs (mouth, pharynx, nose, thorax, etc.) to the central nervous system, while the visceral efferent fibers return impulses from the central nervous system to smooth muscles, cardiac muscle, and body glands.

The visceral efferent fibers of the thoracolumbar region and the sympathetic ganglia near the spinal cord form the sympathetic nervous system.

This system is divided into various branches and plexuses. The branches include spinal nerve branches, cranial nerve branches, arterial branches, and visceral branches. The plexuses (a tangle of nerves) include the cardiac plexus, the celiac plexus, and the pelvic plexus.

The visceral efferent fibers of the cranial and sacral portion of the spinal cord form the parasympathetic nervous system; its ganglia are located near specific viscera. As with the sympathetic system, the parasympathetic system is divided into various branches and plexuses.

WHERE TO EXAMINE

Like the nervous system itself, its examination encompasses all parts of the body, from the concentration of cranial nerves in the face and upper body to the permeation of the nervous network throughout the entire muscular system and body.

WHAT TO EXAMINE WITH

Although most of the neurologic examination depends on the clinician's skills and attentiveness, there are several pieces of equipment which may prove useful adjuncts (see Fig. 17-5). Many of these have already been mentioned in the preceding text. A reflex hammer of appropriate size (both a pediatric and adult size will be useful to the practitioner who deals with children from birth to 18 years). Even though the side of the hand can be used to obtain knee jerks, it is almost impossible when trying to obtain the triceps, biceps, or brachioradialis reflexes. Other necessary items for performing a complete neurologic examination are closed vials of peanut butter, orange extract, or other easily recognizable odors; as well as a safety pin; cotton balls; two test tubes filled with hot and cold water; a tuning fork; containers of salt and sugar and an applicator stick for applying them

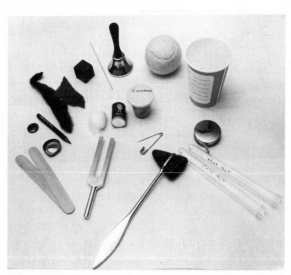

Figure 17-5 Equipment needed to do a complete neurological examination.

to the tongue; a tongue blade for obtaining the gag reflex; an ophthalmoscope; a tape measure for comparing symmetry of muscle pairs; some objects of various shapes and textures (coins, bottle caps, different types of material); and an audiometer or other instrument or means for assessing hearing.

HOW TO EXAMINE AND WHAT TO EXAMINE FOR

A complete neurological examination is rather complex and time consuming, and the nurse will probably not wish to include the total system in every physical examination. However, it is vital that the nurse be familiar with it, since it should be done if there is any questionable neurological history or significant physical findings. The nurse will always, however, wish to incorporate one test for each part of the neurologic examination into every physical; if these few items are questionable, a more extensive workup should be done.

Traditionally, the neurological examination is divided into six tests: tests for cerebral function, for cranial nerve function, for cerebellar function, for motor system function, for sensory system function, and for reflex actions. This outline works very well for adults and older children, but the nervous system of younger children is less mature and much more difficult to evaluate. The authors will follow the traditional outline in discussing the neurological examination, but will give specific references to the younger child and infant when possible.

Tests for Cerebral Function

Tests for cerebral function can be divided into those which test generalized types of functions and those which test specific functions. Generalized cerebral function is manifested in general behavior; level of consciousness, orientation, intellectual performance (including knowledge, judgment, calculation, memory, and thought content); and mood and behavior. These functions are more difficult to assess in a young child than in an adult.

Knowledge of normal development and previous knowledge of the child's behavior are the most important aids in evaluating generalized cerebral funtions. The one best test for these functions is a good developmental test. State of consciousness can be evaluated, although the important clues for a young child are primarily motor rather than verbal. (Is the infant or young child lethargic, drowsy, or even stuporous?) Excessive drowsiness, for instance, may indicate a metabolic problem, hypothalamic disease, or a diffuse brain tumor. Excitation or hyperactivity are also important. In the infant, orientation may be roughly assessed by recognition of the mother's face and later of familiar objects and people. Acute disorientation may result from inflammatory, toxic, metabolic, or traumatic brain disorders. Insidious loss of orientation may result from brain tumors. Generally, disorientation as to person or place is more serious than disorientation as to time. This is particularly true in children, since the time concept comes relatively late in the developmental sequence.

Immediate recall refers to brief retention of an idea, sound, or object. In general, a child of 4 years can be expected to repeat three digits or sounds after the examiner (e.g., "Johnny, see if you can say these numbers exactly as I do; now listen carefully '4 . . 2 . . 1'; OK; now you do it"). A child of 5 years can generally repeat four digits and a child of 6 years will usually be able to repeat five digits correctly. Loss of immediate recall is most often due to generalized cerebral disease or diseases of the primary projection area of the cortex. It is important to make sure that the child is neither too anxious nor failing to pay attention.

Recent memory refers to memory which is required to hold an idea or image slightly longer. The child is shown an object and told that he will be asked later to tell what it was. About 5 minutes later, the examiner should ask him to recall what the object was.

Remote memory refers to memory which holds for longer periods of time. The child may be asked what he had for dinner last night, for instance. An older child might be asked his address or birthday.

Specific functions of the cerebral cortex should also be tested when possible. There are three such localized functions. *Cortical sensory interpretation* refers to the ability to recognize objects through the different senses. *Cortical motor integration* refers to the integrative ability necessary to perform purposive, skilled acts. The lack of this ability is called *apraxia*. Finally, language both written and spoken is a specific function of certain areas in the cerebral cortex. In both spoken and written language the child is required to have the ability to communicate by receiving and expressing ideas or commands. Lack of any of these abilities is called *aphasia.*

Many tests for these abilities can be incorporated into the developmental screening examination. Others can be turned into games which the child will enjoy. The ability to recognize objects through the different senses, for instance, can be tested with various games. The game of "find it" can be played to detect difficulties in visual perception; "Johnny, we're going to play a game to see how good you are at finding things. I'm going to put these five things out on my desk and when I name one you have to hand me that very one. OK? Now, hand me the apple." The examiner must be careful not to have the child himself name the object, since this involves not only recognition, but expressive language skills. *Stereogenesis* is the ability to recognize an object from its feel. This can also be assessed through games; "Now, Joanne, we're going to play another game. When you close your eyes, I'm going to put one of these three things in your hand; then I'm going to take it back, and when you open your eyes you must tell me which one it is." Objects such as bottle caps, coins, and buttons work well for this purpose. Children with cerebral palsy have particular difficulty with this sense. Difficulties with this sense also may be due to peripheral neuropathy, parietal lobe disorders, or posterior column disease.

Graphesthesia is the ability to identify shapes traced by the examiner on the palm or back of the child's hand. School children will usually be able to identify the numbers 0, 7, 3, 8, and 1; younger children do better when the examiner draws either geometric figures or parallel and crossing lines. This is done twice and the child is asked whether they are the same or different. It is usually best to do this first with the child's eyes open and then with them closed, to make sure he or she understands the game. If the test is consistently failed or if there is a great difference between the ability of the two hands, the results are most suspicious. Very young children who are still having difficulty with the concepts of "same" and "different" will be difficult to test accurately.

Kinesthesia is the ability to perceive weight or direction of movement. Children under about 5 years of age are developmentally too immature to be able to compare weights, but school-aged children should be able to do so fairly well. The child's directional sense is tested by playing the "up, down game." The child closes her eyes and must tell the examiner whether her finger is up or down. The examiner passively manipulates the digits to either an up or down position. Care must be taken to handle the digit by the sides so that the weight of the examiner's fingers does not give a clue. The younger children will again be too immature to have the concepts of up and down. Texture discrimination can be tested in the "rough, smooth game," in which the child closes his eyes and tells the examiner whether a piece of cloth (wool or silk) is rough or smooth.

Auditory agnosia is tested for by having the child identify sounds, such as a bell, a hand clap, or a knock on wood, with his eyes closed.

Problems of visual agnosia usually originate in the occipital lobe; problems of auditory agnosia, in the lateral and superior portions of the temporal lobe; tactile agnosia, in the parietal lobe; and agnosia of body parts and relationships, in the posteroinferior areas of the parietal lobe.

Cortical motor integration is tested by having the child perform a semicomplex skill, such as folding a piece of paper and sealing it in an envelope. Again, the developmental level must be kept in mind, and this type of integration is usually evident when doing any of the standard developmental screening tests.

Language is also usually tested with a developmental screening device. In the younger child, only spoken language will be tested. Screening tests for both speech and articulation are important, and the nurse should be familiar with them. Articulation requires fine motor coordination and can reflect neurologic difficulties. Separate tests for receptive and expressive abilities of speech are best for the neurologic evaluation of a child.

Although speech cannot be evaluated in the very young infant, the quality of his cry can have great neurologic significance. The normal cry should be loud and angry sounding. A high-pitched, whiny cry may indicate a central nervous system disorder, while a shrill, penetrating, high-pitched cry may be a result of intracranial damage. A cry that sounds like a cat screeching, especially in combination with microcephaly, micrognathia, oblique epicanthal folds, hypertelorism, or low-set ears, may indicate a chromosomal defect called *cri-du-chat* (cat's cry) *syndrome.* A weak cry, hoarseness, or aphonia is another danger sign the examiner should be alert for.

This group of functions is closely related to specific areas of the cortex. *Visual receptive aphasia (alexia)* is influenced by lesions of the occipitotemporal junction, while defects in the superior temporal cortex may result in *auditory receptive aphasia.* The lateral part of the temporal lobe may produce *nominal aphasia,* or inability to name objects, while lesions above the Sylvian fissure may cause difficulties in expressive language, which may be discovered with a speech-screening test. Difficulties in the occipital cortex may cause *visual agnosia,* while problems with tactile perception may result from lesions in the contralateral parietal lobe. Defects located in the nondominant parietal lobe may cause graphesthesia (see above).

Tests for cerebral function are difficult to perform on the infant, although levels of consciousness and general behavior should always be assessed.

Assessment of Cranial Nerves

The next section of the neurologic examination is the assessment of cranial nerve function. There are 12 pairs of cranial nerves and their anatomic location has already been discussed. The method of evaluating their function will be discussed in this section.

The test for the first cranial nerves (olfactory nerves) is concerned with the sense of smell. The child is asked to identify familiar odors; peanut butter, oranges, or onions are a few which are usually familiar to young children. Each nostril is occluded in turn and closed vials of the peanut butter, orange, or onion extract are opened under the patient's nostril. Defects in either the olfactory bulb and tract or in the olfactory receptors in the nasal mucosa itself can interfere with smell. Many nonneurologic factors, such as colds or allergies, can also interfere with this sense. Some very young children may be able to smell accurately, but may not be able to name the smell.

The second cranial nerves (optic nerves) are tested first by visual acuity screening tests as discussed in Chapter 16 and also by the test for visual fields. In this test, the examiner asks the child to cover each eye in turn and look at the examiner's nose. It is very difficult to get small children to maintain their stare at the examiner's nose, and sometimes a bright sticker or other object stuck on the end of the nose will help the child keep the eyes focused steadily. While the child is looking at the nurse's nose, the nurse starts at the periphery of each quadrant of vision and brings a finger in towards the center, asking the child to say when he can first see the finger (see Fig. 17-6). The examiner should stand 3 feet away, keeping his or her own right eye closed when the child's left eye is closed. In this way, the nurse can compare his or her own visual fields with those of the child. The finger should be midway between the child and the nurse's own face. After assessing the limits of the child's visual fields, the nurse should recheck findings by asking the child to say when the nurse's finger is moving and when it is still. This should be done in eight positions: at 12 o'clock, 1:30 o'clock, 3 o'clock, 4:30 o'clock, 6 o'clock, 7:30 o'clock, 9 o'clock, and 10:30 o'clock. This procedure can be done more effectively if the examiner stands behind the child and slowly brings the finger from behind into the visual field of the child at each of these eight points. This method of assessing visual fields, however, necessitates a second person standing in front of the child to make sure the eyes do not move. Normally, visual fields extend

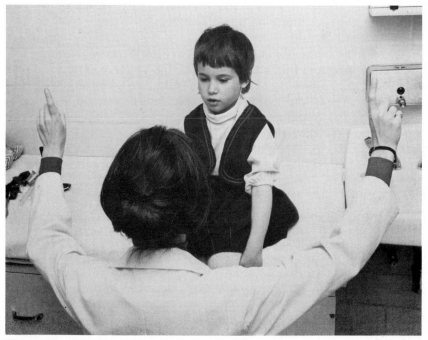

Figure 17-6 Examiner checking peripheral fields.

60° on the nasal side, 100° on the temporal side, and 130° vertically. This angle is estimated by counting the straight-ahead visual point as 0°. This would result in an object directly above, below or to either side of the head as being 90°. Care must be taken to repeat this test in all eight quadrants because specific defects will show up as very localized limitations of visual fields. For instance, a lesion of one optic tract will result in blindness in the opposite half of both visual fields, while defects in the temporal lobe may result in blindness in the upper quadrants on the side contralateral to the defect. A parietal lobe impairment can produce similar contralateral blindness in the lower quadrants of both eyes, while a lesion located in the occipital lobe may cause blindness in the contralateral half of each eye, both upper and lower quadrants. It is easy to see from this how important it is to test separately all quadrants of vision of each eye. The specific losses can also be important clues as to where a lesion is impinging on the optic tract. For instance, if a defect is seen in only one eye, the lesion is anterior to the optic chiasm; if it is on the temporal side of both eyes, the lesion is in or close to the chiasm; if the temporal half of one eye and the nasal half of the other eye show blindness, the lesion is posterior to the optic chiasm. Funduscopic examination can be included at this point, and is discussed earlier in Chapter 5, "The Eye."

Cranial nerves III, IV, and VI (oculomotor, trochlear, and abducent) can be tested as a unit, since they all supply the various muscles which rotate the eyeball; the oculomotor nerve supplies the superior rectus, inferior rectus, medial rectus, inferior oblique, and levator palpebrae, as well as the muscles of the iris and ciliary body; the trochlear nerve innervates the superior oblique; and the abducent controls the lateral rectus muscle. The child is asked to follow the nurse's finger as it moves to all 8 quadrants of vision. Any unequal movement of the pupils should be noted; at all times the pupillary light reflex should appear in corresponding spots on the two pupils. The eyes should also be observed for nystagmus. Very slight nystagmus, particularly at the far corners of the eyes, can be normal, but any sustained nystagmus should be referred. The pupillary examination, both direct and consensual, is also discussed in the chapter on the eyes.

The fifth cranial nerve (trigeminal nerve) has both a motor and a sensory division. The motor division innervates the masseter, temporalis, and pterygoid muscles, and its functions can be tested by asking the child to bite hard on a tongue blade while the nurse tries to pull it away; the jaw muscles are tense at this time and are palpated for symmetry and strength of contraction. Then, with the jaw relaxed and slightly open, the middle of the chin is tapped sharply with the reflex hammer. A sudden slight closing movement is the response expected in the normal child. This test is often difficult because it is hard for many children to relax their muscles when told to do so, and most will be unable to relax their jaws, thus invaldating the test. Further testing of these muscles can be performed by palpating the jaws when the child is asked to clench his teeth and evaluating symmetry of jaw strength or by pushing the lower jaw first to the left and then to the right, each time asking the child to resist the nurse's push and again evaluating how equal the strength is on both sides.

There are three parts of the sensory division of the fifth cranial nerve: the opthalmic, maxillary, and mandibular. All are tested through various sensations. Wisps of cotton, warm and cold test tubes, and the point of a pin are used on the forehead, cheeks, and jaw to test for presence of sensation. The child is asked to close her eyes and tell the examiner when the gremlin touches her. This is done in all three areas on both sides. Presence and symmetry of response are noted. The corneal reflex is also tested by touching the tip of a wisp of cotton to the cornea (see Fig. 17-7). The normal response is a blink. (Care must be taken to touch only the cornea.) Some examiners also touch the buccal mucosa inside the cheeks with a tongue blade to ascertain touch sensation in this area.

The seventh cranial nerves (facial nerves) also have both a sensory and motor division. The sensory division innervates the sense of taste on the anterior two-thirds of the tongue, part of the sensation from the external ear canal and also the lacrimal, submaxillary, and sublingual glands. The motor division innervates most of the facial muscles. It is tested in the game "make a face," in which the nurse asks the child to make exactly the same

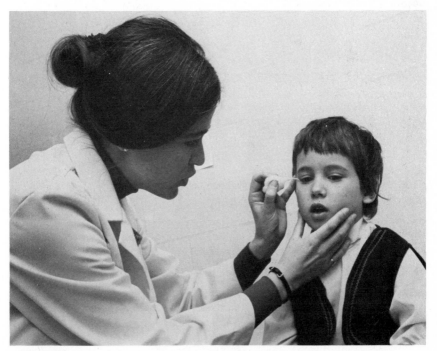

Figure 17-7   Examiner testing the corneal reflex with a wisp of cotton.

faces as he or she does; the nurse then looks at the ceiling, wrinkles the forehead, frowns, blows out the cheeks, purses the lips, smiles, and raises the eyebrows. The child's face is observed for any asymmetry that might indicate paralysis (minor asymmetry is almost always present and should be considered normal). The child is then asked to close his eyes and to keep them closed, even though the examiner will try to force them open. The examiner then pushes upward on the eyebrows while the child attempts to keep his eyes tightly shut. Equality of strength is noted. The sensory division can be tested by having the child stick out his tongue and to identify the taste of salt and sugar on the anterior sides of it. Some examiners also include sour substances (lemon juice or vinegar) and a bitter taste (quinine) but this is probably not necessary unless a sensory question exists about the function of these nerves (see Fig. 17-8). Care must be taken to have the child keep his tongue out until the testing of each substance is finished or the substances will dissolve and travel to both sides of the tongue. It is helpful to have these substances dissolved in water before applying them with a cotton swab to the tongue. A glass of water should be taken between the salt and sugar.

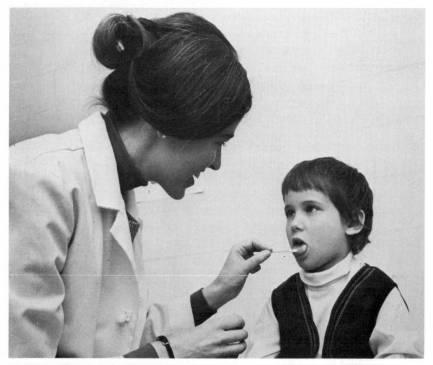

Fig. 17-8 Examiner testing child's taste for salt and sugar.

The eighth cranial nerve (acoustic nerve) also has two divisions, the cochlear and the vestibular. The test for vestibular function is not routinely performed. It involves injecting 5 to 10 ml of ice water into the ear canal. Vertigo and nystagmus are expected to occur. This test is impractical for the nurse-examiner and if there is any indication that it should be done, the child should be referred. The cochlear division of the acoustic nerve is concerned with acuity of hearing and sound conduction. An audiogram or hearing screening test should be done and the nurse should be familiar with this procedure (see Chapter 16). A tuning fork may also be used for the *Weber* and *Rinne tests* (see Fig. 17-9). In the Weber, the vibrating tuning fork is placed in the middle of the head and the child is asked if he hears it louder in either ear or if it is the same in both ears. Normally, it will be the same in both ears. This decision is frequently hard for a child to make, particularly if she does not yet have the "same-different" concept, and her response is not always reliable. In the Rinne test, the vibrating fork is placed first on the mastoid process behind the ear and the child is asked to tell the nurse when she can no longer hear the sound; at that point, the fork is brought around in front of the ear (not touching the child) and the child is asked if she can hear it then. Since air conduction should be about three times better than bone conduction, the child should reply that she does hear it when placed in front of her ear, even though the sound carried through the bone conduction from the mastoid process has stopped. This test seems to be easier than the Weber for most young children.

Cranial nerves IX and X (the glossopharyngeal and the vagus) are tested together. Both are involved in innervating the muscles in the mouth and throat area, although the distribution of the vagus extends further than this. The examiner should note any hoarseness of the voice, the ability to swallow, the movement of the uvula (when stoked with a tongue blade on each side of the uvula, it should rise and deviate to the stimulated side), the gag reflex and any dysarthria, dysphagia, or regurgitation of liquids through the nose.

Cranial nerve XI (accessory nerves) innervates the muscles of the upper shoulder. It is tested by checking the strength and symmetry of the sternocleidomastoid and trapezius. The child is asked to turn his head to one side; the examiner then pushes the child's chin in the same direction in which his head is turned while the child tries to push as hard as he can against this pressure. This will cause the sternocleidomastoid muscle on the opposite side to stand out, and it can be easily palpated. The process is then repeated on the other side. The trapezius is tested by having the child try to push the shoulders up against the examiner's hands while the examiner exerts pressure in a downward direction. Again, the muscles will tense and stand out where they can be easily inspected and palpated (see Fig. 17-10).

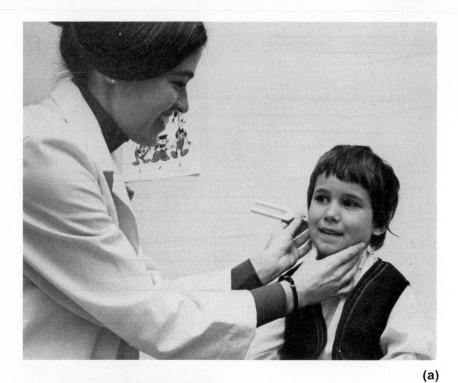

(a)

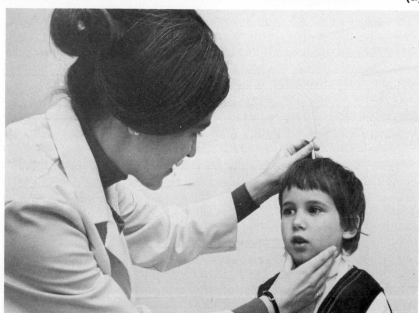

Figure 17-9   Examiner doing *(a)* the Rinne and *(b)* the Weber tests.   **(b)**

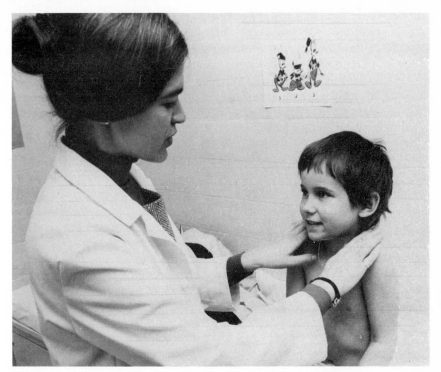

Fig. 17-10 Examiner testing the strength of the trapezius muscle.

Finally, the twelfth cranial nerve (hypoglossal nerves), which innervates the muscles of the tongue is tested by first asking the child to stick his tongue out as far as he can. it should be observed for tremors or fasciculations. The nurse then places the tongue blade against one side of the tongue and pushes it in the other direction, instructing the child to try to push the stick away. This is then repeated on the other side, and the symmetry of the muscle strength of each side of the tongue is assessed.

Most of these tests will be extremely difficult to do on the child under 2, although some symmetry of various muscles can be assessed by watching the child's movement. Even with an infant, some of the sensory tests, such as response to pain and touch, can sometimes be performed.

Tests for Cerebellar Function

The cerebellum functions primarily in regard to balance and coordination. In a child this may be reflected in the quality of skilled activity he is able to perform. A developmental screening tool may be the most effective way to assess this quality. Motor skills, such as dressing, undressing, and buttoning, can be observed, as can block stacking, putting a raisin in a bottle, and throwing and kicking a ball. Handling a pencil is also important. When he draws a plus sign (+), can he cross the midline in one movement, or must he stop at the middle and change the pencil to the other hand? This kind of detail can be important in assessing the neurologic status of a child.

Other specific tests also are used. Can the child touch his nose first with a finger of one hand, then with the other, and finally with each hand in succession while his eyes are closed? Can he touch his finger to his nose and then to the examiner's finger, back to his nose and again to the examiner's finger in a new position? This sequence is done more rapidly the second and third time. There are no exact standards for this test, which are age-specific, but consistent past-pointing should arouse suspicion. The nurse will gain a general idea of how well each age group is able to do this after working with many children (see Figs. 17-11 and 17-12).

The child can be asked to pat her knees with the palm of her hand and then with the back of her hand. Again, this should be repeated several times fairly rapidly (see Fig. 17-13).

He can also be asked to touch each finger to the thumb of the same hand in rapid succession (see Fig. 17-14). He can further be asked to run each heel down the contralateral shin and to draw a figure 8 in the air with his foot while lying on his back.

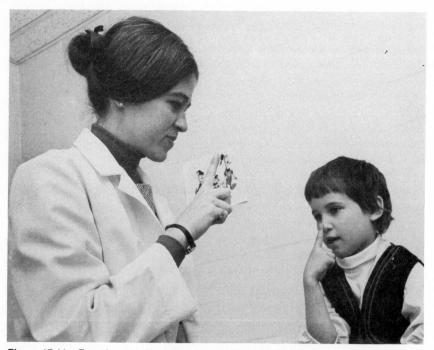

Figure 17-11 Examiner testing child with finger-to-nose test.

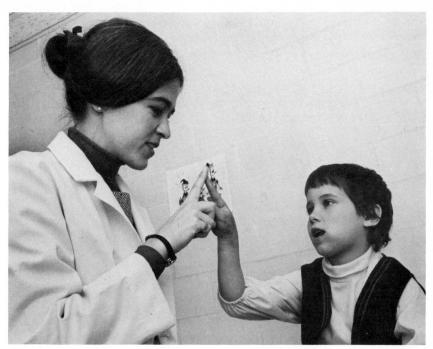

Figure 17-12 Examiner testing child with finger-to-finger test.

When erect, she can be asked to stand straight, with feet together and eyes open and then closed. Walking in her normal gait with her eyes open and then closed and finally walking tandem may also be helpful (see Fig. 17-15). Many types of abnormal gait may indicate neurologic problems. Lesions in the cerebellar lobe may cause staggering and falling. This is different from the gait in which the child lifts her feet very high, placing them down with great force; this kind of abnormality is usually due to posterior column disease. Toe drop in which extreme plantarflexion is present will cause a similar gait. Hemiplegia, scissors gait, and the broad-based gait of muscular dystrophy should all be noted, although they are not specifically due to cerebellar disease or malfunction. Any abnormal gait should be referred; in order to do this effectively, the nurse must be well aware of developmental changes in gait such as the wide-based gait of the new walker or the knock-kneed gait of the preschooler.

Standing on one foot is another test for cerebellar function which is often useful (see Fig. 17-16). By the age of 4, a child should be able to do this for about 5 seconds; by the age of 6 he should be able to do it for 5 seconds with his arms folded across his chest; and by 7 he should be able to do it for 5 seconds with his eyes closed. In an infant, cerebellar function is more difficult to evaluate, although coordination such as that seen in the

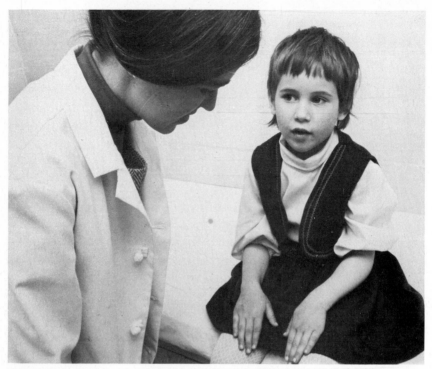

Figure 17-13 Child patting her knees with her hands.

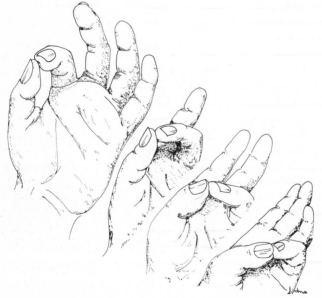

Figure 17-14 Child attempting finger-to-thumb test.

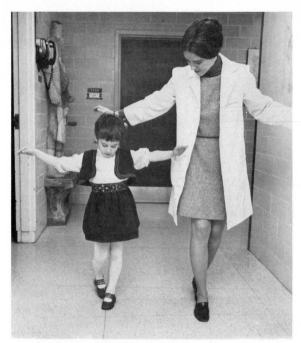

Figure. 17-15 Child walking tandem.

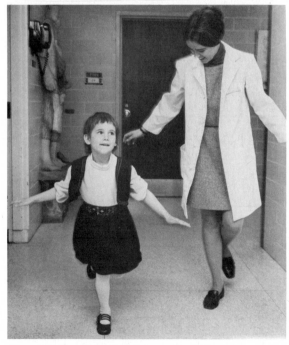

Figure 17-16 Child standing on one foot.

sucking-swallowing movements and reaching and grasping development, are important.

Tests for Evaluating the Motor System

Evaluation of the motor system is an important part of the neurologic examination. Particular attention is paid to four aspects of the motor system: muscle size, muscle tone, muscle strength, and abnormal muscle movements.

Muscle size should be assessed as part of the physical examination of all children. Either hypertrophy or atrophy of the muscles should alert the examiner to the possibility of muscular dystrophy, particularly if it is coupled with a wide-based gait, difficulty in going up or down stairs, muscle weakness, or the characteristic method in which children with muscular dystrophy arise from the recumbent position, that is, by placing their hands on their legs and literally climbing up themselves. Generalized wasting can result from anterior horn cell disease, while localized wasting accompanied by a characteristic "rubbery" feel to the muscle mass can occur with lower motor neuron disease. If there is any suspicion of abnormality in muscle size, corresponding muscles should be measured with a tape measure at comparable places of both limbs. Any but very slight asymmetry should be considered abnormal, and the child should be referred to a physician.

Muscle tone is next evaluated through both passive range of motion and active motion. During passive range of motion, any involuntary resistance, spasticity, flaccidity, or rigidity should be noted, as should an increase or decrease in the expected range of motion. Assessment of muscle tone can be one of the most valuable clues to neurologic difficulty in the infant. For the first 2 months, an infant's muscle tone is expected to be primarily of the flexor type. After 2 months, extension gradually becomes more pronounced, beginning with the head and extending slowly to the feet. As the child's muscles enter this stage of extension, spasticity may begin to appear in the case of an infant with cerebral palsy. Spasticity is one of the earliest signs of most types of cerebral palsy, and certain maneuvers should be routinely done in order to elicit early signs of spasticity. When the examiner pushes the infant's head forward, a child with beginning signs of cerebral palsy will frequently resist this pressure and extend his neck back against the examiner's hand. Another useful sign is for the examiner to flex the infant's legs onto his abdomen and then quickly release them. In an infant with cerebral palsy, the legs may jump quickly back into extension and then adduction, perhaps even crossing. Any kind of crossing of this type, frequently referred to as "scissoring," should make the examiner highly suspicious. Another sign often encountered in an infant in the early stages of cerebral palsy is that when it is in the prone position and the examiner lifts his head, the infant will fail to extend his arms in the protective mechanism most infants display.

Muscle tone in infants is often most obvious from abnormal posturing, and the physical examination of an infant should always be begun by observing his resting posture for a few minutes. The normal posture of a newborn is generally one of symmetry with limbs semiflexed and hips slightly abducted. The details will be influenced by the position he had assumed in utero. There are several abnormal postures which should serve as red flags to the examiner. The first of these is called the frog position in which the hips are held in abduction and are almost flat against the table while the hips are positioned in external rotation. This may be normal in a breech presentation, but in a vertex presentation, this should call for further neurologic investigation. It can be a sign of hypotonia, the so-called "floppy infant syndrome." Opisthotonus, the position in which the back is arched and the neck is extended, may also be normal if there was a face presentation at birth, but can have serious neurologic implications. Undue rotation of the head, extension of an arm, a hand held over the head, an infant who constantly holds both hands in front of the mouth, or a strikingly asymmetrical posture are examples of postures that may be clues to neurologic problems.

Muscle tone should also be assessed by holding the infant in certain positions. In ventral suspension, the examiner can support the baby with the hand held under the infant's chest, thus allowing an excellent view of the way the baby controls his head, trunk, arms, and legs (see Fig. 17-17). A full-term infant should be expected to hold his head at a 45° angle or less from the horizontal line; his back should be straight or slightly flexed, arms flexed at the elbows and partially extended at the shoulder, and knees partly flexed. The floppy infant will have greater head lag than normal, a limp, floppy trunk, and dangling arms and legs (see Fig. 17-18).

The examiner should pull the infant by his wrists from a supine position, lying on the table, to a sitting position. Even in premature infants,

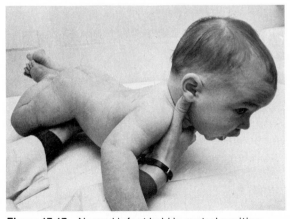

Figure 17-17 Normal infant held in ventral position.

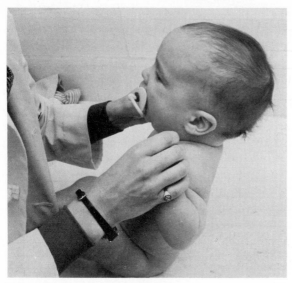

Figure 17-18   Testing for head lag in a normal newborn.

there will be some flexion of the head; usually in full-term infants, the head will be kept almost in the same plane as the body until the child reaches the sitting positon; at this point, the head will balance for a second or two in line with the body and then bounce forward. The head of a floppy baby will lag notably, and will never balance atop the neck. In view of the importance of muscle tone in the neurologic assessment of the infant, the two maneuvers just described should be routinely incorporated into every physical examination of a young infant.

Muscle strength is evaluated next. This is usually tested by having the child push against some resistance offered by the examiner (see Fig. 17-19). For instance, strength of the flexor muscles of the fingers may be estimated by extending the child's fingers while he tries to resist and keep them flexed. He is then asked to keep them straight even though the examiner will attempt to flex them. With his arms straight out in front of him, the examiner will try to push them apart while the child attempts to keep them together; then with the arms extended to either side, the examiner tries to push them together while the child tries to resist this movement. Strength of various muscle groups can be checked in this same general way. Some can be checked by active movement without resistance; for instance, strength of the abdominal muscles can be assessed by having the child do several sit-ups. Muscle strength in the infant and toddler is slightly harder to assess, but can be judged fairly well from the newborn's suck and general motor activity and later by the speed with which motor skills develop.

The last part of the assessment of the motor system involves observation of various abnormal muscle movements. Swift jerking movements may

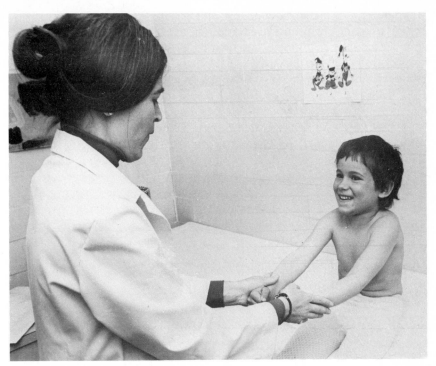

Figure 17-19 Examiner testing arm strength.

be associated with extrapyramidal syndromes, while the slow, worm-like, irregular movements may be a sign of athetoid cerebral palsy. Usually this type of movement does not develop until about the 18th month or so. Any kind of twistings, tics, choreiform movements, or tremors should be noted. Involuntary movements are more difficult to assess in the very young child, but an attempt should be made. Tremors are relatively common in the newborn, and if they are of high frequency and low amplitude, even though the child is not crying, they may be normal for the first few days. After the 4th day, this would be suspicious if it should occur anytime except during vigorous crying spells. Low-frequency, high-amplitude tremors are always suspicious, as are constant overshooting of movements, unusual rhythmic twitchings of the face, facial movements that seem to indicate paralysis, constant facial frowning, or tonic or clonic convulsions. Abnormal gaits have been previously discussed.

Tests for Evaluating the Sensory System

After an evaluation of the motor system, it is important to assess the sensory system. This is done in much the same way as when assessing the sensory division of some of the cranial nerves. There are two main divisions of tests used to assess the sensory system: those concerned with primary sensation and those concerned with cortical and discriminatory forms of sensation. In testing for primary sensation, all parts of the body can be tested, but a complete neurologic examination demands that at least the face, trunk, arms, and legs be tested and the borders of the various forms of sensation should be mapped out for each of them. At least five types of sensation can be tested: superficial tactile sensation, superficial pain, temperature, vibration, deep pressure pain, and some would include motion and position, which have already been discussed under the section on cerebellar functions. Normal sensitivity to superficial tactile sensation varies with the specific area of skin involved; therefore, symmetrical areas should be compared. With some types of damage to the sensory cortex, the child may be able to feel, but not be able to localize the feeling; it is wise, therefore, to have the child point to the spot where he feels the wisp of cotton, while keeping his eyes closed. Superficial pain should be tested by alternating the sharp and blunt ends of a pin and asking the child to tell you which it is with her eyes closed. In certain conditions, such as tabes dorsalis or peripheral neuritis, the child will at first perceive dullness and then have an afterimage of sharpness. Again, it is most important to compare sides. Sensitivity may be found to be normal, reduced, or increased, but there are no objective standards for this and the judgment must be made after the examiner has tested many children and becomes subjectively familiar with the range of normal. If there is a deficit, temperature will usually be found to be defective also, since distribution of these two senses is very similar. If the results of the tests for pain are equivocal, temperature will frequently be a more satisfactory standard. Temperature should be tested with test tubes filled with warm and cold water. The nurse must be careful to recheck frequently the temperature of the tubes, since the heat dissipates quickly.

The sense of vibration is also tested by means of a tuning fork, although it is really pressure receptors which are involved. The greatest sensitivity will be found between 200 and 400 cycles/second. A large tuning fork should be used since the vibration delay is slower than that of a small one, making it more useful. The sternum, elbows, knees, toes, and iliac crest should be tested. The examiner tells the child to say when the vibration stops. At that point, the examiner places the fork on his own body in an analogous area to see if he can still feel it. The patient's sides can also be compared in this way.

Deep pressure pain can also be tested. This should not be done unless there is definite indication that it is necessary, since rapport with the child frequently will be lost. Deep pressure pain can be tested over the eyeballs, testes, achilles tendon, and calf and forearm muscles.

Cortical and discriminatory forms of sensation can include two-point discrimination, point localization, texture discrimination, stereognostic sensation, graphesthesia, and the extinction phenomenon. In this discussion, the authors have chosen not to include texture discrimination, stereognostic sensation, and graphesthesia because they have been covered under cerebral functions.

Two-point discrimination is the ability to tell without visual clues whether there are one or two points pressing on the skin (see Fig. 17-20). In the "mosquito game," the child is asked to close the eyes and tell whether he feels two mosquitoes or only one. Body areas differ in how sensitive they are to two-point discrimination. For instance, the average person can first distinguish two separate stimuli on his tongue when they are only 1 mm apart; on the fingertip, the stimuli need to be 2 to 8 mm apart; on the chest and forearm the normal individual will first sense two separate points at a distance of 75 mm. These are adult standards; there have been no standards worked out specifically for children, but the authors' clinical experience suggests that the distances are probably similar.

Point localization is similar to two-point discrimination, except that only one point is used. The child is asked to close her eyes and point to the spot where she feels something touch her. This can be incorporated into the testing for primary sensation by having the child point to the spot where the test tube or wisp of cotton or pin touches her.

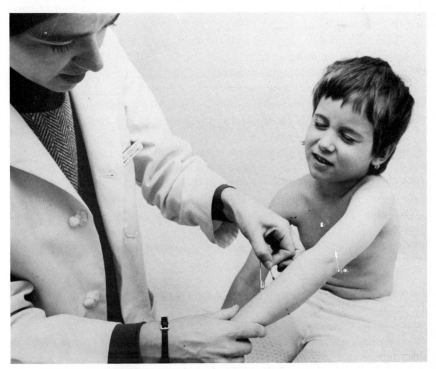

Figure 17-20 Examiner testing for two-point discrimination.

Finally, the extinction phenomenon is tested. This is the situation in which two homologous parts are touched simultaneously; the child should be expected to know that there are two separate spots. Certain defects in the parietal lobe will cause the individual to experience only one stimulus even though two separate places are actually touched. The nurse should touch either the child's hand or cheek or both several times while his eyes are closed. He should be able to respond by telling where the touch is felt. For developmental reasons, this test is not always accurate under 6 years of age.

It is obvious that all these tests can easily be made into games and the children usually enjoy them immensely.

Very little of this testing is applicable to toddlers and infants. At times one can tell if a child this age responds to pain and touch but, in general, testing is unreliable.

Assessing the Reflexes

The final traditional division of the neurologic examination to be discussed in this section is the assessment of reflexes. Reflexes are specific muscular responses to specific stimuli. They can be of various types. For adults and older children, they can be divided into three types: superficial, deep, and abnormal. For infants and very young children, some additional miscellaneous reflexes will be discussed.

There are many superficial reflexes, and four common examples will be given here. The abdominal reflexes are four in number. They consist of a movement of the abdominal musculature in the direction of a stimulus. They are obtained by stroking the four quadrants surrounding the umbilicus lightly with a pin or sharp point. This can be done in such a way that the scratches form either a square or a diamond on the abdomen (see Fig. 17-21). The expected response is for the umbilicus to move toward the quadrant which was stroked. In a newborn infant, this response is usually weak the first 2 days, but almost always present for the first 10 days. In general, however, there is a great variability in this response and total lack does not indicate a pathologic condition. Asymmetry of response can be a danger sign, but in the clinical experience of the authors, asymmetry is frequently seen, probably as a result of an asymmetrical stimulus.

The cremasteric reflex is another superficial reflex relevant only in boys. The stimulus consists of stroking an inner thigh with a sharp object such as a pin. The expected response is for the testis on that side to be drawn from the scrotum up into the abdomen. This is a fairly reliable reflex, and its absence should make the investigator think of conditions such as spinal cord lesions. This response can also be elicited by cold or fear.

The plantar grasp reflex consists of a plantar flexion of the feet in response to the stimulus of pressure against the balls of the feet. This

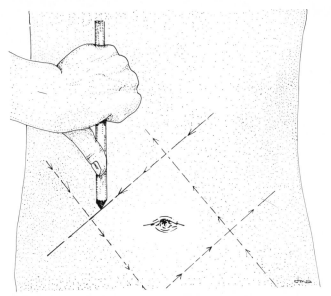

Figure 17-21 Examiner testing abdominal reflexes.

sometimes is elicited by mistake when the examiner attempts to elicit a Babinski reflex on a young infant. The plantar grasp reflex can also be absent as a result of spinal cord lesions. It is normally present until about 3 months of age.

The final example of a superficial reflex is the gluteal reflex. To obtain this, the nurse spreads the buttocks of the child and scratches the perianal area. The expected response is a quick contraction of the anal sphincter. If it causes low back pain, the examiner should worry about compression of the cauda equina.

Deep tendon reflexes are theoretically possible in any large muscle area; when the tendon is struck, contraction of the muscle is expected. Only the five most common reflexes will be discussed here: the biceps, triceps, brachioradialis, Achilles, and patellar. The biceps reflex is obtained by flexing the child's arm over the examiner's arm while the examiner's thumb is pressed against the biceps tendon in the antecubital space (see Fig. 17-22). A tap of the reflex hammer onto the examiner's thumb should result in a quick, sharp contraction of the biceps. The triceps reflex is elicited again with the child's arm in the flexed position. This time, the reflex hammer is struck directly onto the triceps tendon behind the elbow (see Fig. 17-23). The authors find this reflex easiest to elicit if the child's upper arm is held straight out from the body and his lower arm is allowed to dangle loosely

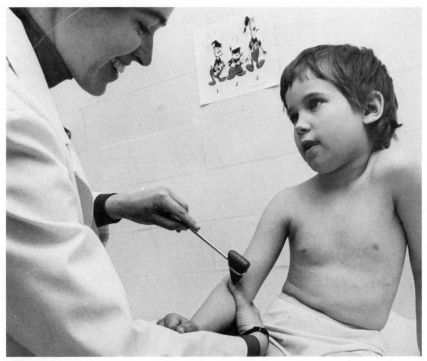

Figure 17-22 Examiner testing the biceps reflex.

toward the floor. The expected response is contraction of the triceps, which should extend the elbow. The brachioradialis reflex is initiated by a sharp tap of the reflex hammer to the styloid process of the radius; this should result in flexion of the elbow and pronation of the forearm (see Fig. 17-24). The patellar reflex is obtained by striking the tendon immediately below the patella (see Fig. 17-25). This should result in extension of the knee, with a kicking action. This reflex can be strengthened by having the child lock the fingers of both hands and pull as hard as he can in an outward direction. Finally, the Achilles reflex is obtained by tapping the Achilles tendon while the child's foot is held in the examiner's hand (see Fig. 17-26). Plantar flexion of the foot is expected. If the nurse-examiner has difficulty in obtaining the desired response, she should try different spots on the Achilles tendon and vary the degree of flexion of the child's foot.

All reflexes should be evaluated as to their symmetry and strength, but there are some reflexes which just by their presence indicate abnormality. One of the most useful in older children is the Babinski reflex. The stimulus for the Babinski reflex is stroking the lateral aspect of the sole of the foot with a relatively sharp object, such as a pinpoint or fingernail (see Fig.

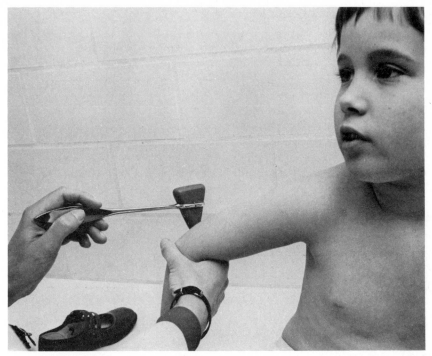

Figure 17-23 Examiner testing the triceps reflex.

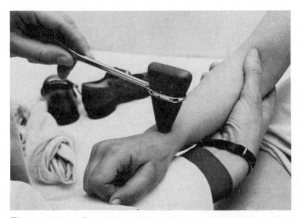

Figure 17-24 Examiner testing the brachioradialis reflex.

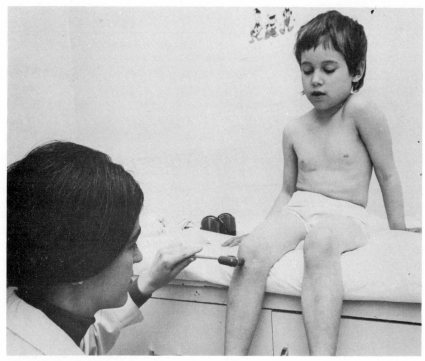

Figure 17-25 Examiner testing the patellar reflex.

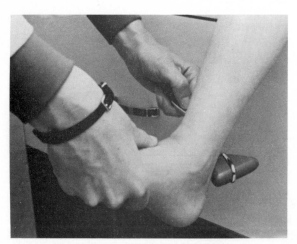

Figure 17-26 Examiner testing the Achilles reflex.

17-27). The stroke should begin at the heel, come up toward the little toe and across toward the big toe. The normal response is an incurving of the toes toward the stimulus. The abnormal response is a fanning of the toes, particularly of the big toe. Fanning is abnormal only after the child has begun to walk. This is a very significant reflex when it can be elicited. As pointed out before, however, the difficulty is that particularly on a young child the pressure used when applying the stimulus may cause the plantar flexion reflex to be elicited, thus invalidating the response. The other abnormal reflexes elicit the same response as the Babinski, but different stimuli are used. The Chaddock reflex is elicited by stroking the lateral aspect of the foot directly under the lateral malleolus; the Oppenheim reflex is elicited by running the thumb and index finger briskly down the anteromedial surface of the tibial bone; and the Gordon reflex is elicited by tightly squeezing the belly of the calf muscle; the responses to all these reflexes are evaluated in the same way as the Babinski reflex.

These reflexes are also useful in assessing toddlers and infants; however, in infants, there are a host of other reflexes. Results of most of them are quite variable, and their usefulness is as yet not certain. However, a brief description of each will be given here along with a discussion of what is known about their significance when this is applicable.

Chvostek's reflex is elicited by briskly tapping the index finger over the parotid gland. In certain conditions, such as tetanus and hypoglycemia, or in infants born of diabetic mothers, a facial twitching may occur.

The lip reflex is elicited by tapping the upper or lower lip sharply; the expected response is for the lips to pouch out or protrude. This response is impossible to achieve if the infant is crying or sucking.

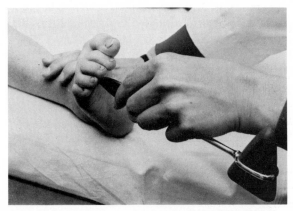

Figure 17-27 Examiner testing the Babinski reflex.

The glabella reflex is obtained by tapping briskly on the glabella (the bridge of the nose). Normally the eyes will close tightly. The examiner should watch for lack of symmetry, possibly indicating paralysis.

The optical blink reflex can be elicited by shining a light suddenly at the baby's open eyes. The eyes should shut quickly, often accompanied by a quick dorsal flexion of the head. Absence of this response may indicate poor or no light perception.

The acoustic blink reflex is similar, but is elicited by a loud clap of the examiner's hands about 30 cm from the child's head. Care should be taken to avoid producing an air current which will strike the face. This is often hard to elicit the first 2 or 3 days of age, and if there is no response, it should be repeated a few days later. If there is still no response, the question of auditory problems arise. Because the infant quickly gets used to this clapping after two or three times, he can be expected to fail to respond if the stimulus is continued.

The tonic neck reflex is one of the more important reflexes. It can be considered both a posture and a reflex. The posture consists of turning the face to the side with the jaw over one shoulder. The arm and leg on the jaw side (the side toward which the face is pointing) will extend while the opposite arm and leg flex (see Fig. 17-28). This is the classic "fencer position." If the child is not lying in this position, the maneuver of turning his head to the extreme right or left should elicit it. This response will sometimes be present at birth, but its peak incidence is at about 2 to 3 months. An infant who never exhibits it should not be considered abnormal. The nurse should worry, however, about a child who displays this behavior constantly, particularly before 2 to 3 months of age, and who seems "locked" into this position. She should also worry if it lasts to a very late age; it would certainly be considered abnormal past 6 months, and if it were seen very often at 4 or 5 months, suspicion should be aroused. While a child is in this position, it is impossible for her to grasp with the arm extended toward the face side, and, of course, she cannot see the arm that is behind her head. Consequently, it is almost impossible for her to develop eye-hand coordination. It also seems to be impossible for most of these babies to bring their hands to midline or into their mouths; consequently they are not usually able to roll over. The developmental ramifications of this problem are obvious.

Recoil of the arm is also an important reflex. To elicit this, the examiner should extend both of the infant's arms simultaneously by pulling them out by the wrists. The examiner then quickly lets go and observes the response. Normally, both arms should flex briskly at the elbows; this response should be strongest in the first 2 days of life, but it should persist through the entire neonatal period. The examiner should watch for asymmetry. In hypotonic or apathetic babies, there may be no response at all.

An attempt should also be made to elicit ankle clonus. This is done by pressing the thumbs sharply against the soles of the infant's feet, dorsiflex-

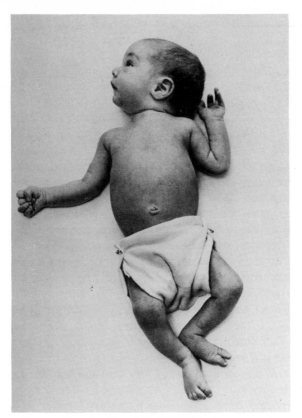

Figure 17-28 An infant displaying the tonic neck reflex. (*Source: Mead Johnson, A Clinical Review of Concepts and Characteristics in Infant Development, vol. II, p. 1, 1972.*)

ing the entire foot. The examiner then quickly releases this pressure and watches for clonus. Minor clonus may be normal, but any sustained clonus is suspect and further investigation is necessary.

The palmar grasp reflex is also tested. The examiner's fingers are pressed into the infant's palms from the ulnar side, being careful that the dorsal side is not stimulated. The normal response is for the infant's hands to grasp the examiner's fingers. The examiner should watch for symmetry, being careful that the baby's head is in midline or a normal asymmetry may be felt. If the response is weak, the examiner should get the infant to suck, since sucking facilitates the grasp. This response is weaker during the first 2 days, and then becomes and remains strong until about 3 months. It should then gradually be replaced by a voluntary grasping.

A magnet reflex is elicited by light pressure to the soles of the feet. The legs should extend toward the pressure while the examiner inspects for asymmetries. This response may be absent in cases of lower spinal cord damage or may be weak with a breech presentation with flexed legs or in babies with sciatic nerve damage. A breech presentation accompanied by extended legs may have a stronger magnet response. This response may be normally more difficult to elicit in the first 2 days.

The crossed extensor reflex is obtained by extending one leg passively while pressing the knee of that leg to the table. With a pin, the sole of this foot is pricked. The response expected is for the other leg to extend and adduct slightly. This reflex is weak the first 2 days, but fairly constant after that; it may be absent in infants with spinal cord lesions and may be weak in those with peripheral nerve damage.

The withdrawal reflex is elicited by pricking the soles of the feet, one at a time. The leg of the foot which is pricked will flex at the hip, knee, and ankle. This response should be constant for the first 10 days, but it may be absent in cases of damaged spinal cords and weak in babies who have sciatic nerve damage or in those who have been delivered by breech presentation with their legs extended (in this case, the response may even be reversed and the baby will be seen to extend his leg rather than withdraw it). Again, asymmetries should be watched for.

The rooting reflex is well known to nurses. When the corners or the middle of the upper or lower lip are touched, the head should turn in the direction of the stimulation. If the upper lip is touched, the mouth should open and the head bend backward; if the lower lip is touched, the mouth should open while the lower jaw drops. The baby will often turn in the other direction when satiated. This response will usually be less vigorous the first 2 days of life, but if it is absent later, suspicion should be aroused that the baby may be in a depressed state, particularly if barbiturates have been used by the mother.

Sucking is another well-known reflex and vital to life. While the infant sucks on the examiner's finger, four aspects of the sucking reflex should be noted. The action of the tongue should be felt to push the finger up and back, the rate should be fairly good, the pressure or strength should be noted, and the pattern of grouping in the suck should be noted. This is less intense in the first 3 to 4 days. Barbiturates, sometimes transmitted in the breast milk, will depress sucking.

The masseter reflex is elicited by placing one index finger on the lower chin of the infant and tapping it sharply with the index finger of the other hand. A quick contraction of the masseter muscle will lift the chin; this can frequently be felt better than it can be seen. It will normally be weak in the first 2 days, but should be present for the first 10 days; its absence may mean brainstem lesions or lesions of the fifth cranial nerve.

The Moro reflex is probably the most important reflex in the young infant and should always be tested (see Fig. 17-29). There are several ways of eliciting a response, but the most effective way is to hold the baby by supporting the trunk with one hand (the baby is lying on his back) and supporting the head and neck with the other hand. When the neck is relaxed, the head is dropped backward a few centimeters. The expected response is an abduction of the arm and shoulder; an extension of the arm at the elbow; an extension of the fingers, with a C formed by the thumb and index finger; and later, an adduction of the arm at the shoulder. The response may have to be repeated three or four times for the examiner to be able to observe all components. It is expected to be present from birth to 3 or 4 months. If it lasts longer than 4 months, one should suspect a neurologic defect; if it lasts longer than 6 months, it should definitely be considered abnormal. It may be absent in the first weeks if there has been heavy sedation or cerebral trauma. If the response is present and then disappears, it may be one of the earliest signs of kernicterus. Again, the practitioner should watch for asymmetry.

Bauer's reflex is elicited with the infant lying prone. The examiner presses gently on the soles of the feet, and the baby should attempt to make crawling movements. This is difficult to get in the first 2 to 3 days.

Galant's reflex is seen when the examiner scratches a pin along the side of the spinal column, about 3 cm from midline, from the shoulder to buttocks (see Fig. 17-30). The trunk should curve to the side of the scratch. If there is a spinal cord lesion, there will be an absence of response below the level of the lesion. This response is easiest to obtain at about 5 to 6 days of age.

The placing reflex may be difficult to elicit in the first 4 days. The examiner holds the baby upright in such a way that the dorsal side of the foot is gently touching the edge of the table. The infant's knees and hips should flex and the foot should rise and be placed on the table. This response is absent in paralysis.

The stepping reflex is similar but has some differences. With the baby upright, the soles of the feet should touch the table surface. Alternating stepping movements should result. This is harder to elicit in the first 2 to 3 days and fades about the third or fourth week. It may be absent with breech delivery or with depression.

The rotation test is also done with the baby in the upright position facing the examiner. The examiner then spins around in such a way that she and the baby are spinning together in first one direction and then the other. When the baby's head is not held, it should turn in the direction toward which the baby is turning. When the head is restrained, the eyes should turn in that direction (the "doll's eye maneuver"). This is a vestibular reflex and may be abnormal if a vestibule of the ear is defective or a muscle paralysis exists.

The Landau reflex is obtained with the baby's abdomen supported on the examiner's hand, and his head and legs extending over either side of the hand. From 6 to 8 months until 3 years of age, the expected response is for

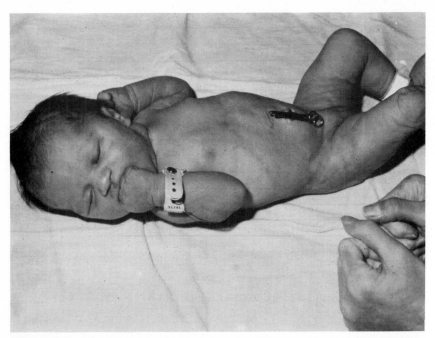

(a)

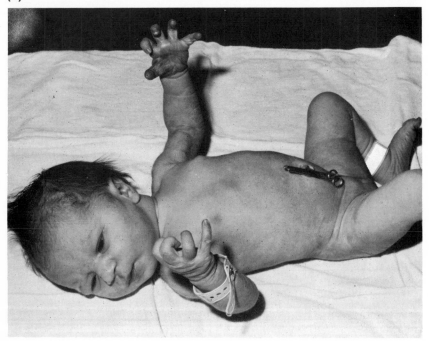

(b)

Figure 17-29 (a and b) An infant demonstrating a complete Moro reflex. (*Source: Clausen et al., Maternity Nursing Today, pp. 676, 677, and 679. Reproduced by permission of the publisher.)*

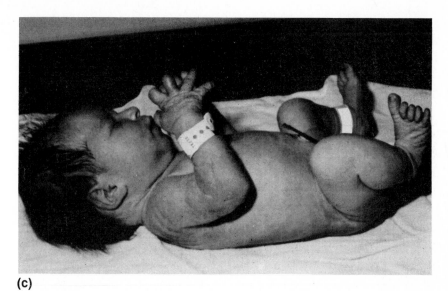

(c)

Figure 17-29 (c) An infant demonstrating a complete Moro reflex. (*Source: Clausen et al., Maternity Nursing Today, pp. 676, 677, and 679. Reproduced by permission of the publisher.*

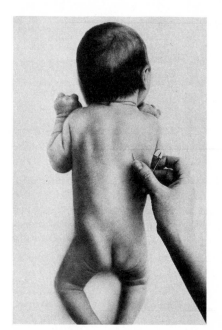 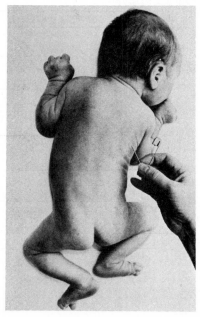

Figure 17-30 The examiner testing Galant's reflex. (*Source: Mead Johnson, A Clinical Review of Concepts and Characteristics in Infant Development, vol. II, p. 3, 1972.*)

the child to lift his head and extend his spine and legs. Lack of this response may be an indication of cerebral palsy.

The parachute reflex is one in which the infant is held prone and lowered slowly toward a surface. Normal babies will try to protect themselves by extending their arms and legs; children with cerebral palsy will often fail to do this. This response is normally present from 4 to 6 months on.

Positive supporting reactions are also important reflexes. When the ball of the foot touches the table, the baby will usually extend his legs and bear some weight. Infants who do extend their legs, but also cross them should be suspected of being afflicted with cerebral palsy.

Another important reflex is the neck righting reflex which is elicited by turning the head to one side. Normally, the body should follow in this same direction anytime between the age of 3 months and 3 years. Many children with cerebral palsy cannot execute this maneuver and, consequently, never learn to turn over.

The protective side turning reflex is elicited by placing the baby in the prone position with the head in midline. Normal babies will protect themselves by turning their head to the side. Certain children with early signs of cerebral palsy will fail to do this.

Neurological "Soft" Signs

No discussion of a neurologic examination could be complete without mention of the "soft" signs so frequently referred to in pediatric neurology. Yet such a discussion is very difficult because of the controversy that exists in the literature regarding such signs. Different clinicians define these signs differently, and, in fact, some do not believe that they exist at all. Even those who believe they do exist do not agree as to exactly what they are or what they mean. In general, the term is used to refer to signs which are minimal and whose significance is not known. Clumsiness, hyperkinesis, language disturbances, perceptual developmental lags or inconsistencies, motor overflow, mirroring movements of the extremities (e.g., when one hand performs a motor task, the child cannot keep the other hand still), mixed or confused laterality, articulation defects, disturbance in balance, and short attention span are all examples of specific signs which some clinicians consider "soft." If these are associated with school difficulties, further investigation is necessary. Usually such problems appear in preschool children; if these signs are indeed predictions of future school problems, it would be desirable to intervene at that point. Although many clinicians feel this is the case, it certainly has not been firmly proved. The nurse-practitioner will probably want to read some of the articles in the bibliography and decide what his or her own policy will be in this regard.

BIBLIOGRAPHY

Alexander, M, and M. Brown: "Physical Examination: Neurological Examination," *Nursing '76,* vol. 6, no. 7, pp. 50–55, July 1976.

Mechner, Francis: *"Patient Assessment: Neurological Examination,"* *American Journal of Nursing,* vol. 75, no. 11, pp. 1–24, September 1975.

GLOSSARY

abducent nerves   the sixth cranial nerves which innervate the rectus lateralis muscle of the eye and cause the eye muscles to rotate laterally

accessory nerves   the eleventh cranial nerves which innervate parts of the pharynx, larynx, esophagus, trapezius, and sternocleidomastoid muscles

acoustic nerves   the eighth cranial nerves composed of a cochlear branch concerned with hearing and a vestibular branch concerned with sensory functions and equilibrium

aqueduct of Sylvius   the drainage system communicating between the third and fourth ventricle

arachnoid   a web-like, avascular membrane lying between the dura mater and the pia mater, separated from the dura mater by the subdural space and from the pia mater by the subarachnoid space

association fibers   a group of fibers in the centrum ovale which connect different portions of the cortex to each other

auditory psychic area   the area of the brain involved in recognizing and integrating sound stimuli with past experience

auditory sensory area   that area of the brain involved in integrating sound stimuli into pitch, quality, and loudness

axon   an extension of a neuron whose function is to transmit impulses from the cell body outward to the rest of the body

basal ganglia   the innermost layer of the brain

Broca's area   that region involved in controlling the ability to articulate speech

central nervous system   the part of the nervous system comprising the brain and spinal cord

centrum ovale (white matter)   the layer of the brain directly beneath the cortex which contains projection fibers, commissural fibers, and association fibers

cerebellum   the second largest part of the brain located between the occipital lobes of the cerebrum and the brainstem which functions in controlling balance, movement, and posture

cerebrum   the largest portion of the brain, containing the two hemispheres

commissural fibers   a group of fibers in the centrum ovale which connect the two hemispheres through the corpus callosum, anterior commissure, hippocampal commissure, fornix commissure, and posterior commissure

corpus callosum   that part of the brain which connects the two hemispheres of the cerebrum

cortex   the outer layer of an organ; the outer layer of the brain

cranium the bony encasement of the brain; the skull

dendrite one of several extensions from the neuron whose function is to receive impulses and transmit them to the cell body

diencephalon that part of the cerebrum which contains the thalamus, pineal body, hypothalamus, and parts of the third ventricle

dura mater tough, fibrous connective tissue which lies directly beneath the periosteum of the cranium

encephalon the brain

facial nerves the seventh cranial nerves which innervate the anterior two-thirds of the tongue, the external acoustic meatus, soft palate, and pharynx, as well as the secretions from the submandibular, sublingual, lacrimal, and palatine glands

glossopharyngeal nerves the ninth cranial nerves which innervate the tongue and pharynx

hypoglossal nerves the twelveth cranial nerves which innervate the tongue

hypothalamus a small mass of gray matter located directly beneath the thalamus whose functions are involved in temperature control, water balance, and some digestive activities

medulla oblongata a continuation of the spinal cord located between the pons and the cerebellum, which serves to transmit impulses to the spinal cord and is concerned with circulation and respiration

medulla spinalis the spinal cord

meninges the three membranes covering the brain and spinal cord

mesencephalon that small, constricted region of the cerebrum which joins the pons and cerebellum to the diencephalon

myelinated describing or pertaining to certain nerves which are protected by a myelin sheath

neuron the basic unit of the nervous system

oculomotor nerves the third pair of cranial nerves involved in the movement of the eye within its socket

olfactory nerves the first cranial nerves involved in the sense of smell

optic nerves the second cranial nerves involved in vision

parastriate area (visual psychic area) that area of the brain involved in recognizing, integrating, and associating visual images with past experiences

parietal area that area of the brain involved in integrating several types of stimulation from various sensory areas

peripheral nervous system the autonomic nervous system composed of the sympathetic and parasympathetic systems

pia mater the deepest layer of the meninges, composed of delicate highly vascular tissue, which attaches directly to the gray matter of the brain

pineal gland a small gland lying posterior to the thalamus which is more active in childhood than in adult years, and whose exact function is unknown

pons a ventral protuberance of the brainstem, which serves as a neural transmission center

postcentral area the area of the brain which receives stimuli from the spinal cord and controls the sensory area of the body

precentral cortex (motor area) that area of the surface of the brain, located on the superior portion of each hemisphere, which controls voluntary muscle contraction

premotor area the area of the brain involved in suppressing motor activity as well as exerting some control over circulation, respiration, and pupillary reaction

projection fibers a group of afferent and efferent fibers in the centrum ovale which connect the cortex, brain, and spinal cord

proprioception the awareness of one's own bodily posture and movement

striate area that area of the brain involved in integrating visual stimuli for size, form, motion, and color

telencephalon that portion of the cerebrum which contains part of the wall of the third ventricle

thalamus a large mass of gray matter forming the lateral wall of the third ventricle, which functions in the transmission of sensory impulses to the cortex

trigeminal nerves the fifth cranial nerves which innervate the sensory portions of the face, the mucous membranes, and internal structures of the head as well as the muscles of mastication

trochlear nerves the ninth cranial nerves which innervate the obliquus superior oculi muscles of the eye and control ocular movement

unmyelinated a term referring to certain of the nerves which are not protected by a myelin sheath

vagus nerves the tenth cranial nerves which innervate the skin of the posterior surface of the external ear, the external acoustic meatus, the pharynx, larynx, bronchi, lungs, heart, esophagus, stomach, kidneys, and intestines

ventricles of the brain a system of small cavities in the brain, consisting of two lateral ventricles, a third ventricle, and a fourth ventricle

Neuromuscular Examination: Cerebral Function*

Generalized function	Yes	No	Not appli-cable	Describe (where appropriate)	Significance
Normal developmental level					
Normal developmental behavior					
Normal state of consciousness					
Normal immediate recall					
(4-year-old can remember 3 digits) (5-year-old can remember 4 digits) (6-year-old can remember 5 digits)					Any abnormality requires a complete neurological examination. If the complete examination reveals several abnormalities a referral to a physician is indicated.
Normal recent memory (about 5 min)					
Normal remote memory					
Specific functions					
Cortical sensory interpretations					
Normal stereogenesis bilaterally					
Normal graphesthesia bilaterally					

	Yes	No	Not applicable	Describe (where appropriate)	Significance
Normal kinesthesia bilaterally					
Normal texture discrimination bilaterally					
Normal auditory discrimination bilaterally					Any abnormality requires a complete neurological examination. If the complete examination reveals several abnormalities a referral to a physician is indicated.
Normal cortical motor integration					
Normal language development (spoken)					
Normal language development (written)					

Neuromuscular Examination: Cranial Nerves

	Yes	No	Not applicable	Describe (where appropriate)	Significance
I Olfactory					
Identifies smells bilaterally					
II Optic					
Normal visual acuity					Any abnormality requires a complete neurological examination. If the complete examination reveals several abnormalities a referral to a physician is indicated.
Normal visual fields					
60° nasally					
100° temporally					
130° vertically					

*These charts are meant to be used by beginning students as they perform their first physical assessments. Each item should be examined on the child and then checked off on the checklist. The significance of the items follows in the right-hand column.

Neuromuscular Examination: Cranial Nerves

III, IV, VI Oculomotor, trochlear, and abducent	Yes	No	Not applicable	Describe (where appropriate)	Significance
Pupillary constriction (direct)					
Pupillary constriction (consensual)					
Pupillary constriction (accommodation)					
Symmetrical movement to all six points					
Nystagmus					
V Trigeminal					Any abnormality requires a complete neurological examination. If the complete examination reveals several abnormalities a referral to a physician is indicated.
Normal jaw muscle strength					
Normal forehead, cheek, and jaw sensation					
Normal corneal reflex bilaterally					
VII Facial					
Normal "make a face"					
Normal facial muscle strength					
Normal taste (anterior tongue)					

VIII Acoustic

Normal audiogram

IX, X Glossopharyngeal, vagus

Normal swallow

Normal gag reflex

Normal uvula movement

Normal taste on posterior tongue

XI Accessory

Normal, symmetrical trapezius strength

Normal, symmetrical sternocleidomastoid strength

XII Hypoglossal

Lack of tremors in tongue

Normal symmetrical tongue strength

Any abnormality requires a complete neurological examination. If the complete examination reveals several abnormalities a referral to a physician is indicated.

369

Neuromuscular Examination: Cerebellar Function

	Yes	No	Not appli-cable	Describe (where appropriate)	Significance
Fine motor skills Developmentally appropriate					Any abnormality requires a complete neurological examination. If the complete examination reveals several abnormalities, a referral to a physician is indicated.
Finger-nose Normal with eyes open					
Normal with eyes closed					
Finger-finger normal					
Finger-thumb normal					
Heel-shin normal					
Tandem normal for age					
Stands on one foot (5 seconds for 4-year-old with arms extended) (5 seconds for 6-year-old with arms crossed) (5 seconds for 7-year-old with eyes closed)					
Position sense normal					

Neuromuscular Examination: Motor System

Muscle group		Normal muscle size	Normal muscle tone	Normal muscle strength	Normal movement	Describe	Significance
Neck							
Upper arm	(R)						
	(L)						
Lower arm	(R)						
	(L)						
Wrist	(R)						Any abnormality requires a complete neurological exami- nation. If the complete examination reveals several abnormalities, a referral to a physician is indicated.
	(L)						
Fingers	(R)						
	(L)						
Thigh	(R)						
	(L)						
Calf	(R)						
	(L)						
Ankle	(R)						
	(L)						
Toes	(R)						
	(L)						

371

Neurological Examination: Sensory System

Primary sensations	Yes	No	Not appli-cable	Describe (where appropriate)	Significance
A. Superficial tactile sensation normal (cotton wisp)					
1. Face					
2. Trunk					
3. Arms					
4. Legs					
B. Superficial pain (pinprick) normal					
1. Face					
2. Trunk					Any abnormality requires a complete neurological examination. If the complete examination reveals several abnormalities a referral to a physician is indicated.
3. Arms					
4. Legs					
C. Temperature sensation normal (hot and cold test tubes; done only if super-ficial pain test raises questions)					
1. Face					
2. Trunk					
3. Arms					
4. Legs					

D. Vibration sensation normal (low-frequency tuning fork)
1. Sternum
2. Elbows
3. Knees
4. Toes
5. Iliac crest

E. Deep pain (not routinely done) normal
1. Eyeballs
2. Achilles tendon
3. Calf
4. Forearm

Cortical and discriminatory sensations

A. Two-point discrimination normal
B. Point localization normal
C. Extinction phenomenon
1. Cheek/cheek normal
2. Cheek/hand normal
3. Hand/hand normal

Any abnormality requires a complete neurological examination. If the complete examination reveals several abnormalities a referral to a physician is indicated.

373

Neuromuscular Examination: Reflex Function

Superficial reflexes	Yes	No	Not applicable	Describe (where appropriate)	Significance
Upper abdominal					
Lower abdominal					
Plantar Right					
Left					
Cremasteric Right					
Left					
Deep reflexes					Should be neither hypo- nor hyperreflexive (this is a subjective decision based on experience). Asymmetricality indicates further evaluation.
Biceps Right					
Left					
Triceps Right					
Left					
Brachioradialis Right					
Left					

Patellar (knee)		
Right		
Left	Not tested	Should be neither hypo- nor hyperreflexive (this is a subjective decision based on experience). Asymmetricality indicates further evaluation.
Achilles		
Right		
Left	Not tested	

Abnormal reflexes

Babinski		
Right		
Left	Not tested	
Chaddock		
Right		
Left	Not tested	Before walking, the normal response is a fanning of the toes. After walking fanning is an abnormal response and needs further evaluation.
Oppenheim		
Right		
Left	Not tested	
Gordon		
Right		
Left		
Chovstek's reflex		Abnormality requires further investigation.

Infant Neuromuscular Examination: Cerebral Function

	Yes	No	Not appli-cable	Describe (where appropriate)	Significance
Normal developmental level					A standardized test usually used.
State of consciousness					
Lethargy					If not just satiation, a referral is needed.
Hyperactivity					Referral or consultation may be indicated.
Cry					
Cat's cry					"Cri-du-chat," a genetic defect with mental retardation.
Hoarse cry					May indicate cretinism.
High-pitched cry					May indicate microcephaly or other neurological problems.
Normal cry					

Infant Neuromuscular Examination: Cranial Nerves

	Yes	No	Not appli-cable	Describe (where appropriate)	Significance
I Olfactory					Not usually tested in infants although they will visibly react to *very* strong odors
II Optic					
Follows well for age					Any abnormalities require further investigation.

III, IV, VI Oculomotor, trochlear, and abducent

Pupillary constriction (direct)		
Pupillary constriction (consensual)		
Symmetrical eye movement to all 6 directions (2 diagonal and 1 horizontal)		
Nystagmus		

V Trigeminal

Normal jaw muscle strength		
Normal forehead, cheek, and jaw sensation		

VII Facial

Normal facial movements		

VIII Acoustic

Turns to noisemakers		

IX, X Glossopharyngeal, vagus

Normal swallow		
Normal gag		

Any abnormalities require further investigation.

Infant Neuromuscular Examination: Cranial Nerves

XI Accessory	Yes	No	Not appli-cable	Describe (where appropriate)	Significance
Good shoulder strength					Any abnormalities require further investigation.
XII Hypoglossal					
Good tongue movements and swallow					

Infant Neuromuscular Examination: Motor System

	Yes	No	Not appli-cable	Describe (where appropriate)	Significance
Neck control adequate for age					Abnormalities require a thorough investigation.
Hypotonic baby					
Rigid muscle tone					

Infant Neuromuscular Examination: Reflex Function

Superficial reflexes	Yes	No	Not appli-cable	Describe (where appropriate)	Significance
Upper abdominal					Hyper- or hyporeflexia, absent or asymmetrical reflexes require further investigation.

Lower abdominal				
Plantar				
Right				
Left				
Cremasteric				

Deep reflexes

Biceps				
Right				
Left				
Triceps				
Right				
Left				
Brachioradialis				
Right				
Left				
Patellar				
Right				
Left				
Achilles				
Right				
Left				

Hyper- or hyporeflexia, absent or asymmetrical reflexes require further investigation.

Infant Neuromuscular Examination: Reflex Function (Continued)

Abnormal reflexes	Yes	No	Not applicable	Describe (where appropriate)	Significance
Babinski Right					
Left					In an infant below the age of walking, the normal response is a fanning of the toes; in an older infant this response would be abnormal and indicate a need for referral.
Chaddock Right					
Left					
Oppenheim Right					
Left					

Infantile Reflexes

	Yes	No	Not applicable	Describe (where appropriate)	Significance
Crossed extension					
Withdrawal					See accompanying chart for appropriate ages for appearance and disappearance of any specific reflexes. Any reflex which lasts too long or does not appear on time requires further investigation.
Automatic sitting					
Primary righting					
Galant					

Rooting				See accompanying chart for appropriate ages for appearance and disappearance of any specific reflexes. Any reflex which lasts too long or does not appear on time requires further investigation.
Sucking				
Grasp				
Tonic labyrinth				
Asymmetrical tonic neck				
Symmetrical tonic neck				
Moro				
Positive supporting				
Landau				
Neck righting				
Rooting (asleep)				
Head raising (prone)				

Source: These checklists are printed with permission from Blue Hill Videotape Incorporated and are part of a more complete programmed learning approach to the physical examination, which includes a workbook and series of videotapes. The materials can be purchased from Blue Hill Educational Systems, Inc., 52 South Main Street, Spring Valley, New York 10977.

Chapter 18

Screening Tests

In the assessment process, most clinicians feel that 80 percent of the important data is found through history taking, 15 percent through physical examination, and 5 percent through screening and laboratory work. This chapter will discuss some of the more common screening and laboratory techniques used in ambulatory pediatrics. In this field the nurse will be involved with a multitude of tests; some the nurse will perform, some the nurse will train others to perform, some the nurse will simply order performed and interpret the results, and some the nurse will neither order nor interpret, but should be familiar with. This chapter will look closely at some of the more common tests encountered in the outpatient setting and discuss the nurse's role with regard to them.

Tests can generally be categorized as either screening or diagnostic tests, both of which the nurse uses frequently. The general purpose of screening tests is to provide a quick, inexpensive measure which can be used with a large population to discover who is most likely to have a certain condition. Only those found to be most likely to have the condition need be tested by the more expensive and time-consuming diagnostic tests. For instance, all children should have vision screening tests, but only the few who fail such tests need to see a specialist for more extensive testing. Screening tests can have both false positive and false negative results; in other words, some children will pass a screening test even though they have the condition for which they are being tested, and some will fail the test even though they do not have the condition for which they are being tested. In the case of vision screening, for instance, some children will fail the test, but when referred to the ophthalmologist, they will be found to have no real vision problem; other children may have a vision problem but be able to pass the screening test and hence not get the visual correction which they need. False positive tests cause overreferral; false negative tests cause underreferral. In general, it is better to overrefer than to underrefer, since, in this way, few children with problems will be missed. A large degree of overreferral may be detrimental, however, since it is wasteful of time and money and may be disturbing to the parents.

Diagnostic tests are employed when there is enough evidence to indicate that a child is very likely to suffer from a certain condition; this evidence may be provided by a screening test or may be directly evident because of the signs and symptoms presented by the child.

Of the many screening and diagnostic tests available, only the more common are discussed in this chapter; the nurse is referred to complete laboratory guides or other reference books for explanation of the less common tests. This chapter will be concerned with common measurements and with vision, hearing, speech, blood, and urine tests.

COMMON MEASUREMENTS

Taking measurements is a routine procedure which is frequently underrated. This chapter will discuss the importance of some of these measurements and how they are taken and recorded; it will include height, weight, head circumference, temperature, pulse, respiration, blood pressure, and some special measurements.

It is usually the job of the nurse to see that these measurements are taken as well as to interpret them, i.e., decide whether they are normal or need further investigation. One important difference between children and adults is that children grow and develop very rapidly, and this growth and development must be constantly evaluated. Physical measurements of a child reflect the rate of growth; a failure in growth, an acceleration in growth, or any change in growth pattern may be the first clue to serious problems. Taking measurements is easy but extremely important, and measurements must be taken correctly and accurately. Sloppy procedures, lack of recording, or inaccurate interpretation may cause serious problems to be neglected.

RECORDING

Keeping records of measurements is of extreme importance. Isolated heights and weights are useless; it is the rate of growth and change that is important. Measurements must, therefore, be taken periodically and plotted on a graph to be useful. There are many ways to record measurements. Some clinics will record them at the top of the chart page for each visit as well as plot them on a graph kept elsewhere in the chart. The best graphs are set up to show percentages, with the mean and standard deviations above and below the mean. Thus a child's measurements are both plotted and recorded as being at the 90th percentile, 50th percentile, or 3d percentile. Measurements can be taken in pounds and ounces or kilograms and grams or feet and inches or meters and centimeters. Many clinics are revising their procedures to include measuring equipment in the metric system and metric graphs for plotting.

SPECIFIC MEASUREMENTS

Height

Height is an extremely important measure of skeletal growth and should be followed carefully from birth to adulthood. Height is usually measured at every well-child visit.

The method of measurement varies with age. Some authorities feel that it is so difficult to get an accurate measurement during the first year that they omit that measurement or take it only a few times during the first year. However, most clinics require that the height be measured at every well-child visit. Measuring the height of a young child is best done by two people with the child lying down. One person secures the head, and the other secures the feet; a mark is made at head and heel. Then the child is removed and the distance measured with a metal tape measure. Some clinics have a sliding measuring board on which the child's head is placed at the headboard and the movable end stretched to touch the child's heel (see Fig. 18-1). Other clinics have a tape measure fastened to a wooden board, and the child is placed on the board and measured from head to foot. The older children are more easily and accurately measured, since they can stand, in their stocking feet, on a standard, balanced adult scale with a built-in tape measure. If one of these scales is not available, a tape measure can be attached to a wall and the child instructed to stand straight against the wall. It is important that the tape measure begins at the child's heels and is not displaced by a baseboard. When measuring, always use a flat, hard surface to reach from the top of the child's head to the wall so that you are not guessing or adding height because of the hair (see Fig. 18-2).

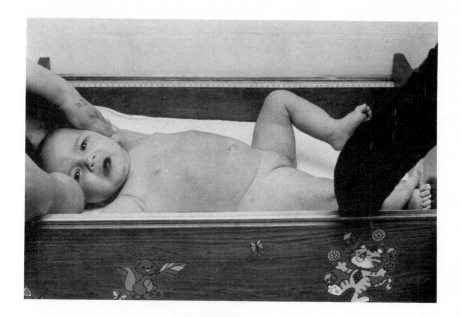

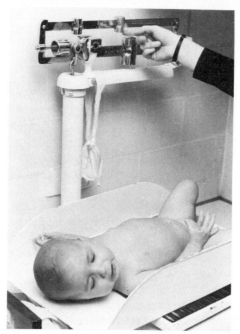

Figure 18-1 Infant being measured for height and weight.

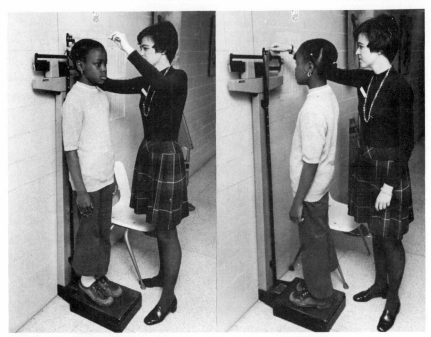

Figure 18-2 Older child being measured for height and weight.

Once the measurement is taken, it must be plotted on a graph (see Figs. 18-3 to 18-6). Height is generally a familial trait, and if parents and grandparents are tall, the child is likely to be tall also. If a child is born with a height at the 25th percentile, he will usually continue to fall at the 25th percentile most of his life. The value of the graph is that it enables the examiner to detect sudden changes in percentile. If the child's height increased to the 50th percentile or dropped below the 3d percentile, further investigation would be indicated. Some slight irregularities are frequently seen on the graph when the child matures to the standing measurement. Indication (on the graph) of the change in method helps reduce the confusion. Unusually tall stature may be due to heredity, overnutrition, or occasionally overstimulated growth hormones. Abnormally short stature can be due to malnutrition, growth hormone deficiencies, chronic infections, allergies, or distinct diseases such as kidney or heart problems. Short stature may also be inherited.

Weight

Weight is another extremely important index of the child's general growth and nutritional status. The child should be weighed at every visit from birth to adulthood. Since weight can fluctuate suddenly and drastically, it is usually measured at both well-child and sick-child visits. At sick-child visits it is often used as an indicator of fluid loss.

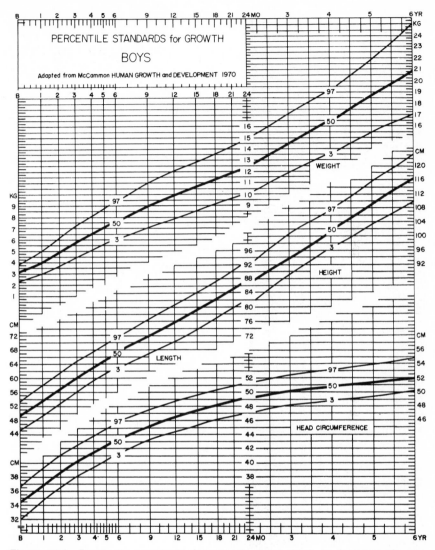

Figure 18-3 Percentile standards for growth—boys, birth to 6 years. (*Source: Robert McCammon, Human Growth and Development, 1970. Reproduced by permission.*)

The method and equipment for weighing varies with age. Infants should have all their clothing removed, including diapers, and be placed in a lying position on a regular baby scale. The scale must be balanced first with the scale paper in place. By the time children are walking they can usually be weighted on the adult standing scale. Depending on the situation, all clothing except underpants or just heavy outer clothing and shoes may be removed.

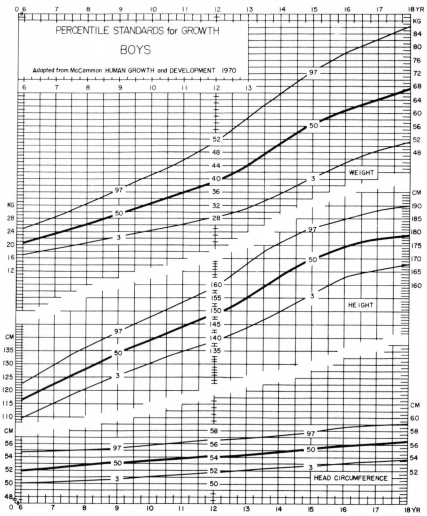

Figure 18-4 Percentile standards for growth—boys, 6 to 18 years. (*Source: Robert McCammon, Human Growth and Development, 1970. Reproduced by permission.*)

As with height, once the measurement is taken, it is plotted on a graph to show the child's long-term weight pattern. Weight should generally follow the same percentile, and sudden drops or increases warrant further investigation. Percentile increases may indicate overnutrition or, rarely, endocrine disorders. Drops in weight percentile can indicate chronic disease, acute infection, dehydration, emotional problems, or malnutrition.

There are some general rules concerning weight measurements. An average infant is born weighing 3500 g ($7\frac{1}{2}$ lb) and is expected to lose 10 per-

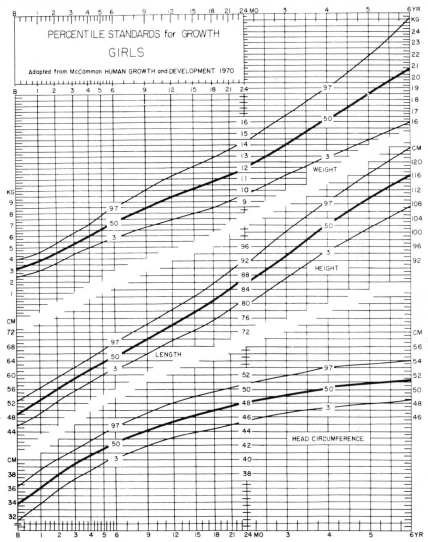

Figure 18-5 Percentile standards for growth—girls, birth to 6 years. (*Source: Robert McCammon, Human Growth and Development, 1970. Reproduced by permission.*)

cent of this weight during the first few days of life. This means an infant could lose up to 350 g (12 oz) during this time. Normally infants will regain their birth weight by the 10th to 14th day. Infants generally gain 30 g/day (1 oz/day) for the first 6 months. After that, growth is slower, and from age 2 to 10 the child will gain an average of about 5 lb per year.

The growth graphs (Figs. 18-3 to 18-6) are taken from the National Research Council and are the best to date on overall growth curves. They

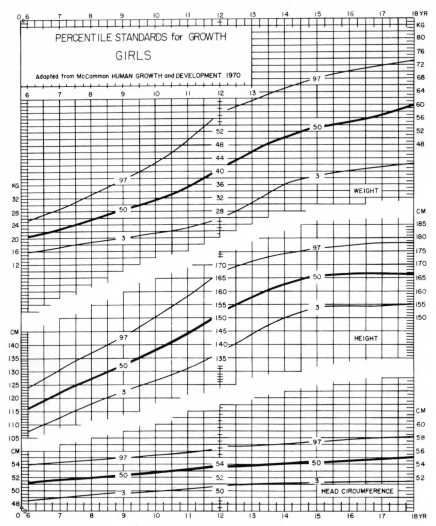

Figure 18-6 Percentile standards for growth—girls, 6 to 18 years. (*Source: Robert McCammon, Human Growth and Development, 1970. Reproduced by permission.*)

were based on white, middle class children over a 20-year period. There is much concern that these charts do not meet the needs of different cultural and ethnic groups and studies are beginning to look at some of these populations. Presently there are no good national standards for these populations and the studies on Puerto Ricans, blacks, Mexican-Americans, Orientals, etc., are beginning with small regional studies.

Head Circumference

The brain grows very rapidly during the first year of life, and the best way to evaluate this growth is to plot periodic measurements of the circumference of the skull. Most clinics include head circumference measurements at every well-baby visit during the first year and some clinics continue into the second and third year. The most reliable tape to use is a metal or paper one, since cloth tapes have a tendency to stretch and give an inaccurate reading. The tape is placed around the broadest part of the head, which is usually over the forehead and occipital protuberance. For greatest accuracy, the tape is placed three times, with a reading taken at the right side, at the left side, and at mid-forehead; the greatest circumference is plotted (see Fig. 18-7).

An infant's brain is one-fourth the adult size and will grow to ninetenths of its final size by the age of 6. In general, a newborn's head circumference is equal to or slightly larger than the chest circumference, and this ratio will continue until the child is 2 years old, when the chest circumference becomes greater than the head size.

As with height and weight, the head circumference measurements must be plotted on a graph. Most clinics use a centimeter graph because it is more

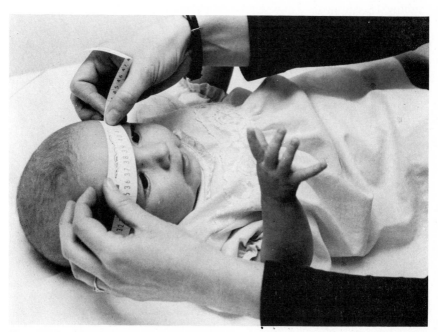

Figure 18-7 Measuring head circumference.

accurate. A child with a weight and height in the 50th percentile will usually have a head circumference in the 50th percentile. Marked differences should be investigated. A circumference which increases more rapidly than is expected according to the graph should be further investigated for hydrocephaly, while a graph showing no growth or little growth may indicate microcephaly. Some specific indications of the various relations between these measurements are discussed in Brown and Murphy (1975).

Temperature

Temperatures are not routinely taken on all children. For well-child visits, they are usually omitted, but they must be part of the workup of every sick child. Oral thermometers are usually long and slender, and rectal thermometers are short with a stubby bulb end. Some clinics are beginning to use electronic thermometers because they are accurate and take less time to register. These have a small box which is the measuring device with a probe and disposable cover. The probe may be placed either orally or rectally, and some can be taped into place in the rectum or axilla for constant monitoring, as in the newborn nursery (see Fig. 18-8). One of the newest thermometers is the Clinitemp Fever Detector which is a black flexible strip of plastic that is held firmly to the forehead (for 60 seconds) until it registers a reading. Thermometers may be Fahrenheit or Centigrade, with a range of 94 to 110°F and 32 to 43°C (see Table 18-1).

The choice of thermometer depends on the child's age. If there is any possibility that they will bite the thermometer, young children must have

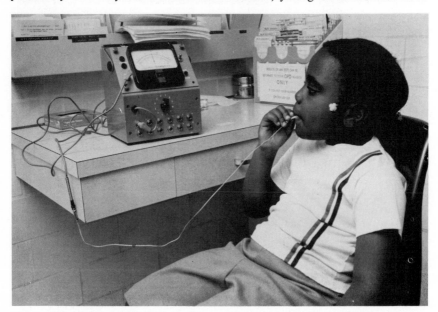

Figure 18-8　Child's temperature being recorded by electronic thermometer.

Table 18-1 Temperature Conversions

Centigrade	Fahrenheit
35.0	95.0
35.5	95.9
36.0	96.8
36.5	97.7
37.0	98.6
37.5	99.5
38.0	100.4
38.5	101.3
39.0	102.2
39.5	103.1
40.0	104.0
40.5	104.9
41.0	105.8
41.5	106.7

their temperature taken rectally. Children with a stuffy nose must also have their temperature taken rectally since an oral thermometer may interfere with breathing. The child is generally placed across the parent's lap with the child's head hanging on one side and the legs dangling on the other. The diaper or panties are removed, and if necessary, the mother can restrain the child with one arm across the shoulders and one hand firmly on the buttocks. The well-lubricated rectal thermometer is inserted approximately 1 in into the rectum (see Fig. 18-9). One study indicated that the thermometer must stay in place for 4 minutes to obtain an accurate reading. If the room temperature is at least 72 °F, the time may be cut to 2 to 3 minutes.

In the newborn nursery the first temperature is usually taken rectally; after that, axillary readings are taken. An oral thermometer is placed under the infant's arm in the axillary area, and the arm is held securely against the body for 4 to 5 minutes. This method is not as reliable with older children because they are more difficult to restrain.

Older children can have their temperature taken orally as long as they are not suffering from some respiratory illness which forces them to breathe through the mouth. Generally by the time children are 6 years old they can understand the instructions for the oral procedure. Some younger children can understand and be trusted, but it is important to be sure that the child will not bite the thermometer. The child should be seated and given an explanation of what is expected before the thermometer is placed under the tongue. One study reported that it took 8 minutes in a room of 65 to 75 °F to obtain a stabilized oral temperature.

For ambulatory care, the temperature is usually charted on the top of the day's sheet, but not usually graphed. The normal oral temperature is 95 to 99 °F (or 35 to 37 °C). Rectal temperatures are normally 1 ° higher than

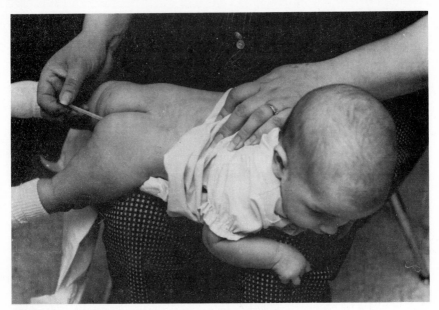

Figure 18-9 Infant's temperature being taken rectally.

oral, and axillary temperatures are normally 1° lower than oral. Thus it is important to record both the temperature and the method of obtaining it. Mild fever in children may be produced by excitement, eating, and vigorous exercise. Significant fever may be caused by bacterial or viral infections, dehydration, tumors, poisoning, convulsions, and some chronic conditions. A low temperature is seen if the child is in shock or has been chilled, or in some infants with infections.

Pulse

Since the pulse rate usually reflects the heartbeat directly, it is one way of evaluating the state of the circulatory system. The pulse rate should be taken at every visit to the clinic.

The pulse can be palpated in the dorsal pedalis, femoral, and radial areas, and palpated and auscultated in the apical area. The pulse is checked for rate, rhythm, and quality of beat. A comparison of radical and femoral pulses is extremely important. A more detailed description of these assessments can be found in the chapter on the heart.

The pulse is usually recorded at the top of the day's chart page. For ambulatory care it is not usually graphed.

Respiration

Observation of the rate, rhythm, and depth of a child's inspiration and expiration is important. Respirations should be checked at every clinic visit and especially at sick-child visits. Newborn infants have very irregular breathing, and their respiration is best obtained while they are resting or asleep. Sometimes palpation and auscultation of the chest make the counting easier. Because of the irregularity of respiration in an infant, it is important to count the rate for a full minute. Older children can be observed as they sit quietly on the examining table, or the respirations can be counted as the examiner listens to the lungs during the examination. For observations the upper clothing must be removed. Children should be unaware of the observations since knowledge of the fact that their breathing is being observed may cause them to alter their respirations.

Respiration rates are recorded at the top of the chart for the day's use but are not generally graphed in the pediatric clinic. An increased respiration rate is sometimes found with an increased pulse rate, fever, fulminating infection, or respiratory distress. A more complete discussion of respiration is found in Chapter 10.

Blood Pressure

Blood pressure is the indirect measurement of pressure exerted against the arterial walls during ventricular contractions and relaxations. It should be measured at every well-child visit; however, accurate measurements of an infant's blood pressure is difficult to obtain, and the American Academy of Pediatrics recommends beginning the procedure when the child is around 3 years of age. Since recent studies (Botwin, 1976) have shown an increased prevalence of hypertension in children, some pediatricians disagree, and think it should be done on every child at every visit. In this way, the examiner learns to become proficient at the procedure and also knows the limitations imposed by the equipment and age of the child. This measure is discussed further in Chapter 11.

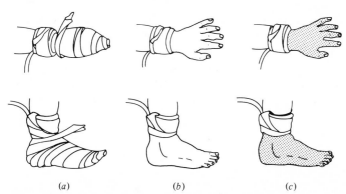

(a) (b) (c)

Figure 18-10 Diagrams of the technique of blood pressure measurement by the flush method. (*Source: Printed by permission of Charles C Thomas Publisher, Problems of Blood Pressure in Childhood, by Arthur J. Moss and Forrest H. Adams, 1963, p. 28.*)

Special Measurements

Occasionally there is a need for special measurements, such as sitting height and chest circumference. In children with growth problems it may be useful to compare their sitting height with their standing height. The child should be seated on a firm surface against a wall; the distance from the level of the head to the level of the buttocks is measured with a metal tape measure. By adulthood, sitting height equals one-half of standing height; these adult proportions should be reached around 10 years of age. At birth, the sitting height is 70 percent of standing height; this decreases to 60 percent by the time the child is 2 years old.

The chest circumference is usually measured at birth only, unless the child is showing signs of growth problems. To measure the chest circumference, the tape measure is placed around the chest and across the nipple line. At birth, the chest circumference should be 32 to 35 cm, or 2 cm less than the head circumference. The chest circumference then increases quickly and equals the head circumference until the age of 2; after that, the normal chest will be larger than the head.

It is important to have the average childhood norms available for comparison and graphs are an easy way to observe this growth (see Figs. 18-11 to 18-22).

DEVELOPMENTAL TESTING

Some of the most useful of the screening tests available to the nurse working in ambulatory pediatrics are those designed to assess the developmental skills of children. There are several popular screening tests used in pediatrics as well as a wide variety of diagnostic tests used for evaluating children's development.

It is important to remember the limitations of screening tests. For example, the Denver Developmental Screening Test does not tell the examiner that the child has cerebral palsy, mental retardation, minimal brain damage, or any other syndrome, only that the child is slow in one of the four large areas sampled. Once this slowness is discovered, the examiner should take a more careful history; perform a more detailed physical examination, including a complete neurological examination; make special arrangements for any additional indicated tests; and get consultation for the child.

Selected Screening Devices

Several developmental tests are popular in pediatrics because they are simple to administer, inexpensive, easily scored, accurate, and reliable in isolating children who need further evaluation. The *Denver Developmental*

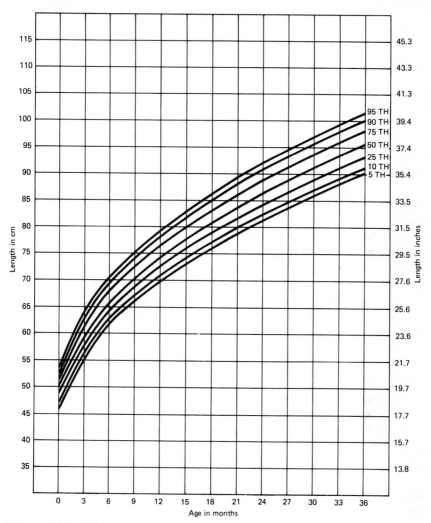

Figure 18-11 Girls' length by age percentiles: ages birth–36 months. (*Source: Monthly Vital Statistics Report, vol. 25, no. 3, pp. 6–17, June 22, 1976, National Center for Health Statistics, Rockville, Md.*)

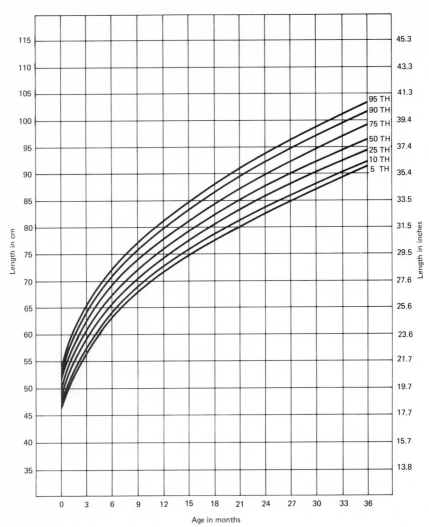

Figure 18-12 Boys' length by age percentiles: ages birth–36 months. (*Source: Monthly Vital Statistics Report, vol. 25, no. 3, pp. 6–17, June 22, 1976, National Center for Health Statistics, Rockville, Md.*)

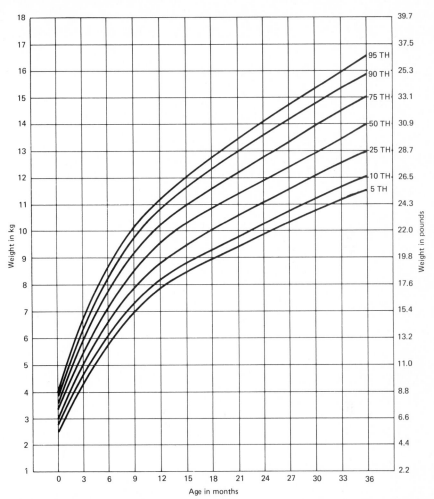

Figure 18-13 Girls' weight by age percentiles: ages birth–36 months. (*Source: Monthly Vital Statistics Report, vol. 25, no. 3, pp. 6–17, June 22, 1976, National Center for Health Statistics, Rockville, Md.*)

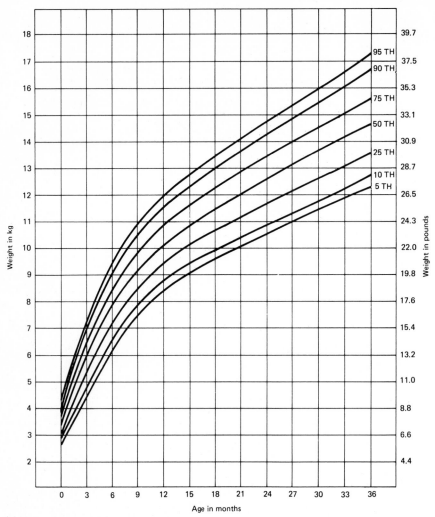

Figure 18-14 Boys' weight by age percentiles: ages birth–36 months. (*Source: Monthly Vital Statistics Report, vol. 25, no. 3, pp. 6–17, June 22, 1976, National Center for Health Statistics, Rockville, Md.*)

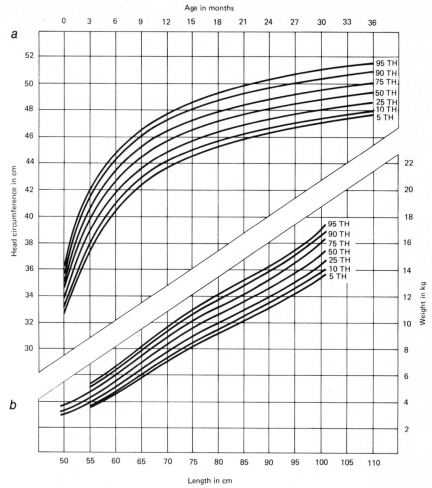

Figure 18-15 *(a)* Girls' head circumference by age percentiles: ages birth–36 months. *(b)* Girls' weight by length percentiles: ages birth-36 months. (*Source: Monthly Vital Statistics Report, vol. 25, no. 3, pp. 6–17, June 22, 1976, National Center for Health Statistics, Rockville, Md.*)

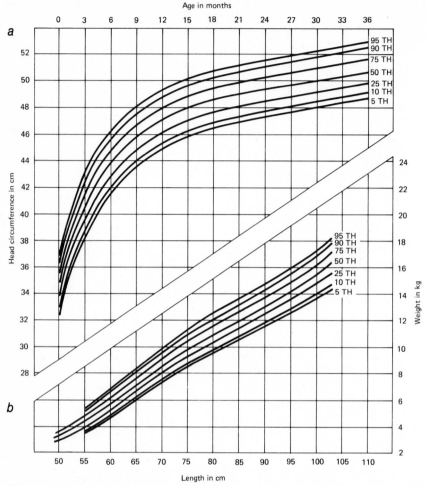

Figure 18-16 *(a)* Boys' head circumference by age percentiles: ages birth–36 months. *(b)* Boys' weight by length percentiles: ages birth–36 months. (*Source: Monthly Vital Statistics Report, vol. 25, no. 3, pp. 6–17, June 22, 1976, National Center for Health Statistics, Rockville, Md.*)

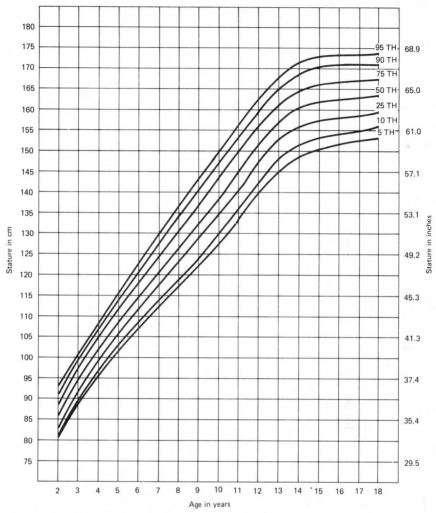

Figure 18-17 Girls' stature by age percentiles: ages 2 to 18 years. (*Source: Monthly Vital Statistics Report, vol. 25, no. 3, pp. 6–17, June 22, 1976, National Center for Health Statistics, Rockville, Md.*)

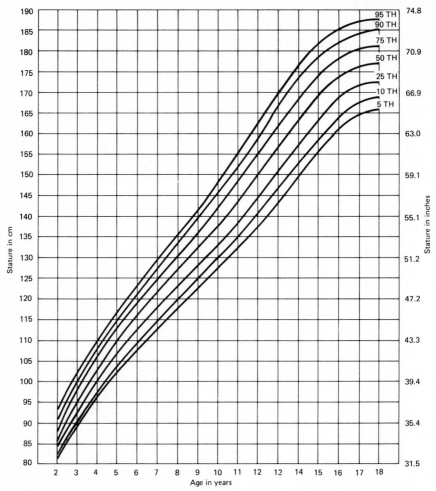

Figure 18-18 Boys' stature by age percentiles: ages 2 to 18 years (*Source: Monthly Vital Statistics Report, vol. 25, no. 3, pp. 6–17, June 22, 1976, National Center for Health Statistics, Rockville, Md.*)

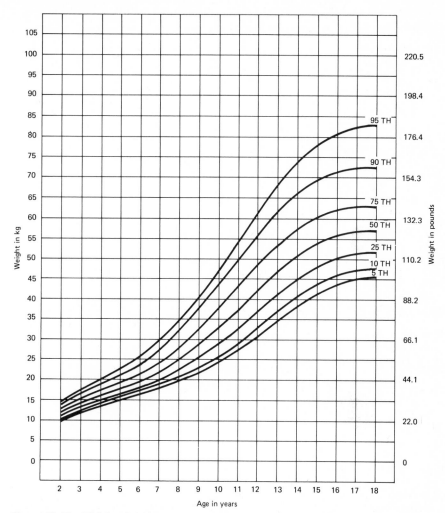

Figure 18-19 Girls' weight by age percentiles: ages 2 to 18 years. (*Source: Monthly Vital Statistics Report, vol. 25, no. 3, pp. 6–17, June 22, 1976, National Center for Health Statistics, Rockville, Md.*)

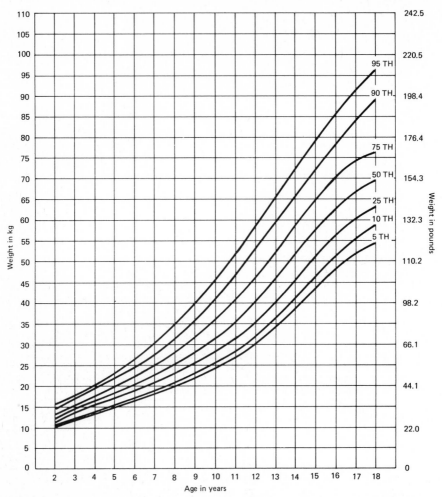

Figure 18-20 Boys' weight by age percentiles: ages 2 to 18 years. (*Source: Monthly Vital Statistics Report, vol. 25, no. 3, pp. 6–17, June 22, 1976, National Center for Health Statistics, Rockville, Md.*)

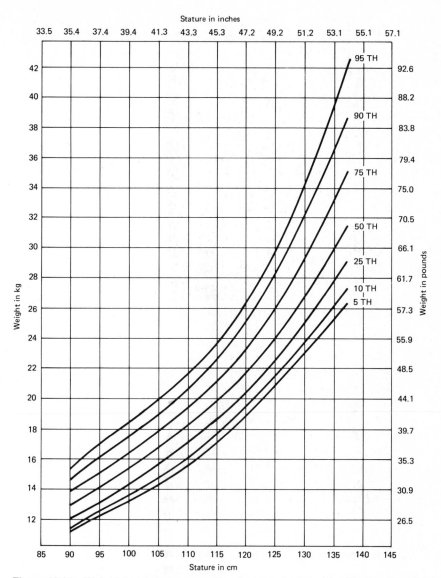

Figure 18-21 Weight by stature percentiles for prepubertal girls. (*Source: Monthly Vital Statistics Report, vol. 25, no. 3, pp. 6–17, June 22, 1976, National Center for Health Statistics, Rockville, Md.*)

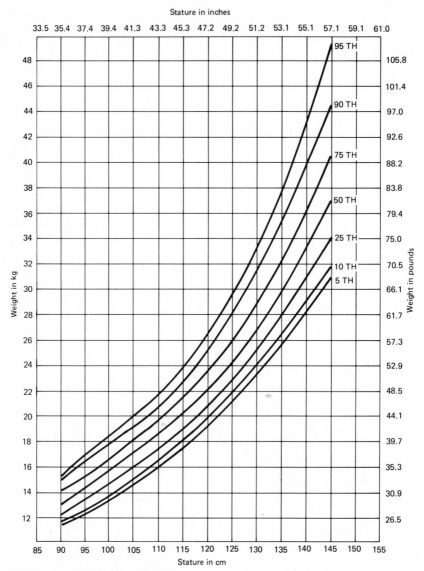

Figure 18-22 Weight by stature percentiles for prepubertal boys. (*Source: Monthly Vital Statistics Report, vol. 25, no. 3, pp. 6–17, June 22, 1976, National Center for Health Statistics, Rockville, Md.*)

Screening Test (DDST) was developed to screen young children for early detection of lags in developmental levels. Originally the test was standardized on 1036 children (Frankenberg, 1971). A good correlation between another 236 children (Frankenberg, 1971). A good correlation between specific sections of the DDST and related psychological tests have been shown. As a result of extensive research, the test forms and scoring have been revised several times.

The standardized equipment includes a tennis ball, eight colored blocks, a rattle, a bell, a pencil, a bottle, raisins, red wool, a pad of test forms, and a manual (see Fig. 18-23).

The information evaluated by the test is divided into four categories: personal-social, fine motor development, language, and gross motor development. Appropriate age levels from birth to 6 years are listed across the top and bottom of the score sheet, and the specific items to be tested are represented by horizontal bars below these age levels. Various points on the bar represent the ages at which 25, 50, 75, and 90 percent of the children pass that item. The area between the 75 and 90 percent is colored a solid blue to emphasize the skills which are particularly relevant to each age. All the bars are labeled with the item to be checked, e.g., "sits, looks for yarn,"

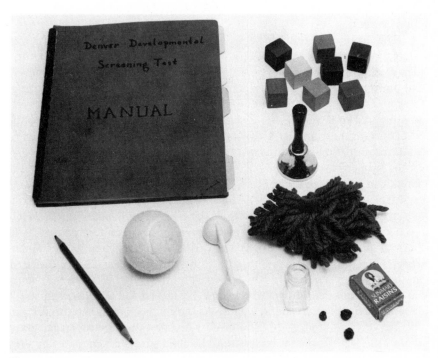

Figure 18-23   Materials used in the Denver Development Screening Test.

"hops on one foot," "walks well." If more explanation is needed to perform an activity, a small number appears to the left of the bar and the examiner can turn the form over for additional information. Since the test relies solely on the examiner's observations of the child and the parent's report, activities must be performed exactly as the instructional booklet describes. The examiner may not improvise by substituting a beach ball for the tennis ball or by making up new prepositions or definitions. This kind of improvisation invalidates the test.

Before administering the test, it is important that the examiner explain to the parent that the DDST is not an IQ test, but only a developmental screening device to estimate the child's level of maturation in his use of muscles, language, and some social activities. The parent should also be warned that the examiner will be asking the child to perform some activities which are too advanced for his or her age and that the child will probably be unable to accomplish certain tasks.

The examiner, parent, and child should be seated comfortably at a desk or table. To help make the testing more pleasant, the DDST should be adminstered before any painful procedures, such as shots or curetting. It is important to allow time for the child to relax in the examining room and grow accustomed to the examiner before the beginning of the exam. The examiner should start with some easy items so that the child begins with a feeling of success.

The examiner should begin by asking the child's birthday and calculating the age in months, days, and years. If the child was premature, the age is adjusted accordingly. The examiner locates the age across the top and bottom of the score sheet and draws a vertical line from top to bottom to represent the child's chronological age. All items crossing that line are administered to the child. Items that do not have an R before them must be performed to the examiner's satisfaction. If the child refuses to do an activity, the examiner may request help from the parent by instructing him or her on the proper way to adminster the test. If neither the examiner nor the parent can encourage the child to perform the activity, the examiner places an R (for "refuse") on the bar. As each item is administered, the examiner marks the bar with P (for "pass"), R, or F (for "fail")(see Fig. 18-24).

Once all the items have been administered, the examiner must interpret the results and give some explanation to the parent. There is some controversy over how much or how little to tell the parent. Some feel it is enough to say, "Your child has done well on the DDST." However, many parents are more curious, and the DDST can provide an opportunity for helping the parent understand what tasks the child can or cannot perform at this age. For example, a 10-month-old who shows no thumb-finger grasp might benefit if the parent understood the child's readiness and began placing some small items (dry cereal, raisins, or small blocks) in front of the child for practice in reaching and grasping.

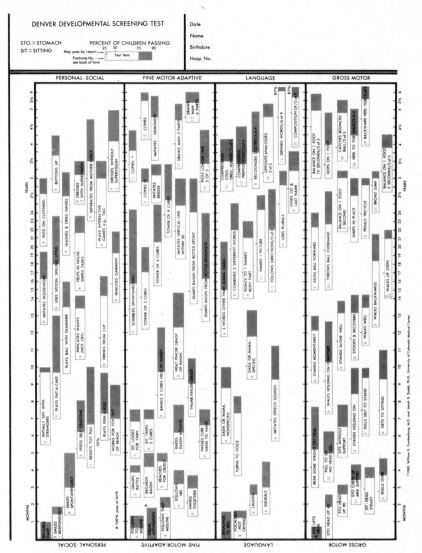

Figure 18-24 The Denver Developmental Screening Test. (*Source: Printed by permission of Charles C Thomas Publisher, Problems of Blood Pressure in Childhood, by Arthur J. Moss and Forrest H. Adams, 1963, p. 28.*)

With each standardization of the DDST the scoring and interpretation have been modified and redefined, and it is important that the examiner follow the directions found in the manual carefully.

The examiner must remember that the DDST is a standardized screening test and that if the results are to have any validity, the items must be done exactly as the test booklet dictates. For instance, it is not permissible to ask the child, "Which line is bigger?" instead of "Which line is longer?"

or to substitute larger, plastic blocks for the set of small, wooden blocks. As the examiner becomes familiar with one age group, the test moves more smoothly and rapidly. However, when in doubt about administering the item or scoring a certain response, the examiner should consult the instruction booklet and follow the directions exactly.

The DDST can take from 5 minutes for an infant to 20 minutes for a 5-year-old and if used properly can give valuable information about the child's developmental level. It is well worth the examiner's time to become familiar with the test and proficient in administering it, although many clinics hire a technician to actually administer the test, and the nurse's responsibilities are then to make sure that it is done accurately and to interpret the results.

Because many clinics did not have enough time to administer the DDST, a shorter "prescreening test" was developed to discover those children most likely to have developmental delays. This test, the *Denver Prescreening Developmental Questionnaire* (PDQ), consists of 97 questions divided by age, in a questionnaire form to be filled out by the parent.

Standardization of the PDQ was done on 1155 parents of varied ethnic, occupational, and education backgrounds. These results correlated with the DDST results at a level of 93.3 percent and continued standardization is presently being done.

The PDQ is available in five forms: one for the 3- to 5-month-old child, one for the 9- to 12-month-old child, one for the 16- to 24-month-old child, one for the 3- to 4-year-old and one for the 5- to 6-year-old child.

The parent answers 10 questions appropriate to the child's age while they are waiting for their health care visit.

The PDQ has several advantages: it is inexpensive, requires no extra space, and demands a minimal amount of time and personnel. It can only be used by those parents who read and write English. Hopefully, it will soon be available in other languages.

Since the PDQ is a modification of the DDST, it assesses the same four types of development; personal-social, fine motor-adaptive, language, and gross motor. For example, a question the parent of a 4-year-old child might be asked is "Does your child put an 's' at the end of his words when he is talking about more than one kind of thing, such as, blocks, shoes or toys?"

When using the PDQ, the examiner determines the child's age in the same manner as is done with the DDST. Questions appropriate for that age are indicated in the questionnaire. For example, a 4-year-old child's parent would answer questions 67 to 76. The parent simply circles one of the four answers provided for each question:

YES —CHILD CAN DO NOW or HAS DONE IN THE PAST

NO —CHILD CANNOT DO NOW, HAS NOT DONE IN THE PAST or YOU HAVE ANY DOUBT ABOUT CHILD'S ABILITY

R —CHILD REFUSES

NO OPP—CHILD HAS NOT HAD THE CHANCE

Nine or ten passes is considered normal; a child with seven or eight passes should repeat the PDQ one month later. At this time, if there are eight or less passes, the DDST should be administered. With six or less passes, the DDST should be performed at that time or as soon as possible. If the findings on the DDST are questionable or abnormal, the child should be further evaluated.

As with the DDST, the PDQ is frequently handed out by a clerk or technician as the family arrives. The nurse is responsible for interpreting the results and making a decision about any needed follow-up.

Another valuable screening tool for verbal intelligence is the *Peabody Picture Vocabulary Test.* It is to be used on children from $2\frac{1}{2}$ years old to adulthood.

The test was standardized on 4000 children ranging in age from $2\frac{1}{2}$ to 18 years, and reliability testing was done not only on children with normal intelligence but also on children with mental retardation, language difficulties, emotional problems, and motor disabilities. Validity was tested by comparison with the Stanford-Binet and Wechsler scales; correlations with these two tests were .50 and .71, respectively.

The material kit includes a booklet of pictures, manual of directions, and 50 scoring sheets (see Fig. 18-25). The test takes about 15 minutes to administer.

The Peabody Picture Vocabulary Test is to be given on an individual basis (not to a classroom of children). The examiner and child should have a quiet room with a table and chairs. Past information needed includes the child's name, birthdate, date of testing, age, home language, and the reason for administering the test. The "Series of Plates" booklet is placed in front of the child. The score sheet contains a list of 150 words; however, the top of the score sheet suggests starting points for various age levels. For instance, a $3\frac{1}{2}$-year-old child might be started at picture 15; the examiner would read the stimulus word "pulling," and ask the child to point to the picture best describing that word. The child should point to the picture of the girl pulling the wagon. The word stimulus becomes more difficult and less concrete as the test progresses. It is not a timed test; therefore children may take as long as they like to give an answer. However, after a minute it is wise to offer encouragement by saying, "Try one. Point to one of them." If the child first chooses one picture and then selects a different one, the final response is the one that counts.

The examiner keeps score of the correct and incorrect responses by recording the number of the response picture beside the correct answer and marking through the geometric symbols when an incorrect response is given. Pluses and minuses are not used since the child might interpret the results and thus become discouraged during the testing. The test is terminated when the child gives six incorrect responses to eight consecutive pictures (see Fig. 18-26).

The test manual is needed for the final scoring and interpretation of the examination. Once the child has established a base line for eight consecutive correct answers and a ceiling of six incorrect answers, the raw score is obtained by taking the ceiling item (the last word presented) and subtracting the number of incorrect responses. Thus, if item 49 was the last one presented and the child had 9 incorrect responses, the raw score is 40. The raw score is then located on tables in the manual to obtain the intelligence quotient, percentile score, and mental age. The final scores may then be interpreted according to classifications found in the manual.

Intelligence quotients	Percentage included	Classification
125 and above	5	Very rapid learners
110–124	20	Rapid learners
90–109	50	Average learners
75–89	20	Slow learners
Below 75	5	Very slow learners

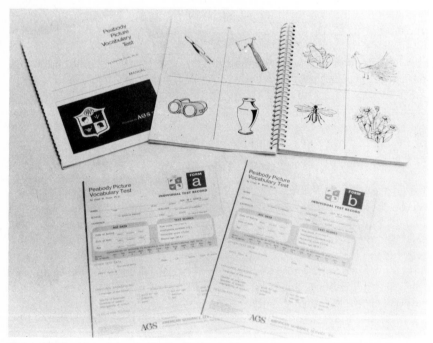

Figure 18-25   Materials used in the Peabody Picture Vocabulary Test.

1. Try to get child to smile by smiling, talking or waving to him. Do not touch him.
2. When child is playing with toy, pull it away from him. Pass if he resists.
3. Child does not have to be able to tie shoes or button in the back.
4. Move yarn slowly in an arc from one side to the other, about 6" above child's face. Pass if eyes follow 90° to midline. (Past midline; 180°)
5. Pass if child grasps rattle when it is touched to the backs or tips of fingers.
6. Pass if child continues to look where yarn disappeared or tries to see where it went. Yarn should be dropped quickly from sight from tester's hand without arm movement.
7. Pass if child picks up raisin with any part of thumb and a finger.
8. Pass if child picks up raisin with the ends of thumb and index finger using an over hand approach.

9. Pass any enclosed form. Fail continuous round motions.
10. Which line is longer? (Not bigger.) Turn paper upside down and repeat. (3/3 or 5/6)
11. Pass any crossing lines.
12. Have child copy first. If failed, demonstrate

When giving items 9, 11 and 12, do not name the forms. Do not demonstrate 9 and 11.

13. When scoring, each pair (2 arms, 2 legs, etc.) counts as one part.
14. Point to picture and have child name it. (No credit is given for sounds only.)

15. Tell child to: Give block to Mommie; put block on table; put block on floor. Pass 2 of 3. (Do not help child by pointing, moving head or eyes.)
16. Ask child: What do you do when you are cold? ..hungry? ..tired? Pass 2 of 3.
17. Tell child to: Put block on table; under table; in front of chair, behind chair. Pass 3 of 4. (Do not help child by pointing, moving head or eyes.)
18. Ask child: If fire is hot, ice is ?; Mother is a woman, Dad is a ?; a horse is big, a mouse is ?. Pass 2 of 3.
19. Ask child: What is a ball? ..lake? ..desk? ..house? ..banana? ..curtain? ..ceiling? ..hedge? ..pavement? Pass if defined in terms of use, shape, what it is made of or general category (such as banana is fruit, not just yellow). Pass 6 of 9.
20. Ask child: What is a spoon made of? ..a shoe made of? ..a door made of? (No other objects may be substituted.) Pass 3 of 3.
21. When placed on stomach, child lifts chest off table with support of forearms and/or hands.
22. When child is on back, grasp his hands and pull him to sitting. Pass if head does not hang back.
23. Child may use wall or rail only, not person. May not crawl.
24. Child must throw ball overhand 3 feet to within arm's reach of tester.
25. Child must perform standing broad jump over width of test sheet. (8-1/2 inches)
26. Tell child to walk forward, ◁◯◑◯◯◯▶ heel within 1 inch of toe. Tester may demonstrate. Child must walk 4 consecutive steps, 2 out of 3 trials.
27. Bounce ball to child who should stand 3 feet away from tester. Child must catch ball with hands, not arms, 2 out of 3 trials.
28. Tell child to walk backward, ◀◯◑◯◯◯ toe within 1 inch of heel. Tester may demonstrate. Child must walk 4 consecutive steps, 2 out of 3 trials.

DATE AND BEHAVIORAL OBSERVATIONS (how child feels at time of test, relation to tester, attention span, verbal behavior, self-confidence, etc,):

Figure 18-25 *(continued).*

The Peabody Picture Vocabulary Test is useful for school nurses evaluating school-age children, as well as for nurses in ambulatory clinics who can incorporate this tool into their routine assessment of children over 2 years of age.

Another popular screening tool is the *Developmental Test of Visual-Motor Integration,* also known as the Beery or VMI, which is designed to assess the visual perception and motor behavior of children between the ages of 2 and 15 years. It is generally given to preschoolers and early school-agers. The test has been standardized and its validity compared with that of similar tests; correlations with these tests have averaged around .89.

Plate No.	Word	Key Resp. Errors*	Plate No.	Word	Key Resp. Errors*	Plate No.	Word	Key Resp. Errors*
1	car	(4)__ ○	26	teacher	(2)__ ♡	51	submarine	(4)__ □
2	cow	(3)__ □	27	building	(3)__ ☆	52	thermos	(4)__ △
3	baby	(1)__ △	28	arrow	(3)__ ◇	53	projector	(3)__ ✇
4	girl	(2)__ ✇	29	kangaroo	(2)__ ○	54	group	(4)__ ♡
5	ball	(1)__ ♡	30	accident	(3)__ □	55	tackling	(3)__ ☆
6	block	(3)__ ☆	31	nest	(3)__ △	56	transportation	(1)__ ◇
7	clown	(2)__ ◇	32	caboose	(4)__ ✇	57	counter	(1)__ ○
8	key	(1)__ ○	33	envelope	(1)__ ♡	58	ceremony	(2)__ □
9	can	(4)__ □	34	picking	(2)__ ☆	59	pod	(3)__ △
10	chicken	(2)__ △	35	badge	(1)__ ◇	60	bronco	(4)__ ✇
11	blowing	(4)__ ✇	36	goggles	(3)__ ○	61	directing	(3)__ ♡
12	fan	(2)__ ♡	37	peacock	(2)__ □	62	funnel	(4)__ ☆
13	digging	(1)__ ☆	38	queen	(3)__ △	63	delight	(2)__ ◇
14	skirt	(1)__ ◇	39	coach	(4)__ ✇	64	lecturer	(3)__ ○
15	catching	(4)__ ○	40	whip	(1)__ ♡	65	communication	(2)__ □
16	drum	(1)__ □	41	net	(4)__ ☆	66	archer	(4)__ △
17	leaf	(3)__ △	42	freckle	(4)__ ◇	67	stadium	(1)__ ✇
18	tying	(4)__ ✇	43	eagle	(3)__ ○	68	excavate	(1)__ ♡
19	fence	(1)__ ♡	44	twist	(2)__ □	69	assaulting	(4)__ ☆
20	bat	(2)__ ☆	45	shining	(4)__ △	70	stunt	(1)__ ◇
21	bee	(4)__ ◇	46	dial	(2)__ ✇	71	meringue	(1)__ ○
22	bush	(3)__ ○	47	yawning	(2)__ ♡	72	appliance	(3)__ □
23	pouring	(1)__ □	48	tumble	(2)__ ☆	73	chemist	(4)__ △
24	sewing	(1)__ △	49	signal	(1)__ ◇	74	arctic	(3)__ ✇
25	wiener	(4)__ ✇	50	capsule	(1)__ ○	75	destruction	(4)__ ♡

Figure 18-26 The Peabody Picture Vocabulary Test.

The work kit includes a manual, a package of test booklets, and score sheets; the examiner provides pencils (see Fig. 18-27). The test takes about 20 minutes to administer.

The test booklet consists of nine pages of drawings; each page contains six squares with designs drawn in the top three. Children should be seated comfortably at a table and the test booklet and pencil placed in front of them. They are then directed to copy each of the designs on that page. They may not repeat the form or erase their original work. Only one trial is allowed for each design. Children are asked, "Can you make one like that?" while the examiner points to the first design. The examiner must not trace the design or give it a name. If children understand the task, they are allowed to work on each form until they fail three consecutive designs. If children do not understand the instructions after the first design, the examiner may continue to ask, "Can you make one like that?" and point to each following design. Children should begin with the simple designs and work toward the difficult ones. Although the test is not timed, children should not be allowed to struggle too long over any one design, but should be encouraged to move on.

The test is interpreted by following the criteria set up for each design in

Plate No.	Word	Key Resp.	Errors*	Plate No.	Word	Key Resp.	Errors*	Plate No.	Word	Key Resp.	Errors*
76	porter	(3)___	☆	101	graduated . .	(3)___	△	126	dormer	(2)___	◇
77	coast	(2)___	◇	102	hieroglyphic .	(2)___	✛	127	coniferous . .	(2)___	○
78	hoisting	(4)___	○	103	orate	(1)___	♡	128	consternation	(4)___	☐
79	wailing	(1)___	☐	104	cascade	(3)___	☆	129	obese	(3)___	△
80	coil	(2)___	△	105	illumination .	(4)___	◇	130	gauntlet	(4)___	✛
81	kayak	(3)___	✛	106	nape	(1)___	○	131	inclement . .	(1)___	♡
82	sentry	(2)___	♡	107	genealogist .	(2)___	☐	132	cupola	(1)___	☆
83	furrow	(4)___	☆	108	embossed . .	(2)___	△	133	obliterate . . .	(2)___	◇
84	beam	(1)___	◇	109	mercantile . .	(4)___	✛	134	burnishing . .	(3)___	○
85	fragment . . .	(3)___	○	110	encumbered .	(2)___	♡	135	bovine	(1)___	☐
86	hovering . . .	(2)___	☐	111	entice	(4)___	☆	136	eminence . . .	(4)___	△
87	bereavement	(3)___	△	112	concentric . .	(3)___	◇	137	legume	(3)___	✛
88	crag	(4)___	✛	113	vitreous . . .	(3)___	○	138	senile	(4)___	♡
89	tantrum	(2)___	♡	114	sibling	(1)___	☐	139	deleterious .	(2)___	☆
90	submerge . .	(1)___	☆	115	machete . . .	(2)___	△	140	raze	(4)___	◇
91	descend	(3)___	◇	116	waif	(4)___	✛	141	ambulation .	(2)___	○
92	hassock	(2)___	○	117	cornice	(1)___	♡	142	cravat	(1)___	☐
93	canine	(1)___	☐	118	timorous . . .	(3)___	☆	143	impale	(2)___	△
94	probing	(1)___	△	119	fettered	(1)___	◇	144	marsupial . .	(4)___	✛
95	angling	(1)___	✛	120	tartan	(2)___	○	145	predatory . . .	(3)___	♡
96	appraising . .	(3)___	♡	121	sulky	(3)___	☐	146	incertitude . .	(1)___	☆
97	confining . . .	(4)___	☆	122	obelisk	(4)___	△	147	imbibe	(2)___	◇
98	precipitation	(4)___	◇	123	ellipse	(2)___	✛	148	homunculus .	(3)___	○
99	gable	(1)___	○	124	entomology .	(2)___	♡	149	cryptogam . .	(4)___	☐
100	amphibian . .	(1)___	☐	125	bumptious . .	(4)___	☆	150	pensile	(3)___	△

Figure 18-26 (continued).

the instruction manual. To obtain a valid score, the criteria must be followed exactly; the test booklet should be examined with the individual score criteria and each form passed or failed accordingly. A raw score is calculated by adding all the correct answers up to the three failed designs. The manual provides a table to find the age equivalent score from the raw score. By comparing the child's age equivalent score with his or her chronological age and by observing the child during the examination, the examiner can assess the child's visual-motor behaviors.

These are a few of the most widely used screening tools available today. Additional tools are continually being developed; it is important that the examiner regularly evaluate newer, more refined devices as they become available.

Additional Developmental Tests

While the previously discussed tests can easily be used as screening tests and given in a relatively short period of time, the nurse may need more information about a particular child or may be doing more sophisticated screening on a smaller number of children. The following developmental tests are not screening tools in the usual sense, but within special situations one or two of

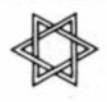

Figure 18-27 The Beery test score sheets. (Source: Printed by permission of the Follett Educational Corporation.)

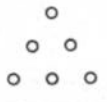

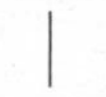

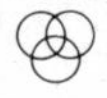

No.	Form	Pass or Fail (P-F)	Observations and Comments
1			
2			
3			
4			
5			
6			
7			
8			
9			
10			
11			
12			

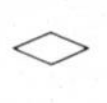

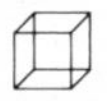

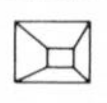

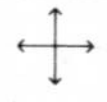

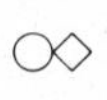

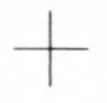

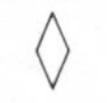

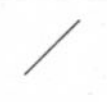

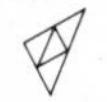

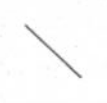

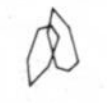

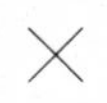

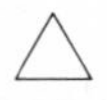

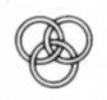

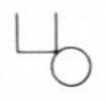

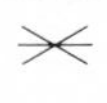

No.	Form	Pass or Fail (P-F)	Observations and Comments
13			
14			
15			
16			
17			
18			
19			
20			
21			
22			
23			
24			

418

them might be utilized in such a manner. There are a great many such developmental tests, and the following is only a sampling of some of the more frequently used ones. Only the briefest description is given here. For more detail or for information on the many other tests available, the reader is referred to the bibliography at the end of this chapter. If the nurse needs to become proficient at administering one of these tests, he or she should seek out the nearest testing center and ask for a demonstration and help in learning the specific test. Scoring will be mentioned, but due to the wide range of interpretation the nurse must be careful in reaching decisions of normality or abnormality.

The *Bender Visual-Motor Gestalt Test* tests perceptual ability and spatial relationships of individuals between the ages of 4 and adulthood. The early standardization included only 474 adults between the ages of 15 and 50 years. Only as recently as 1964 was the test standardized on children. Over the years many modifications of the test have been made. Presently the test consists of a series of nine designs which the child is asked to copy. The test kit includes a design booklet, paper, pencil, manual, and score sheets. Generally it takes 10 to 15 minutes for the child to be shown the designs and copy them. From the nine designs, 105 items are scored, and the score is compared with scales provided in the manual.

The *California First-Year Mental Scale,* also known as the Bayley mental scales, tests infants between the ages of 1 month and 18 months. The early standardization was on 54 middle-class children between 1 month and 21 months. The test is divided into several sections: postural development, motor development, perception, attention span to objects and humans, language, object manipulation, understanding commands, and problem solving. Many of the tasks are taken from the Gesell scales. Once a raw score is obtained, the test provides an estimated mental age.

One of the more popular infant tests is the *Cattell Infant Intelligence Scale.* It is used on children between the ages of 3 months and $2\frac{1}{2}$ years to determine their intelligence quotient. Many standardizations have been done, but the original covered 274 children in a longitudinal study with 1346 actual tests given. It was found to have very high correlations with other tests on children after the 9th month of age. Items were picked from other tests to provide a continuity between tests for very young infants and tests for the older child. All the items are grouped by age, and each age is tested in five areas. The test includes material such as rattles, a toy, a cup, cubes, a spoon, peg board, paper and pencil, picture cards, an instruction manual, and score sheets. The child is placed in a high chair or on the mother's lap or examining table. The examiner places certain objects in front of the child and asks for certain responses, either motor or verbal. Usually the test takes around 20 to 30 minutes. Scoring is done by placing a plus or minus beside each task on the score sheet and adding all pluses to find the raw score, which is applied to a formula to obtain the basal age, mental age, and intelligence quotient of the child.

The *Developmental Screening Inventory for Infants* (DSI) is used on infants between the ages of 4 weeks and 18 months. The test is taken from Gesell and is divided into categories of adaptive behavior, language, personal-social tasks, and gross and fine motor behavior. Materials for the test include a cup, embroidery hoop, bottle, round candies, picture book, crayon, paper, and blocks. The infant is placed on the examining table or sits on the parent's lap while different objects are presented; the examiner observes for specific responses. Scoring is separate for each category tested.

The *Full-Range Picture Vocabulary Test,* or Ammons vocabulary test, tests for daily, used vocabulary. It was set up to test children between the ages of 2 and 17 years and standardized on 589 children within that age range. Validity was tested by a comparison with the Stanford-Binet test. Materials include a series of 16 drawings, an instruction manual, and score sheets. The test comes with two forms, each containing 85 words. As the examiner pronounces the word, the child must point to the drawing best describing the word; the entire test takes from 10 to 15 minutes. Scoring is based on the norms given in the instructional manual.

One of the most familiar tests is the *Gesell Developmental Schedules.* Originally it was standardized on 107 children, and there has been much controversy over the small sample, the economic status of the children (all middle class), and the low correlations with standard IQ tests. Standardization continues, and it is still a widely used and imitated test. There are two forms: the infant schedule and the preschool schedule. The infant schedule tests the child from 4 weeks to 1 year of age and is divided into four large areas: motor, adaptive, language, and personal-social. The preschool schedule tests the child from 15 months to 6 years and has the same categories. Kits for both tests include a baby ring, blocks, bottle and pellet, book, cup, paper, pencil, picture cards, ball, instruction booklet, and score sheets. Much of the examination depends on the observations of the tester. With infants, the examiner simply places the baby on the examining table or mother's lap, presents certain items, and watches the response. With older children, the examiner may show certain items or ask for certain tasks and the child responds or performs appropriately. As each task is completed, the examiner assigns a plus for correct and a minus for incorrect responses. The final raw score is applied to an algebraic formula to obtain percentile and rank.

The *Goodenough-Harris Drawing Test* may be used for children between the ages of 3 and 15 years to assess intelligence and personality traits. In 1950 it was standardized on 2975 children across the United States. Materials are simple, with only a test booklet, pencil, and instruction manual. The test is not timed, but generally takes around 15 minutes and may be given individually or in groups. Older children may fill in their own background information (name, sex, date, grade, age, birthdate, father's occupation). Children are told to draw three pictures in the spaces provided: a man, a woman, and a self-portrait. Younger children may need a rest period between pictures. Using the manual, the examiner scores each individual figure according to specific standards supplied in the manual. Specific items on the figure are given a score of 1 if drawn according to specification; the raw score is applied to a formula to obtain a standard score and percentile.

The *Illinois Test of Psycholinguistic Abilities* (ITPA) was developed to test language development in children between the ages of $2\frac{1}{2}$ and 9 years. It was standardized on 700 children within the age range of the test. The test is divided into nine large areas: automatic auditory-vocal, visual decoding, motor encoding, visual-motor sequencing, auditory-vocal association, vocal encoding, auditory-vocal sequencing, visual-motor association, and auditory decoding. Materials include an instruction manual, test sheets, and certain objects (cup, ball, block, etc.), and a picture book. The ITPA can be given only individually. The examiner follows instructions in showing the child certain objects or pictures and asking for specific responses. The raw scores of each section are converted into profile scores and plotted on a percentile graph.

The *Marianne Frostig Developmental Test of Visual Perception,* called simply Frostig, is used with children between the ages of 3 and 8 years to isolate perceptual problems. Standardization began on 1800 schoolchildren between the ages of 5 and 9 years and continues today. Studies show a reliability of .80 on a test-and-retest basis. A validity of .44 to .50 is found if the scores are compared with teacher ratings; a somewhat lower validity (.32 to .40) appears when scores are compared with scores from the Goodenough-Draw-a-Man Test. There is still much controversy over the standardization.

The test is divided into six large areas: eye-hand coordination, figure-ground discrimination, constancy, spatial position, spatial relations, and a total score called a *perceptual quotient.* Materials include demonstration cards, instruction manual, score sheets, and administration sheets. The test is not timed, but generally requires 30 to 45 minutes. The child should be comfortably seated at a desk or table and given a pencil and the administration sheets. The examiner introduces each section of the demonstration cards and gives instructions. The child is asked to accomplish certain tasks such as drawing lines between two boundaries or connecting dots on the page. The raw score is obtained by using the booklet, which gives the criteria for each task. The perceptual quotient and perceptual age are obtained from the raw score.

The *Minnesota Preschool Scale* is used to test the nonverbal, verbal, and intelligence quotient of children between the ages of 3 and 6 years. It was standardized on 900 children, and when the two forms of the test were given 1 week apart, the reliability ranged from .68 to .94. Equipment for the test includes test cards, a large doll, a small doll, a large ball, a small ball, a watch, scissors, pencils, paper, 12 cubes, secured and loose cubes, a key, a penny, cardboard, and a cardboard clock. The child is presented with one of the test items at a time and asked certain questions, such as: "What is this?" A raw score is obtained by adding the number of correct answers in the verbal and nonverbal sections and applying this to a formula to get the percentile placement and intelligence quotient equivalent. This test is not widely used because of the age limitations.

The *Oseretsky Tests of Motor Proficiency* may be used on children between the ages of 5 and 16 years to assess general coordination, hand coordination, speed, voluntary movements, and synkinesia. The equipment includes wooden boxes, 20 pennies, paper, wooden spool, 40 matchsticks, a rubber ball, a block of wood, a 6-ft-long rope, ruled paper, a wooden hammer, 2 mazes, 36 playing cards, a matchbox, a book, pencils, a wooden sieve, a wooden stick, a stop watch, an instruction booklet, and score forms. It is a timed test. As the child performs the tasks, the examiner puts a plus beside the items correctly done and a minus beside the incorrect responses. If the task requires both hands or feet and the child uses only one, a score of half is given. As with all tests, it is best to begin with tasks that the child can easily do. Items are given until the child fails all the items within one grouping. The raw score is applied to a formula to obtain the mental level and the motor level.

The *Piaget Right-Left Awareness Test* was developed to test handedness of schoolchildren between the ages of 5 and 11 years. It is a simple test in which children are given several verbal commands requiring them to differentiate between their right and left hands. The examiner sits opposite the child and says, "Show me your right hand," or shows the child several objects and asks the child on which side each object is placed. Equipment needed includes a coin, pencil, bracelet, and key. The raw score of the items passed is applied to a grid for appropriate ages for each task.

The *Preschool Inventory* is a simple screening tool to give information on children between the ages of 3 and 6 years and predict that child's probability of success in school. It was standardized on 389 children. Besides the instruction manual and score sheets, the examiner needs three small colored cars, eight large crayons, a box of checkers, and three cardboard boxes. The test is timed. The examiner asks the child to perform certain tasks described in the manual. As the child accomplishes each task, the examiner scores the correct answers. A total raw score of 64 points can be accrued and is converted to a percentile by following instructions in the manual.

The *Preschool Readiness Experimental Screening Scale* (Press) was developed to assess the level of maturation of children between the ages of 4 and 5 years. Validity was originally established by comparing it to the Slossen Intelligence Test. Later (Rogers, 1975) it was administered to 170 children before kindergarten and compared to teacher ratings and the Metropolitan Readiness Test administered after the kindergarten year. It appeared to be a good predictor of kindergarten success. Minimum equipment is needed: the instruction manual, score sheets, tongue blades, paper, and pencil. The test is divided into five large categories (introduction, colors, numbers, general, and drawing), with three questions in each category. The test can be administered during the physical examination of the child or done separately. Either way, it takes about 2 to 3 minutes. The child is simply asked a list of questions, some requiring a verbal response and some a motor response. Scoring is kept simple and ranges from 0 to 10.

A very familiar intelligence quotient test is the *Stanford-Binet Scales.* Originally the Stanford-Binet was standardized on 1500 school and preschool children. Over the years the standardization has continued, and additional studies now include over 3000 subjects tested. The test may be used on individuals from 2 years to adulthood. Originally there were two forms, but recently these have been combined into one form. The test is divided into age levels and several categories: visual perception, visual imagery, visual memory, thinking, memory and attention, abstractions, reasoning, vocabulary, and concepts. Materials include a set of toys (doll, car, scissors, utensils, doll chair, etc.), a test booklet, and score sheets. To administer the test to younger children takes between 40 and 50 minutes, while testing older children and adults may take as long as 60 to 70 minutes. Initial items are chosen slightly below the child's expected level to give a feeling of success. All the items in all the areas are given until the child reaches a ceiling level. As the child responds to the requests, the examiner assigns a plus for correct answers and a minus for incorrect items. It is expected that the child will have a scattering of scores in several different areas. The raw score is applied to a formula to obtain the child's mental age and intelligence quotient.

The *Vineland Social Maturity Scale* is used on individuals from 1 year to adulthood; it assesses the person's independence and self-reliance. Originally it was standardized on 620 children. Test items are arranged according to age and fall into eight categories: general self-help, self-help in eating, self-help in dressing, self-direction, occupation, communication, locomotion, and socialization. Test materials include the instruction booklet and score sheets. The individuals being tested do not have to be present as long as a representative who knows them well answers the questions being asked. Scoring is a complicated process of graduation from "absolutely can do" to "positively cannot do," including "beginning skill," "no opportunity," etc. Each score is given a credit; the total score is converted into a raw score and finally into percentiles and age value.

The *Wechsler Intelligence Scale for Children* (WISC) includes three scales: the WPPSI scale for children from 4 to $6\frac{1}{2}$ years, the WISC scale for children from 7 to 10 years, and the WAIS scale for anyone over 16 years of age. Earlier forms of the test have been standardized. Test materials include the manual, test items, and test score sheets. Generally the test takes one hour to administer, and it should be given individually. The test is divided into two sections. The verbal section includes information, comprehension, arithmetic, similarities, and vocabulary. The performance section includes block design, picture completion, picture arrangement, object assembly, mazes, and coding. The examiner administers each subtest as quickly as the child can respond. Additional information on items or explanation can be asked for if the examiner does not understand the subject's first answer. Scoring is difficult, since the answers are scored not only for correctness but for surrounding responses, e.g., slowness, compulsiveness, lack of organization. The final score gives the child's intelligence quotient.

There are, of course, many more developmental tests available than those listed in this chapter, but this list should give the reader some idea of the wide range of development that can be tested. This list also skips the many fine guides that have been developed to help the examiner look at the child, such as the Yale Developmental Screening tool or the Washington Guide to Promoting Development in the Young Child. Both of these guides take items from standardized tests, but are not standardized themselves as tests. They can, however, give the observer a good deal more organized, detailed information about a child than unplanned, spontaneous observation. Some of the standardized developmental tests mentioned in the chapter are much better than others, and some are more specific than others; the nurse will soon learn her own preference.

VISION TESTING

Vision screening is an extremely important part of the care of children of all ages. Difficulty with vision is both a common and a serious condition. If a child's vision has always been poor or if it has become poor gradually, the child is likely to be unaware that a problem exists. Unless the defect is rather severe, the parents will probably be unaware of it also. Although it is easy to tell if a child is suffering from a very severe degree of poor vision, it is quite difficult to pick up less incapacitating, yet important losses. Preschoolers who have some lessened degree of visual acuity will miss out on many of the experiences that are important in their perceptual and cognitive development. Their eye-hand coordination may be poor; they may not learn to distinguish important aspects of pictures that should lay the foundation for later reading ability. Schoolchildren who cannot see well are missing important parts of their education that they may never be able to make up. Therefore, detecting visual problems is important because of the significance to the individual child and because of the large numbers of children who have such problems. Vision impairment is the fourth most common disability in the United States; it is the leading cause of handicapping conditions in childhood (Krupke et al., 1970). From 5 to 10 percent of the preschoolers in this country have vision problems, while 20 to 30 percent of the school-age children have such problems (Green and Richmond, 1962). Many of these problems are not being currently detected. This is particularly true of the preschool group, in which only 2 percent receive any type of vision examination (Lippman, 1971). The importance of such screening is clear from the fact that although $7\frac{1}{2}$ million schoolchildren suffer from some type of visual difficulty, only one-fourth of these will manifest symptoms (Lippman, 1971). The other three-fourths would never be found without some type of visual examination. The fact that many of these children never are found is evident from the report of Armed Forces rejections in 1964–1965. Of those individuals who were rejected for eye defects, 75 percent had defects that could have been prevented or treated in childhood (Krupke, 1970). Certainly the most dramatic case is that of the child with a minor degree of crossed eyes; if the defect is caught early, the child can have perfect vision for life, but if it is missed, the child may totally lose the vision in one eye by school age. This is certainly a pressing reason for regular vision screening of preschoolers.

Vision is not only very important but also a very complicated function. It deserves careful evaluation at each well-child visit. A thorough history and careful observation are necessary. Methods of screening the six most important aspects of vision will be discussed in this chapter: visual acuity, farsightedness, nearpoint vision, heterophoria, color vision, and visual fields. These will be discussed with regard to methods now available for evaluation at various age levels. First, however, it is important to be aware of some general eye-related complaints that may indicate visual difficulties. Any child who seems to be either inattentive or excessively attentive to visual clues should be suspected of having visual problems. Such children may contort their face, squint their eyes, close one eye, cock their head or thrust it forward, or hold their body tensely while looking at things in the distance. Children who frequently try to brush things away from their eyes or who rub their eyes excessively (some of these children will have recurrent styes as a result) should be examined carefully. A physical finding or history of permanently or transiently crossed eyes demands ophthalmological consultation. Children should be asked whether they can see the blackboard, and they should be observed while reading from the blackboard as well as reading from books. Sitting very close to the television set may be an indication of visual problems although many children with adequate vision seem to do this from habit. At any rate, a careful physical examination and thorough history should accompany visual testing to discover possible eye problems.

Visual Acuity

Visual acuity is arbitrarily defined as the ability to see a standardized symbol at a standardized distance. Classically, this refers to a Snellen "E" or alphabet chart seen at 20 ft. The Snellen alphabet chart is by far the most accurate and should be used whenever possible. Generally it can be used with children above the third grade. It is important that the test be given accurately. Some charts are available which provide adequate illumination, but most charts come without lighting, and the lighting should be tested with a light meter. The light should fall evenly across the chart without shadows or glare and should measure between 10 and 30 footcandles. If lighting in the area is inadequate, it can be supplied by a 75-watt bulb in a gooseneck lamp, situated 5 ft away at a 45° angle. It is important to test children individually so that they cannot memorize the chart while waiting in line. One examiner should be stationed at the chart and one with the child. The examiner usually begins with the 20/30 or 20/40 line and works either up or down depending on how well the child does. Each child should be tested as far down the chart as he or she is able to read. A passing score on a line consists of reading the *majority* of letters on that line; this will differ from line to line since the lines vary in length. It is important to expose the entire line at once rather than a single letter at a time for this age group, since some authorities feel (e.g., Sheridan, 1970) that exposing one letter at a time may allow certain children with amblyopia to be missed. Vision tested by the single-letter method can be as much as $1\frac{1}{2}$ lines better than that tested by exposure of the whole line. The vision of both eyes together will never be poorer than that of either eye singly; for this reason, most authorities suggest not beginning the test with both eyes (it may be necessary with younger children in order to accustom them to the test). Some (e.g., Lippman, 1970), however, do suggest beginning the test with both eyes uncovered, since this may reveal a tropia. If a near and far cover test is done, however (as it should always be), a tropia will be seen anyway. Children should be able to read the 20/20 line by the fourth grade; any who are unable to read this line with either eye should be referred for further examination. Children from the age of 4 years through the third grade, should be able to read the 20/30 line accurately with both eyes, and children younger than this are expected to read the 20/40 line. These standards differ from those available 10 years ago; it has been shown that children's vision is much better than once believed. Any children who do not read the line appropriate for their age with each eye should be referred; furthermore, any children who show a two-line difference between eyes, even though the worst eye is seeing at a level appropriate for the child's age (for instance, a 3-year-old who has 20/20 vision in one eye and 20/40 in the other), should also be referred, since this difference may result in the child suppressing the vision in the poorer eye and eventually losing it completely. For this reason all children should be tested as far down the chart as they are able to see.

If the building in which the testing is being done does not have a space long enough to utilize the 20-ft chart, two alternatives exist. The Snellen chart is made in a 10-ft version which, though less desirable since it has been less thoroughly standardized, is generally quite adequate. A second possibility is to use the 20-ft chart with a mirror. In this situation, the examiner sits next to the child with the 20-ft chart between them. Both the examiner and the child look directly into a mirror 10 ft in front of them in which they can see each other and the chart. This arrangement has certain advantages; only one examiner is necessary, and she can remain close to the child, helping to maintain rapport. If an alphabet chart is used, it must be one specially constructed for use with a mirror; that is, the letters are printed backward so that they appear normally oriented to the child looking in the mirror.

For children who are too young to utilize an alphabet chart, the next best standardized chart is the Snellen E, sometimes called the illiterate E since it does not require knowledge of letters (see Fig. 18-28). Some feel that this is slightly less good, since no curves or complicated letters are used which might detect certain forms of astigmatism. Nonetheless in practice it is almost as good as the alphabet chart. Most E charts have the letter E oriented in four directions: up, down, right, and left. This is important since oblique angles are usually too developmentally advanced for the age

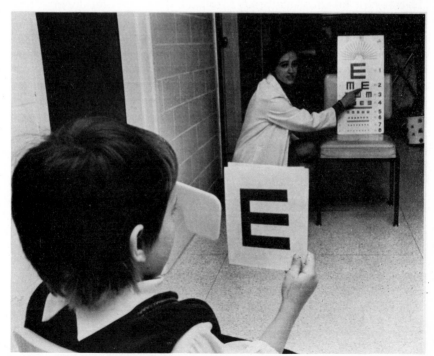

Figure 18-28 Child being tested with the E chart.

of the child who must use the E chart. The mechanics of testing with the E chart are basically the same as those for the alphabet chart. There are some problems, however, usually related to the age group with which this chart is used. One is that certain preschool children are still having difficulties with directionality. Children are generally asked to point a finger, hand, or entire arm in the direction which the E is pointing (or in which the "legs of the table" are pointing). This requires them not only to see the letter, but also to comprehend the idea of direction, to match this direction to the direction of their hand, and to be reasonably agile in making their hand or arm conform to the direction in their mind. In other words, this tests not only vision, but several other complicated skills; when children give an incorrect answer, it is difficult to be sure that it is their vision that is at fault. There are several approaches to this problem. One is to paste colorful, easily recognized pictures (e.g., a dog, a rabbit, a boy, and a girl) on the wall above, below, and at each side of the chart and then ask the child to say which picture the E is pointing to. This, at least eliminates the difficulty in motor maneuvering and in mentally matching the direction of the letter to the direction of an arm or hand. It does not eliminate the basic problem with directionality, however. Another very helpful step is to ask the parent to practice with the child at home the week before the test. This considerably increases the rate of testability. The National Society for the Prevention of Blindness has printed forms of the E chart for use in testing children at home (see Fig. 18-29) which can be sent home the week before the examination. In a clinic situation, it might be wise to institute a system where such a chart with an explanatory letter is automatically sent to the home of children from about 3 years of age on up. Practice in using the chart can also be given in a classroom setting by the teacher or nurse and is sometimes more effective than individual practice. The other difficulty in testing preschool children is the difficulty of gaining rapport. The mirror method described above is particularly helpful in this situation. Children this age may also have difficulty in looking at one letter at a time. For this reason, the National Society for the Prevention of Blindness suggests that single-letter exposure may be used for children below kindergarten. As noted earlier, some authorities disagree, saying this may mask amblyopia. It is important that the nurse record which method was used in testing.

Because the two Snellen charts are the best standardized, it is important to use them if at all possible; the accuracy of the results justify the extra time involved in having the child practice with the parent or in setting up a mirror arrangement or in any other measures that may be useful. If it is impossible to use the Snellen charts, however, the next best tests are those which utilize certain figures from the Snellen. The Landholt rings chart is exactly the same as the illiterate E chart, but uses the letter C instead. The same problems are inherent in it—the problem of directionality and the dif-

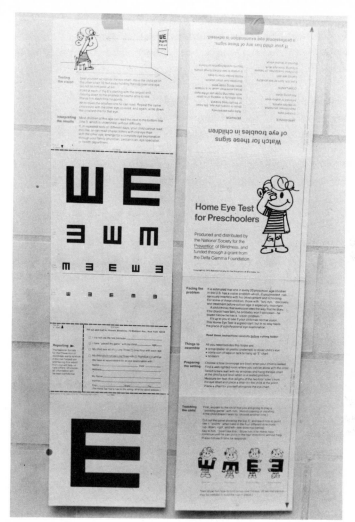

Figure 18-29 E chart for home testing.

ficulty in keeping the child's interest and the authors have found no advantage in it. The Ffooks chart is similar but utilizes a square, circle, and triangle (because these figures are developmentally recognized first). Since they are not the exact letters of the Snellen, their standardization is less accurate. By far the best test the authors have found for younger children is the Stycar test. This test is available in several forms. All forms have letters selected from the standardized Snellen which are recognized at a developmentally early stage. After working with several thousand young children, Sheridan and Gardiner isolated V, A, T, C, O, L, H, U, and X as the most easily recognized letters. The Stycar chart is similar to the Snellen alphabet chart but uses only these letters. Since children are not yet able to name the letters, they are given a card with the nine letters on it. They merely point to the letter which matches the letter being pointed to on the chart. For younger children, the test uses fewer letters: for the 4-year-old, seven letters are used; for the 3-year-old, five letters are used; and for the 2-year-old, only four letters are used. Only a single letter is shown at a time to younger children. This, of course, has the disadvantage of single-letter testing discussed above. Sheridan also suggests that the test be given at 10 ft with the use of a mirror. It has been found that 100 percent of the 4-year-olds are testable with the seven-letter method, 80 percent of the 3-year-olds are testable with the five-letter method, and 30 percent of the 2-year-olds can be tested using four letters. These are extraordinarily high rates of testability for these age groups. Lippman (1970), who compared the E test at 20 ft, the E test at 10 ft, the Allen cards (to be discussed later), the Stycar test, and the Starcar test (to be discussed later), determined that children found the Stycar easiest to learn, that it was highly accurate, and that testability became much higher with the Stycar on the second attempt than it did with the test at 10 ft although they were similar on the first attempt. It seems unfortunate that such a useful test as this is not more widely used in the United States.

If none of the more standardized tests (i.e., the Snellen alphabet, E, Landholt rings, or Stycar) can be used with a child, the next choice is one of the picture charts. These are far less standardized, and therefore far less accurate, and it should seldom be necessary to use them. Not only are they less standardized, but most of them are difficult to use because of the child's lack of familiarity with the pictures used. In Lippman's study (1970) it was found that testability rates are one-third lower with children from lower economic groups than rates from higher economic groups; the pictures used are generally of things a middle-class child rather than a lower-class child would be familiar with. Some of the tests are also put out in color. Although color may add interest, color charts are even less standardized than black-and-white ones. Probably the Allen cards are the best of the available picture tests, since greater effort has been put into their standardization (see Fig. 18-30). The tests consist of a series of black-and-white pictures (e.g., a telephone, a birthday cake, a man on a horse, a Christmas tree) which are shown to a child by an examiner as he slowly comes toward the child. The distance at which the child is first able to recognize three of the pictures is used as the numerator over the denominator of 30. A 3-year-old should achieve a score of 15/30; a 4-year-old, a score of 20/30. Any child who misses the appropriate pictures or who shows a 5-ft difference between eyes should be referred. Examples of other picture charts available are the Osterberg chart (see Fig. 18-30), a Danish chart of black-and-white

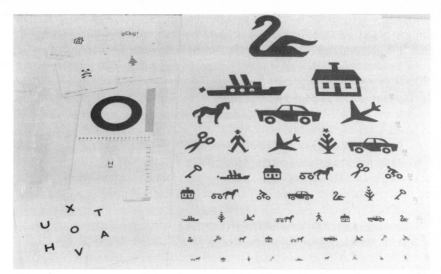

Figure 18-30 Vision testing materials: Allen cards, Osterberg chart, and Stycar test.

figures such as a swan, house, Christmas tree, man, and key; the Kindergarten chart, with colored pictures of a circle, heart, flag, sailboat, and cross; the A.O. and B&L test, which is similar to the Kindergarten chart but has black-and-white pictures; and the California Clown test, in which the clown's hand points in various directions. Other tests which might be considered picture tests are Sjogren's Hand and Withnell's Blocks (see Fig. 18-30). Sjogren's Hand is very much like the illiterate E test. However, in the attempt to turn the E into the more interesting picture of a hand, the standardization has been lost. The child may often determine the correct answer by the thickness of the palm rather than through an ability to distinguish between the fingers. Withnell's Blocks are inexpensive and quite portable. The cards depict one, two, or three rectangles in both horizontal and vertical positions (in order to detect certain types of astigmatism). Although more work has been put into standardizing this particular test, it still lacks the exact standardization of the Snellen, and in addition, it lacks the added interest of picture charts. The child must be able to count up to 3 in order to report how many blocks he sees.

For very young children, not even the picture tests will suffice, and only a rough estimate of their vision can be made. Again the most useful tests for this age group have been popularized by Mary Sheridan. The Starcar is a test devised by her which utilizes two sets of seven small toys—a car, plane, chair, knife, spoon, fork, and doll—one of which the examiner holds at 10 ft against a black background. The child has a similar set of toys (in different colors than the test toys so that the child is unable to match by color) which he holds up to match the one chosen by the examiner. This test cannot be exactly equated with the Snellen standards, but Sheridan advises that the child who can distinguish between the small knife and fork at 10 ft has vision equal to 20/20; a child who cannot distinguish between the large fork and knife should be referred for further evaluation. This is a more difficult test to administer, and the nurse should do it rather than delegating it to ancillary personnel. Sheridan has been able to use this test from about 21 months until the Starcar letters are usable.

For children below 21 months, there is only one rough test available, and again, it is seldom used in this country. This test consists of rolling standard-sized balls across a dark background and seeing whether the child can follow them at a distance of 10 ft. Again it is impossible to equate this test exactly to Snellen standards, but Sheridan says that a baby from 6 to 9 months can be expected to follow the $\frac{1}{4}$-in ball; a 10-month-old will follow a $\frac{1}{8}$-in ball; and by 12 months, the child should follow all balls. This test is more difficult to do monocularly since babies often object to having one eye closed, but it is sometimes worthwhile trying.

Heterophoria

Next to acuity testing, the most important screening test of vision available is the screening test for heterophoria. This is the most serious visual condition, particularly in preschool children, that the nurse is likely to encounter with any degree of frequency. *Heterotropia* refers to the situation in which a child's eyes do not focus together in such a way as to transmit good coordinated binocular vision; *heterophoria* is a tendency, not always overt, toward the same problem. This results from some type of inequality between the eyes or eye muscles which prevents each eye from focusing on exactly the same point at the same time. Sometimes this is obvious, as in cases of severely crossed eyes, but often it is more subtle and requires careful observation and screening procedures to detect. It is extremely important to detect this condition because in some cases if it is undetected, the child will learn to suppress the vision in one eye completely; if not caught until school years, there is a good chance that this vision will never be regained. Neither the child nor the parents will ordinarily be aware of this problem, and therefore routine screening for it is essential. Hatfield (1966) found that 20.9 percent of the eye problems found in his sample of 3-year-olds were problems of this type. Many babies will exhibit intermittently crossing eyes. If such a muscle imbalance is horizontal rather than vertical, if it is not constant, and if it becomes gradually better, it can be considered normal up until the age of 6 months. After this, it may be normal, but should be referred to an ophthalmologist for careful consideration. After this age, any history of eyes which cross when the child is tired or sick or occasionally for unknown reasons should also be referred for ophthalmological consultation. When such crossing is overt and constant, it is referred to as *tropia*. Where there is merely a tendency to such crossing, it is called a *phoria*, and must usually be detected by certain screening methods. These screening methods should be incorporated into every well-child examination. The first of these is called the *corneal light reflex* (or Hirschberg's reflex) and should be done in both a near-point (i.e., about 14 in) and far-point (i.e., about 20 ft) position. The child is asked to look straight ahead at a particular spot designated by the examiner. The examiner then shines a penlight into the child's eyes and notes where the light reflex falls. It should fall on exactly the same position in each eye; any asymmetry should be referred for further consultation. In order to evaluate this carefully, it is important that the child's eyes remain completely still, giving the examiner enough time to determine where the light reflex is falling. This can usually be explained to older children. With young babies, a bright, flashing, moving toy is ideal, since they will generally focus on it long enough for such a determination. It is often wise to turn out the room lights, since overhead lights will also be reflected in the eyes and it may be difficult to tell which light reflex is coming from the room lights and which from the examiner's penlight.

The next test which should also be done at each visit is called the *cover test*. It is another method of making manifest a phoria which cannot usually be seen. This test is also begun by having the child focus on a specified spot, first 14 in away and then 20 ft away. While the child is focusing on the spot, one eye is covered. It is important that the eye be covered completely so that it is unable to focus. It is also important that neither the eye nor the eyelashes be touched, since this will cause the child to blink when the cover is moved, and the examiner will not be able to see the response of the pupil. The cover should be held over the eye from 5 to 10 seconds and then removed fairly abruptly. The examiner then watches the *previously covered eye* to see if it moves. If there is a phoria, the covered eye will have begun to wander when it was unable to focus on the designated spot (i.e., when it was covered), and when the cover is removed, the eye will attempt to refocus with a sharp jerky movement. It is this movement which will indicate to the examiner that the eye has a phoria. This procedure is repeated for both eyes both at the near point of 14 in and the far point of 20 ft. Although a very slight movement can be normal, the authors feel that any movement requires a referral to an ophthalmologist. Since the consequences of underreferral are so grave (i.e., amblyopia with possible irreversible loss of sight in one eye), it is better to err on the side of overreferral.

Farsightedness

Although young children are normally slightly farsighted, some authorities feel that it is important to detect an abnormal amount of farsightedness or *hyperopia*. For preschoolers and schoolchildren through the second grade, this is done by having them read the 20-ft line of the E or alphabet chart at a distance of 20 ft through a +2.25 lens. Normally, a child should be unable to accommodate enough to see this line clearly. If the eyes *do* accommodate, and the child is able to read four of the six symbols correctly, this amount of hyperopia may be an indication that this child is more likely to develop eye fatigue or symptoms of muscle imbalance. Not all ophthalmologists agree that this test is worthwhile for the preschooler, so before initiating this screening it is wise for the nurse to consult with the ophthalmologist in the community to whom children will be referred. This procedure is more commonly accepted for older schoolchildren. Generally it is recommended that a +1.75 lens instead of a +2.25 be used on children in the third grade and older.

Near-Point Vision

Near-point vision refers to the acuity achieved by the eyes at a distance of 13 to 14 in (reading distance). It is almost always the same as acuity at a distance of 20 ft. The primary condition in which a difference will be seen is *presbyopia,* a condition of old age. In young children, accommodative powers are great, and even a child who might have difficulty in reading for longer periods of time will usually be able to adapt for the few minutes necessary for the test. For this reason, the National Society for the Prevention of Blindness does not recommend its routine use. It is possible that a phoria may become manifest during its use, but this should be detected when doing the near-point cover test. Again, this test may be more useful with older school-age children. Most of the charts available for testing acuity at 20 ft are also available in sizes standardized for near-point testing at 14 in.

Color Blindness

Not all clinicians agree that testing for color vision is important. The authors, however, feel that every boy should be tested for color blindness, preferably during kindergarten. Since color blindness is so rare in girls, routine testing of them is probably not necessary. Although color blindness is not correctable, it is important to know that it exists. One reason the authors recommend testing during kindergarten is the increasing use of color in educational materials, for instance Sullivan's *Words in Color* and the Cuisenaire rods used so often today. If the teacher is aware that a child is color-blind, much misunderstanding can be eliminated when using these materials. Awareness of this defect is also important in considering occupational choices since certain occupations rely heavily on color vision. Color testing needs to be done only once, since the results will not change. The classic materials for testing color vision are the *Ishihara* plates, and these are still used with adults and older children. They consist of a series of plates with figures composed of dots hidden in a background of similar dots. The only cue to help the individual distinguish the figure is color. If the person is color-blind, the figure remains hidden. There are four types of plates: the *vanishing-figure* plate, which contains a figure that a person with color vision can see but a person with either red or green color blindness cannot see; the *diagnostic* plates, which contain two hidden figures, one which can be seen only if a person has normal red vision and the other which can be seen only if normal green sensitivity is present; the *transformation* plates, which also have two hidden figures, one which is seen only with normal vision and one which should be seen only with abnormal color vision; and the *hidden-digit* plate, with figures which persons with abnormal color vision can see but which those with normal color vision cannot see. These last two types are not totally accurate, since some people with normal color vision are able to see the figures which should be seen only by color-blind individuals.

An improvement has been made on the Ishihara plates by adding plates to detect difficulties in yellow-blue color vision. These are the AOHRR polychromatic plates, which, although they have just been discontinued, are still used in most places. They are considered to be more valid than the Ishihara, and are 100 percent effective with red-green difficulties and somewhat less effective with blue-yellow defects. The test consists of 24 plates, including 4 demonstration plates and 20 test plates. A quick screening test can be given by selecting only the high- and low-chroma plates. Individuals missing these can be further tested with the more moderately hued plates. It is important to use the lamp which comes with the test since normal room light completely invalidates the findings. These plates are useful with children who have reasonably good figure-ground skill and who can name the letters, numbers, and geometric figures on the plates. For younger children, tracing the figures can sometimes be useful although this requires considerable eye-hand coordination.

For children too young to be tested by these plates, some researchers have used such tasks as matching colored yarns or putting colored table tennis balls in similarly colored muffin tin compartments. Various forms of color wheel matching tests are also used. None of these are accurate. The only other test known to the authors to be constructed specifically for young children is Guy's color vision test (see Fig. 18-31). This test uses the Ishihara plates but provides matching figures that the child can point to rather than actually naming them (the same principle utilized in the Stycar test). Although no research has been done on this test, the authors have found it quite easy to use with young children. However, since only the high-chroma plates are used, it might be possible to miss children with more minor degrees of color defects. For this reason, if Guy's test is given in kindergarten, it might be wise to rescreen children when they are old enough to utilize the AOHRR plates.

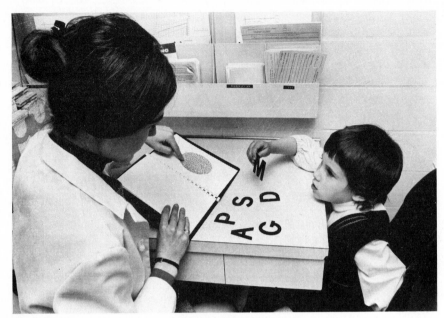

Figure 18-31   Testing for color vision with Guy's color test.

Visual Fields

Testing for visual fields is usually considered part of the neurological examination, although we are including it under visual screening techniques. The object of this screening is to assess the child's peripheral vision. It is possible to have limited peripheral vision due to ocular, neurological, or pituitary problems (usually a pituitary tumor). The procedure for this test begins with the child facing the examiner, about 3 ft away, with the examiner's arms outstretched halfway between the child and herself. The fingers of one or both hands are moved at a spot where the examiner can see and ask the child to say which finger is moving. This should be repeated in all four quadrants of vision, first with both eyes and then with each eye individually. When the eyes are tested individually, the examiner must remember to close his or her own left eye while the child closes the right eye and vice versa. Because there is really no standard, the child's peripheral vision must be compared with that of the examiner. For this reason it is essential to keep the moving finger exactly halfway between the examiner and the child. Roughly, peripheral vision is expected to be 60° on the nasal side, 100° on the temporal side, and 130° in both vertical directions. The only more objective method of measuring peripheral vision is with a machine called a *multiple pattern field screener,* but this is available in very few places.

Testing Infants

When dealing with infants, it is impossible to test specifically all the aspects of vision discussed in this chapter. It is important, however, to be sure that they have at least some vision. Historically, there has been a gradual increase in the awareness of how well infants can see. As we devise better and better methods of assessing infants' vision, it becomes clear that infants have an acuity better than we have realized simply because we have not had adequate methods of testing. This is still true. It used to be thought that an infant had an acuity of 20/670; today it is felt that acuity is actually 20/450. Chances are that it is better than that; we are simply still unable to test it well. For clinical purposes, the nurse should at least be certain that every newborn can see. This can be done in three ways: the following response, the turning-to-light response, and the nystagmus response to an optokinetic drum. The following response consists of just that: following. Even a newborn will show the ability to track a light or bright object for limited distances. An infant who does this certainly is not blind; the nurse does not, of course, know how well the infant sees. If an infant is held face up in the examiner's arms with the back of the head toward a source of bright light, such as a window, the eyes of a normally sighted infant will turn toward the source of light. Again, no measurement of vision is possible, but at least the nurse is assured that the baby can see. A third method of testing for presence of some vision is by using an optokinetic drum. Generally the drum has stripes on it although some have various pictures on them. When the drum is twirled slowly in front of the infant's open eyes, nystagmus will be elicited if vision is present (see Fig. 18-32).

When and Where to Do Vision Screening

A child's first visual examination should be performed soon after birth, usually in the nursery. In the normal newborn, testing methods already discussed are sufficient; in premature infants, periodic visual examinations should be done by an ophthalmologist during infancy and later (the effects of retrolental fibroplasia are not always immediately evident). After that the nurse should make some attempt to assess the child's visual abilities at every well-child visit. The appropriate methods for various age groups have been discussed above. It is also important not to overlook the family's assessment of the child's vision. In very serious visual problems, the parents will often be the first to suspect a problem; in more minor problems they may be unaware of the difficulty.

With children over $2\frac{1}{2}$, it may be possible for the parent to test the child's eyes with an E chart at home long before it is possible for an unfamiliar examiner to test them. The National Society for the Prevention of Blindness has created a card for such testing which parents can use at home (Fig. 18-29). Press (1968) found that more visual problems were discovered

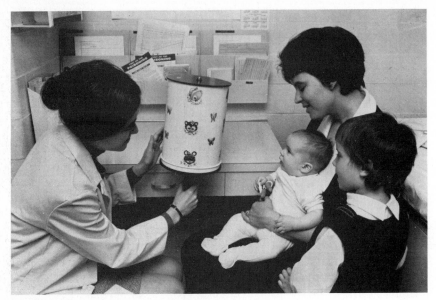

Figure 18-32   Nystagmus test for vision.

by parents than by nurses and that there was only a 4.6 percent rate of over-referrals. Trotter (1966) compared testing by parents with testing by volunteers and found parents much more accurate. Home testing can be an extremely important adjunct to the office visits. At this time, 94 percent of the preschool children in this country have never received a vision screening exam; this situation could be greatly improved by teaching parents to test their own children. Cards for home testing are available at no cost from local chapters of the National Society for Prevention of Blindness.

In addition to testing at every well-child visit, it is usually recommended that schools test children's vision according to the schedule discussed before since many of the children of this age do not see a physician regularly.

HEARING TEST

As with vision screening, a careful evaluation of the child's hearing is an essential part of every well-child visit. Estimates of children in this country with some degree of hearing impairment vary from 2 to 12 percent, and of these, 3 to 5 percent have defects serious enough to interfere with schoolwork (Moghadam et al., 1968). This figure is far greater for those living in poorer socioeconomic conditions, either rural or urban; it is estimated that about 19.8 percent of these children suffer from hearing loss

(Fay et al., 1970). It is important that all nurses be alert to clues indicating the possibility of future language disorders, since hearing and language are so closely related. Children who should arouse the nurse's suspicion include babies who babble normally until about 6 months and then gradually decrease in sound production (even totally deaf babies will babble the first few months); who constantly miss high-pitched consonants and fricatives such as "s," "sh," "ch," "f," "th," and sometimes "k"; who pay little attention to the radio or who turn its volume up above the comfort level of others in the house; who are consistently inattentive to speech; who manifest garbled speech; whose voice quality is poor or whose voice is quite loud or a monotone; who consistently drop word endings; who use mostly vowel sounds after 1 year of age; who do not turn to the source of sound by 4 months, who omit initial consonents after age 3; whose speech is highly unintelligible after age 3; who are not talking at all by age of 2; who are inconsistent in responses to speech or environmental sounds during the first 2 years; who do not understand commands or instructions by 18 months; who do not react with a startle to loud noises during the 1st year; or who do not react to name or commands by 6 to 9 months. Although these behaviors may be normal or may indicate other problems, they should make the nurse highly suspicious about the child's hearing or language development.

Types of Hearing Loss

Hearing loss can be of two types: peripheral and central. Peripheral losses can be either conductive or sensorineural. Conductive losses are the most common in young children. They are caused by some physical obstruction which interferes with the sound waves being conducted from the outside air through the middle ear. Most often, the obstruction is in the form of thick fluid such as exists in serous otitis or glue ear. During the acute phase of otitis media, one-third of children will have some hearing loss, which will last until the infection is completely healed and probably for 1 or 2 weeks after that. Children with conductive losses lose hearing sensitivity equally in all frequencies, although it is sometimes more accentuated in the lower frequencies. Air conduction is poor but bone conduction is normal.

Sensorineural or cochlear hearing loss refers to a loss caused not because of a problem in the middle or outer ear, as is true for conductive loss, but because of a defect in the inner ear, usually with the cilia or fluid system of the cochlea; sometimes damage to the eighth (acoustic) cranial nerve will result in such a loss. This type of loss is usually permanent (or at least has always been considered so until the advent of acupuncture as a possible cure for nerve deafness). It affects primarily high frequencies and results in a general loss of clarity in hearing acuity. Air conduction is equal to bone conduction, and recruitment may be present; recruitment is the abnormal increase in sensitivity to loudness; in other words, a person hears less and less clearly as the sounds become softer and softer until, suddenly, as the lowest hearing threshold is neared, the sounds become disproportionately louder.

Central hearing losses can be either retrocochlear losses, which are uncommon in children, or losses due to brain damage, either generalized throughout the brain or localized to the temporal area.

Causes of Hearing Loss

Hearing loss can appear at birth or later in childhood. It is important to detect hearing loss which is present from birth as soon as possible; many specialists recommend putting hearing aids on children as soon as the loss is detected, sometimes as early as 2 or 3 months to achieve the best results. Hearing losses present at birth may be of a hereditary nature, and a careful family history in this regard should always be taken. Some such hereditary diseases will appear at birth, but most will be progressive and become manifest only gradually. Other congenital problems can also result in hearing losses. Cleft palate is frequently associated with frequent serous otitis media and often results in eventual hearing loss. Children with this defect should have their hearing evaluated regularly. Prenatal infections may result in hearing losses of the sensorineural type in infants. Syphilis and rubella during the first 4 months of pregnancy are well-known causes; other viruses are probably implicated as well. Losses resulting from such prenatal infection may be present at birth, but may not become evident until the child is older; therefore these children should be followed carefully even though as newborns they appear to have normal hearing. Metabolic or endocrine problems in the pregnant woman as well as various kinds of poisoning (quinine, salicylates, alcoholic overdoses) may also cause the newborn to suffer hearing losses. Any pregnant woman who has taken such drugs should have her infant carefully evaluated. Obstetric trauma, birth anoxia, Rh or ABO incompatibility, or kernicterus are other conditions known to be associated with an increased incidence of hearing loss in the newborn. Again, such loss may be present in the newborn, but may not become evident until later.

Other agents can cause hearing loss later in childhood. Most common of these is recurrent, frequent otitis media or serous otitis. Any child with such a history should be evaluated very thoroughly. Labyrinthitis of otitic origin, especially in infants, is often implicated, as are infectious diseases which affect the auditory nerve or organ of Corti (examples of these are measles, mumps, viral neuritis of the eighth nerve, and meningitis and encephalitis, particularly when caused by *Hemophilus* influenza). Drugs may also be etiologic; particularly ototoxic are neomycin, kanamycin, and streptomycin. These drugs may result in immediate loss or may be responsible for a loss which is delayed by 2 to 3 months. A careful history for these drugs should always be taken. Impacted wax is an infrequent but real cause of some conductive loss in older children, as are inflamed adenoids which block the opening to the eustachian tube, often resulting in serous otitis. Progressive inherited deafness may also become evident only in later childhood.

Screening Tests

The nurse working in ambulatory pediatrics must be alert to all such suggestive clues indicating the possibility of hearing loss, but even without such indications, every child deserves a careful hearing evaluation at every well-child visit. The type of evaluation will differ with the age of the child. This chapter will discuss some of the screening tests available for various age groups as well as some of the diagnostic tests which are utilized in the specialist's more thorough evaluation.

Tests used with the school-age child will be discussed first since they are, in general, the easiest to administer and the most clearcut. There are several such tests available, and although the nurse should be aware of them, it is the authors' strong opinion that only an audiometric screening test is adequate for evaluation of school-age children. Certainly some of the commonly used tests are clearly inadequate. Examples of these are coin-click tests, watch-tick tests, and whispered-voice tests. These are all tests in which the examiner roughly compares the patient's hearing with his or her own. They are not standardized, and in the case of a child, in whom accurate hearing is so vital, they can only be considered insufficient. Tuning forks, also, although useful for certain specific purposes, are not adequate for the hearing evaluation of a child.

Tuning-Fork Tests Three tuning-fork tests are commonly used: the Weber, the Rinne, and the Schwabach. The Weber test is performed by striking the tuning fork to make it vibrate and placing the stem in the midline of the scalp. The child is then asked if it is louder in either ear or if it is the same in both. A normally hearing child will hear it equally well in both ears and will usually localize it at the midplane. If the sound lateralized to one ear, a conductive loss may exist in that ear or a sensorineural loss may exist in the opposite ear. In any case, such a child needs further evaluation by an audiologist. This test is usually impossible with preschoolers, who are unable to comprehend the concept of comparing loudness between ears.

The Rinne test is performed by striking the tuning fork until it is vibrating, and then placing the stem on the child's mastoid until he no longer hears it. At this point, the fingers of the fork, which are still vibrating, are placed in midair, 1 to 2 in lateral to the concha and the child is asked whether he can hear them. Since air conduction should be about two times better than bone conduction, the child should be able to hear the fingers of the fork vibrating in the air after he can no longer hear the stem of the fork vibrating on his mastoid process. Any child who is unable to do so should be referred for further evaluation.

The Schwabach test is less commonly used. It consists of comparing the patient's bone conduction to that of the examiner's. The stem of the vibrating fork is placed on the child's mastoid until she can no longer hear it; it is then placed on the examiner's mastoid. If the examiner can still hear the vibration after the child has said she can no longer hear it, the child should be referred for further evaluation. The frequencies usually suggested as best for the tuning forks which are to be used in these tests are the 256, 512, and 1024. These tests give the nurse an idea of the difference between air-conduction level and the bone-conduction level in the child's hearing, but they give no indication of the actual level of hearing which the child has. They should be used only as supplementary to the audiometric screening.

Audiometric Tests Audiometric testing has been used since the early 1900s when the Western Electric Company produced the first multiple mass screening audiometer. It is important that the nurse be familiar with audiometers and certain terminology pertaining to their use although the nurse will generally be responsible only for supervising others in administering the tests. Many types of audiometers are available, and a listing of those which have met the standards of the Subcommittee on Conservation of Hearing of the American Academy of Ophthalmology and Otolaryngology is published regularly in the *Transactions of the American Academy of Ophthalmology and Otolaryngology.* Audiometers are basically similar although there are some differences. They may be either battery-operated or electric, and they may be either the standard type or of special adaptation such as those used only for neonates, those which can be used for automatic screening, and those which can be used for screening with multiple earphones. All will have an on-off button, an output selector which directs the noise to the right or left ear, earphones (red for the right and blue for the left ear), a hearing threshold level to regulate the loudness, a frequency lever, sometimes an air-bone selector, and sometimes a masking device. Machines should be calibrated to the ANSI standards which were adopted in 1969. If old machines are used which are calibrated to the previously used ASA or ISO standards, a conversion table should be attached to the machine and the results translated into the new standards.

It is important that the nurse be familiar with certain terms and abbreviations commonly used in testing hearing so that he or she will be able to record the findings and to understand the recordings of others. The abbreviation for the term *decibel* is dB, which refers to the degree of loudness or intensity of a sound. The abbreviation for *Hertz* is Hg and for *cycles per second,* that is, the pitch or frequency of a sound, is cps. *Recruitment* refers to the abnormal sensitivity to loudness when nearing the threshold; this symptom is caused by damage to the cochlear portion of the ear. *Threshold* is the faintest tone which can be heard 50 percent of the time. *Air conduction* is the conduction of sound from the air through the outer and middle ear; *bone conduction* refers to the conduction of sound through the bone. *Masking* is a noise introduced into the better ear in a situation in which one ear hears considerably better than the other. It is not used in screening. Abbreviations for recording should also be familiar to the nurse. Findings from air conduction are always indicated by a solid line. This line is interrupted by the symbol O for the right ear and X for the left ear; □ is used as a symbol for the right ear masked during air conduction and △ for the left ear masked in air conduction. When air conduction is performed without earphones, as in the case of very young children who are afraid of earphones, it is done in a soundproof room by a specialist who records a blue S for the findings of the left ear and a red S for the findings of the right ear. S stands for *sound field,* the term used for the open, soundproofed room. Bone conduction is indicated by a dotted rather than solid line. In bone conduction, the symbol > indicates the right ear unmasked; < indicates the left ear unmasked; ▶ symbolizes the right ear masked; and ◀ indicates the left ear masked. Although not all these symbols will be used in the type of screening the nurse will usually be involved in, it is important that she be familiar with them since reports from the audiologist will often use them.

The human ear can hear from about 20 to 20,000 Hz, but of these, the most important speech frequencies are 500, 1000 and 2000 Hz; 3000, 4000, and 6000 Hz are sometimes considered important for environmental sounds. Sounds over 6000 Hz are rarely important in human hearing. Many specific audiometric screening tests are available, but all of them specify certain of these important sounds to be tested. Specific directions for the various audiometers come with the machines, but some pointers are important for all of them. Children should always be positioned in such a way that they are unable to see the examiner's hands operating the interrupter switch. The interrupter switch should be used to channel the noise first to one ear and then to the other, always in an irregular pattern so that children are not able to respond to the pattern rather than the actual sound.

Several types of screening tests are used for school-age children. The Massachusetts test uses a multiple-earphone audiometer, and the child is asked to circle yes or no when hearing a sound of 500, 4000, and 6000 Hz. As many as 40 children can be tested at one time, and this test is generally rapid and efficient in fourth grade and above. A similar test is the Glorig Automatic Group Screening Test. This test can be used with as many as 40 children with multiple headphones attached to one machine. It is automatic and requires no trained personnel. It is effective only after the level of about third grade. The Reger-Newby Group Screening Test is operated in the same automatic manner, and the child is asked to count the number of sound spurts heard at each frequency. The Johnston Group-Tone is another multiple-earphone audiometric test. It is constructed in such a way that the child can respond by raising a hand rather than recording an answer as is done in the other tests. Not all earphones receive the sound at the same time, so children are prevented from responding solely on the criterion that children next to them are raising their hand. The advantage to this method is that children who are not yet old enough to write can be tested; the disadvantage is that a trained person is necessary since the test is not totally automatic; it is often found that children below fourth grade are not testable even with this method since they require more individualized attention.

The 1974 National Conference on Identification Audiometry recommended that, whenever possible, individual audiometric tests be given (Fig. 18-33) although it recognized that mass screening was more economical and could be used where economics was the deciding factor. It is also stated that manual rather than automatic machines should be used, particularly for younger children. This body suggested that the frequencies of 1000, 2000, and 4000 Hz be tested at the level of 20 dB (ANSI). If the 400-Hz-level test is failed at the 20-dB level, it can be retested at the 25-dB level. A child who passes the 400 Hz signal at the 25-dB level is considered to have normal hearing.

Diagnostic Testing

Children who fail the screening audiometric test should be rescheduled for a second screening within 1 week; if they again fail, they should be referred to an audiologist who will perform a more definitive threshold audiogram. This test uses the same machine and the same basic principles of audiometric screening but differs slightly in technique and purpose. The goal of the threshold audiogram is to find the child's threshold (i.e., the lowest level at which a sound is audible 50 percent of the time) for each frequency. The Committee on Conservation of Hearing of the American Academy of Ophthalmology and Otolaryngology recommends that this be performed by the ascending technique; that is, the test begins below the level at which the tester expects the child to hear and proceeds to increase the decibels by 10 until the child can hear; the decibels are then decreased in steps of five until the child can no longer hear. This technique, known as the Hughson-Westlake ascending technique, is continued until the child's threshold is discovered for each frequency. This test is much more time-consuming and requires more skill than the screening tests and should probably not be utilized by the nurse if a trained audiologist is available.

Further diagnostic testing may be performed in the form of speech audiometry. In general, speech sounds are not as accurate as pure tones in

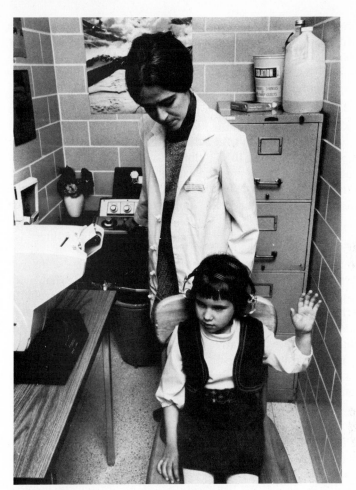

Figure 18-33 Individual audiometric testing.

assessing accurate levels of total hearing ability, but in certain circumstances they may be more accurate since they test the amount of hearing that the child is able to utilize when listening to spoken communication. Usually spondees (i.e., two-syllable words phonetically balanced with random high and low frequencies) are used, although occasionally monosyllables, sentences, and connected discourse are used. Such testing may miss high-frequency losses since the words may be recognized by the frequency vowels, but, as stated before, this may be useful in discovering how well the child has learned to utilize what hearing he or she has. The audiometer necessary for speech audiometry is different from that used for pure tone audiometry and is generally available only in speech clinics. Although one form of speech audiometry, the fading-numbers test, has been used in the past for screening purposes, this is no longer considered adequate and only pure-tone audiometry should be used in screening.

When and Where to Do Hearing Screening

Generally, it is recommended that audiometric screening be scheduled in the school at the kindergarten, first, third, fifth, and seventh grades every year and that it include all transfers to the school during the preceding year no matter what grade they are in. In the clinic situation, hearing evaluation should be done as part of every physical examination, and as follow-up to any disease known to be potentially ototoxic (e.g., measles, mumps, otitis media, any disease with high fever, and upper respiratory infections even without known ear infections); after administration of ototoxic drugs such as streptomycin, kanamycin, and neomycin; and regularly in high-risk groups as discussed earlier.

Testing Preschoolers Preschoolers and toddlers are somewhat more difficult to test, but it is at least as important and maybe more important to be sure these children are hearing well. They are not old enough to be aware of whether they are developing a hearing loss or not, and hearing is crucial to the important skills they are learning, particularly their language skills. Audiometric testing using pure tones is the most accurate measure available, and some mature preschoolers will be able to cooperate easily with this method. Most younger children, however, will need certain modifications. As in vision testing with the E chart, it is worth taking some extra time to help this age group understand the audiometric test since there is no other test as accurate. Patience is usually the most important component to successful testing with this age group. Inclusion of the parent in the testing and asking the parent to practice the testing at home using earmuffs and a whistle the week before the examination are extremely helpful. Sometimes open-field audiometry in which no earphones are used is necessary, but this requires a soundproof room and a skilled audiologist; it is impossible to test the ears separately with this method. But for high-risk children who cannot be tested in other ways or for children about whom the nurse has a question, this may be necessary.

In general, audiologists will attempt to use play audiometry to test children of this age, and many of these techniques can be adopted by the nurse in the clinic setting. The underlying assumption of play audiometry is that the child will be much more responsive if meaning is given to the sound. Some elaborate mechanisms, such as the peep show in which the child can push a button when a sound is on and activate a doll or cause some other interesting visual stimuli or the frequently used pedacoumeter in which seven puppets will pop out if the button is pushed in response to a sound, are available in specialized hearing clinics but seldom if ever in outpatient pediatric clinics. The nurse can attempt on a simpler level, however, to create more interest in the test. This is usually done by having the child use a more interesting response than the traditional hand raising. Sometimes children will enjoy putting a ring on a peg or a block in a box. It is usually best to start without earphones on and with very loud sounds to which the parent responds by putting a block in a box. Then the parent and the child respond together, and the parent guides the child's hand with the block in it into the box at the appropriate moment. Gradually the child is allowed to do this alone. Only when the child understands the game completely are the earphones put on. This may require several sessions, sometimes with practice at home in between visits. An excellent example of this is seen in the film "Too Young to Say," available from the John Tracy Clinic. Speech audiometry is sometimes used for this age group because although it lacks some of the accuracy of the pure-tone testing, it is inherently more interesting to the young child. One picture test consists of four phonetically similar words with matching pictures. The words are filtered through known frequencies and the child is asked to point to the appropriate picture (Bennett, 1951). The more widely used Verbal Auditory Screening for Children (VASC) is a similar test consisting of 12 responses and stimulus pictures. Currently these are not recommended as accurate screening tests.

Experiments have also been done by Downs and the University of Denver in which familiar animal sounds are filtered at specific frequencies and the child is asked to point to the picture of the animal which made such a sound. This test is not commonly available, however.

Mary Sheridan, one of the world's leading authorities on the sensory screening of young children, feels strongly that children of all ages should be tested not only for pure-tone sensitivity, but for hearing of actual speech as well. As discussed previously, it is impossible to standardize speech sounds as accurately as pure tones, particularly without the use of filtered speech monitored by a specialized audiometer. Sheridan, however, has worked extensively with this problem and has devised several spoken tests which are easily administered clinically. These consist of a series of identification tests in which children are asked to point to one of several toys in front of them. For the 3- to 7-year-old, Sheridan devised a seven-toy test, which uses a set of seven toys, the names of which are carefully selected to test an ascending frequency scale of sounds. Starting from the lowest-pitched words, the names are "spoon," "doll," "fork," "car," "knife," "plane," and "ship." The examiner first ensures that the child knows all the appropriate names and then, standing at ear level, 10 ft from the child, names the toys in this order in a moderate tone of voice. The child is asked to point to each toy as it is named. For the younger child (2 to 3 years old), Sheridan devised a six-toy test consisting of a cup, spoon, ball, car, doll, and brick. Again the sounds used in the words appear in an ascending order of frequency. Finally, Sherican reports success using the five-toy test (by omitting the spoon) for children as young as $1\frac{1}{2}$ years.

One of the most exciting technological advances in auditory screening has been the recent introduction of impedance tests. This tests for conductive loss in a more objective and sensitive way than has ever been possible before. An impedance meter is a special machine with an earpiece. One end is placed inside the external auditory canal and the other is attached to the machine. A measured amount of force is then emitted and the resistance encountered is registered. The resistance comes from the tympanic membrane; a middle ear which is filled with fluid, as in the case of serous otitis, will cause the tympanic membrane to be stiffer than normal, and more resistance will be measured on the graph; a middle ear in which the ossicles are missing or broken will result in a very loose tympanic membrane, and less-than-normal resistance will be measured on the graph. This test takes only a few seconds to administer and requires no response or even cooperation from the child; for this reason it is suited for infants and young children. Although it cannot pick up sensorineural deafness, it is exquisitely sensitive to the most common type of ear pathology in young children—conductive loss from serous otitis; in this situation it is much more reliable than the commonly used pneumonic otoscopic tests. It is hoped that impedance machines are now becoming available in outpatient pediatric clinics.

If a child is too young or too immature to be tested by the audiometer through either pure-tone or speech audiometry, the nurse must resort to less standardized techniques.

Testing Infants For toddlers and young infants, one of the more commonly used tests is that devised by Hardy (1959) as a modification from the early work of the Ewings (1944). This is a test in which the child is held in the parent's lap and has his attention visually attracted directly in front of him. A noisemaker is then sounded to one side and the examiner observes whether a head or eye turn localizes the sound. This test is best performed with two examiners, one producing the sound to the side. The sounds produced should be of high frequency (a high-pitched rattle, the unvoiced consonants of "S" or "Sh," or the opening of a small ball of crisp tissue paper), medium frquency (a medium-pitched rattle or a metal teaspoon stirring gently against the rim of a cup), and low frequency (a xylophone, a low-pitched rattle, or the examiner's voice saying "baa," "bu," or "ga"). It is important for the examiner making the noise to stay completely out of view on a level with the child's ear, about 2 to 3 ft behind the child. By 3 months of age localization efforts should begin and the child will turn either the entire head or the eye toward the source of the sound if it is localized at ear level. By 6 months the localization response should be reasonably well developed, and a mere eye turn is not enough; a turn of the entire head is required. At 9 months, sharp localization is expected to sounds produced at the level of the ear or below, and by 1 year, the child should be able to localize either above or below the ear level. This is only a rough test since many frequencies are included in all such noisemakers; Clark (1956) analyzed 24 different such noisemakers and found a minimum of five frequencies in each. Testing of this kind is clearly demonstrated in the film "Auditory Screening of Infants," available from the Maryland State Department of Health, 301 Preston St., Baltimore, Maryland.

A recent development in this area is the manufacture of a device called the Denver Children's Screener Model PA-20 (available at the time of this writing from P.A. Electronics, 1024 Santa Fe Drive, Denver, Colorado 80204 for $250). This is a small box, easily held in one hand, which emits sounds of known frequencies at known decibel levels (available frequencies range from 500 to 600 Hz and decibels range from 30–80 cps). Use of this device enables the examiner to be much more precise in the assessment.

With neonates, testing is even more difficult. Neonatal audiometers such as the Xenith Nemometer and the Vicon Apriton are available. These emit the frequency of 3000 Hz at 80, 90, and 100 dB. They should be held 10 in from the ear. The most consistent reliable response indicating that the infant has heard the noise is an eyeblink, sometimes called the *acousticopalpebral reflex*. A *Moro* or *acoustic muscle reflex* (generalized flexing), an *auditory oculogyric reflex* (a horizontal movement of the eyes in infants over 4 months), an *arousal response* (eye opening, stirring, or limb movement), a cessation of movement or vocalization, or a change of expression are also considered evidence that the infant has heard. It is important that infants being tested be in the "drowsy state," that is, not so active that they are responding to many stimuli and not in such a deep sleep that they will not respond to any stimuli. This kind of testing is quite subjective, and even with training, Moncur (1968) found that 39 percent of the "yes" responses recorded by the examiner came at a time when no sound was even emitted. Downs and Hemenway (1969) screened 17,000 infants of whom 500 failed. Of these 500, only 15 had real hearing problems, and 1 child who passed did have a hearing loss. In spite of the high amount of overreferral and the missed child, Downs and Hemenway feel this procedure is justified, since the PKU test which has been instituted by law finds only 1 in 4000 to 6000.

Attempts have been made to find more objective response criterion. Bartoshuk (1964) used a change in the heart rate in both newborns and fetuses in utero; Heron and Jacobs (1969) used changes in respiration as the response. A "Papousek cradle" has been especially constructed for this purpose; the child is placed in the cradle and actual head turnings to sound are reported to be quite consistent (Bench, 1970).

One of the most exciting recent developments in infant screening for hearing problems is a device called the "crib-o-gram." This is a crib, especially equipped with a sensitizing device which detects and records small movements of the infant. With the infant in a quiet state, sounds of known frequencies are emitted at known decibel levels and any infant response is recorded automatically. This method has great promise since it is much more practical than some of those procedures previously discussed; at least in the early studies, it seems to be a very good detector of hearing problems.

In summary, then, it is important that each child's hearing be tested by the most accurate method available appropriate to his or her age. Children who are high risk because of the situations discussed previously or whose parents are concerned about their hearing deserve particularly careful evaluation. Any child who fails the test or about whom the nurse is uncertain should be referred for more sophisticated evaluation.

SPEECH TESTING

Another very important part of well-child care is the periodic evaluation of speech development. In this chapter, emphasis will be placed upon clinical evaluation of the individual child's speech. It is important to be generally aware of the developmental sequence of vocal sounds from the beginning cry through adultlike speech. This is particularly true of the developmental sequence of the sounds of articulation, which are repeated here for the reader's convenience:

3 to 4 years: lip sounds—"m," "p," "b," "w," "h"
4 to 5 years: tongue contact sounds—"n," "t," "d," "ng," "k," "g," "y"
5 to 6 years: "f"
6 to $6\frac{1}{2}$ years: "v," "th" (voiced, as in "then"), "ch," "sh," "l"
$6\frac{1}{2}$ to 7 years: "z," "s," "r," "th" (voiceless, as in "this")

Knowledge of normal development in this area will help alert the nurse to early danger signs. Even in infants and toddlers some of these dangers signs are already apparent. Some indications that should alert the nurse to evaluate a child carefully are difficulty in sucking, lack of musical inflection in early babbling, not responding with a startle to loud noises during the first year, not looking for the source of moderately loud sounds by eye or head turning by 4 to 8 months, not reacting to one's own name or commands such as "no-no" by 6 to 9 months, inconsistent response to speech or environmental sounds during the first 2 years, excessive drooling, not speaking at all by the age of 2 years, not comprehending commands or instructions by 18 to 24 months, or any expression by the parents that they are concerned about the child's speech or hearing development. Fiedler et al. 1971) found a history of abnormal crying in 19 percent of the children with poor speech and only 1 percent of children with normal speech. He also found a higher incidence of prenatal complications in the children with speech problems. An older child may also present certain signs which should alert the nurse to the possibility of hearing or speech problems. The nurse should evaluate very carefully any child who uses mostly vowel sounds in speech after the age of 1 year, any child in whom the amount of verbalizing decreases rather than increases at any time from birth to 7 years, any child who consistently drops word endings, or any child in whom the voice is a monotone, extremely loud, largely inaudible, or of poor quality.

Causes of Speech Problems

The most common cause of speech problems is mental retardation, while the second most common cause is loss of hearing (this is why many of the early danger signs of lost hearing are the same as those indicating the possibility of future speech problems). Fiedler (1971) found a "poor environment" in 45 percent of the children with speech problems, but in only 15 percent of those without speech problems. Certain anatomical problems can cause poor speech also. Cleft palate is a common etiology for speech problems. This refers not only to overt clefts but to submucous clefts as well. For this reason it is important for nurses always to include a check for submucous cleft in their physical examination of the mouth. This is done by palpating the upper hard palate to make sure it is intact. If a submucous cleft exists, a large notch will be felt (see Fig. 18-34); this can frequently be seen as well if the patient is asked to say "ah." It is important to remember that submucous cleft is frequently associated with a bifid uvula, and any

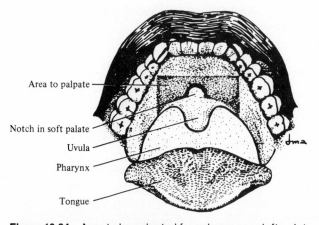

Figure 18-34 Area to be palpated for submucous cleft palate.

child with a bifid uvula should be examined very carefully for the existence of submucous cleft. Children with cranial nerve damage in which they lost control of their uvula or portions of the mouth and throat may also have poor speech, while children with tumors of the larynx may present with persistently hoarse speech. Problems with lip mobility which may be reflected in poor pronunciation of such sounds as "p," "b," "wh," "m," "f," and "v" are seldom organic, but may need a speech specialist to correct them. Difficulties with malocclusion may result in inaccurate articulation of the sounds "s," "z," "sh," "zh," "ch," and "j." Anatomical problems of the tongue are usually problems of either tongue thrust or paralysis of the tongue. Tongue thrust is a controversial subject. Such a condition apparently does exist, but its etiology, normal prognosis, and cure are not clear. This problem is sometimes referred to as *reverse swallowing* and consists of a backward movement of the tongue in the swallowing process, ending with a thrust of the tip of the tongue against the front teeth. Both dental and speech problems may result. This pattern is probably normal in certain very young children, but when it persists into the ages of active speech development, problems can arise: it should always be gone by the time of the eruption of permanent teeth (7 to 9 years) but can cause problems long before this. The nurse can examine for this by placing the fingers over the child's masseters while breaking the lip seal with the thumbs (see Fig 18-35). The child is then asked to swallow, and the nurse feels for a contraction of the muscles of mastication. Normally a significant contraction can be easily palpated; in children with tongue thrust, this contraction is felt either very slightly or not at all. It is interesting to note that this condition is seldom noted in children who have been breastfed for most of their infancy. This has led many to believe that this is caused by certain types of nipples, particularly very long nonpliable nipples. In fact, one of the commercial nipples, Nuk, is said to prevent tongue thrust because of its similarity to the human breast; this has not been proven, however.

Articulation Testing

Although it is important to be aware of all aspects of a child's speech—articulation, lexicon, syntax, and semantics—by far the most clinically useful screening tests are available for articulation. In general, these tests attempt to test individual sounds within the context of other sounds (that is, within words). Sounds are usually tested in three positions: word initial, word medial, and word final. Some tests test several positions in one word; although this is less time-consuming, it requires very good listening ability on the part of the examiner. Probably the least important position is word medial. It has been found that when this position was not tested, only 1 percent of the children with speech defects were missed.

One of the biggest difficulties in administering such tests is accurately

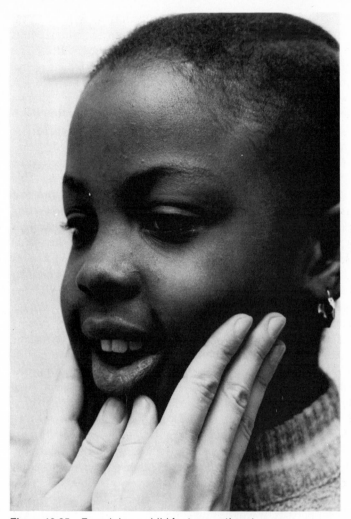

Figure 18-35 Examining a child for tongue thrust.

assessing the sound being tested. It takes some concentration to be able to listen only to the sound being tested and not to be influenced by the surrounding sounds. Although Irwin (1970) has found a very high correlation between examiners, the examiners in his study were speech pathology majors in college who had had a great deal of practice in this kind of listening. It is important for the nurse to be aware of this problem and to be carefully trained, ideally by working with a speech therapist or by obtaining such films as the one which teaches the Denver Articulation Screening Test, available from Laradon Hall, Denver, Colorado. It is easy to assume that you are hearing correctly when you are in fact not doing so.

The screening tests available for assessing speech are of three types: spontaneous, word imitative, and nonsense imitative. In the spontaneous type, the child speaks a familiar word without having heard it first. The most common technique used in this type of test is to present a picture and ask the child to name it. The word imitative test is one in which the examiner says a word and asks the child to repeat it. The nonsense imitative test is one in which the examiner says a nonsense word (such as "shuk" to test the word initial "sh" sound) and asks the child to repeat it. There is controversy concerning which of these types is best. Carter and Back (1958) and Snow and Millisen (1954) have shown that there are fewer errors when children repeat nonsense words than when they repeat real words. This seems to indicate that even though children hear the examiner pronounce a word, if it is a well-known word that they have heard pronounced in a different way before, they will pronounce it the way they are used to hearing it rather than the way the examiner pronounces it. An example of this is the use of the word "mother" in the Denver Articulation Screening Exam. Many black children repeat this word as "mothah," according to their own dialect. This certainly does not indicate that the children are incapable of using a word final "r" sound: it indicates merely that they do not think that sound is appropriate in that word, and they repeat the word with their correction. Carter and Buck (1958) and Snow and Millisen (1954) have further shown that there are fewer errors in imitative testing than in spontaneous testing; that is, it is apparently less difficult for children to imitate a word they have just heard than it is for them to pronounce a word which they know but have not just heard.

The most important attribute of a screening test, however, is its ability to predict future problems. The difficulty lies in the fact that articulation errors, even when age-inappropriate, tend to decrease without any kind of therapy from the first through the third grade. In other words, when a child of this age is found with an articulation defect, it is very possible that it will go away with no help at all. However, if the examiner waits until the third grade and the defect persists, it will be much more difficult to correct than if it had been referred in the earlier years. The problem, then, is determining which types of defect will disappear by themselves. This is not entirely known, and when possible the nurse should refer any child with a problem to a speech therapist. However, the question of how to predict which kinds of articulation problems will disappear spontaneously has been studied and some things are known. Intelligence and social maturity do not seem to have any effect on the disappearance of the problem. It is probable that the more consistent the error, the less likely that it will correct itself. There are also specific types of errors (like lateral lisps) which are less likely to disappear without therapy. Carter and McKenzie (1958) found that when a child made an error on the spontaneous test *which did not correct itself on the nonsense test,* this error was less likely to be outgrown. Steer and Drexler (1960) tested kindergarteners and found that the best predictor of speech errors which would not self-correct were (1) the overall number of errors, (2) the overall number of errors in word-final position, (3) the number of errors of omission in word-final position, and (4) errors in the "f" and "l" sounds (these sounds are particularly developmentally relevant at the kindergarten level). In order to avoid excessive overreferral, then, it might seem best, at least from the information available at this time, to use the comparison of a spontaneous and an imitative nonsense test. Unfortunately, the authors know of no commonly used test of this type suited for the clinical situation. Findings from the Steer and Drexler study are also useful in this regard.

Many types of tests are available for both screening and diagnostic purposes. The most complete and most commonly used diagnostic test is the Templin-Darly Diagnostic Test of Articulation, which is composed of 176 items in both picture card version and reading version. The format for this test is a sentence spoken by the examiner with a missing word to be filled in by the child. A picture to prompt the correct word accompanies the sentence. For instance, the examiner may say, "This is Smokey the _____," and show the child a picture of a bear. A comparable Templin-Darly screening test is also available and consists of 50 items.

Fiedler (1971) has devised a home screening examination which asks the child to perform and includes certain articulation skills and includes a survey of certain pertinent historical information such as pregnancy and labor problems. This test is specific for 3-year-olds. The Predictive Screening Test of Articulation (PSTA) was devised by Van Riper (1969) in order to predict which articulation errors would not correct themselves. It consists of some imitation of nonsense words, some imitation of words in sentences, some tests of recognition of misarticulation, and some items of skill in which the child imitates a rhythm by clapping the hands. Van Riper clearly states that this test is not yet fully tested, and one would assume that he does not yet feel it is adequate for clinical use. The Laradon Articulation Scale also attempts to predict which articulatory problems need therapy, but its predictive powers have not yet been proven. The Carter-Buck tests previously discussed also attempt to be predictive and actually consist of three subtests: one which tests spontaneous articulation, one which tests word imitative articulation, and one which tests nonsense syllable imitative abilities. The score is a comparison of the tests. This test is quite lengthy, however, and certainly cannot be considered a screening test. The Picture Articulation Test by Irwin and Musselman (1962) is quite short since it incorporates several of the sounds being tested into one word. Although the shortness is an advantage clinically, the increased skill required to hear several sounds correctly in one word probably makes this test a poor choice for the nurse working in the ambulatory setting. The Developmental Articulation Test is rather lengthy and has been criticized because it does not contain enough blends. The Deep Articulation Test exists in both picture and written forms and tests sounds in many different contexts. It is quite thorough and lengthy, and must be considered a diagnostic rather than a screening test. Many other tests are available, such as the Arizona Articulation Proficiency Scale, the Photo Articulation Test, and the Meacham Language Development Scale, but none of these are suited to clinic use by the nurse. The test with which the authors have had the most success is the Denver Articulation Screening Exam, which is constructed for use as a screening tool by persons who are not speech therapists. It takes about 10 minutes to administer, and although it comes with pictures to help maintain the child's interest, it is basically a word imitative test; that is, the nurse says the word and the child repeats it. Twenty-two words are used, and only one sound in each word is tested. Again, the authors would like to emphasize that the test may appear deceptively easy, and it is suggested that nurses spend some time comparing their assessment of the sounds with that of a speech therapist or with the films available from Laradon Hall. The test is scored according to percentiles of children who have acquired certain sounds at certain ages. Figure 18-36 and 18-37 show the test itself and the scoring mechanism.

Instructions: Have child repeat each word after you. Circle the underlined sounds that he pronounces correctly. Total of correct sounds is the raw score. Use charts in Fig. 4-20(b) to score results.

Name:

Hospital no.:

Address:

Date: _____ Child's age: _____ Examiner: _____

Raw score: _____

Percentile: _____ Intelligibility: _____ Result: _____

1. table	6. zipper	11. sock	16. wagon	21. leaf
2. shirt	7. grapes	12. vacuum	17. gum	22. carrot
3. door	8. flag	13. yarn	18. house	
4. trunk	9. thumb	14. mother	19. pencil	
5. jumping	10. toothbrush	15. twinkle	20. fish	

Intelligibility: 1. Easy to understand   3. Not understandable
(circle one)   2. Understandable   4. Cannot evaulate
                             half the time

Comments:

Figure 18-36 Denver Articulation Screening Examination Test Form for children $2\frac{1}{2}$ to 6 years of age. (*Printed by permission of Amelia F. Drumwright, University of Colorado Medical Center, 1971.*)

To score DASE words: Note raw score for child's performance. Match raw score line (extreme left of chart) with column representing child's age (to the closest *previous* age group). Where raw score line and age column meet, number in that square denotes percentile rank of child's performance when compared with other children that age. Percentiles above heavy line are *abnormal*, below heavy line are *normal*.

Percentile Rank

Raw score	2.5 yr	3.0 yr	3.5 yr	4.0 yr	4.5 yr	5.0 yr	5.5 yr	6 yr
2	1							
3	2							
4	5							
5	9							
6	16							
7	23							
8	31	2						
9	37	4	1					
10	42	6	2					
11	48	7	4					
12	54	9	6	1	1			
13	58	12	9	2	3	1	1	
14	62	17	11	5	4	2	2	
15	68	23	15	9	5	3	2	
16	75	31	19	12	5	4	3	
17	79	38	25	15	6	6	4	
18	83	46	31	19	8	7	4	
19	86	51	38	24	10	9	5	1
20	89	58	45	30	12	11	7	3
21	92	65	52	36	15	15	9	4
22	94	72	58	43	18	19	12	5
23	96	77	63	50	22	24	15	7
24	97	82	70	58	29	29	20	15
25	99	87	78	66	36	34	26	17
26	99	91	84	75	46	43	34	24
27		94	89	82	57	54	44	34
28		96	94	88	70	68	59	47
29		98	98	94	84	84	77	68
30		100	100	100	100	100	100	100

Figure 18-37 Denver Articulation Screening Examination Percentile Ranking.

To score intelligibility:	Normal	Abnormal
2½ years	Understandable half the time, or "easy"	Not understandable
3 years and older	Easy to understand	Understandable half the time Not understandable

Test result: 1. Normal on DASE and intelligibility = normal
2. Abnormal on DASE and/or intelligibility = abnormal

If abnormal on initial screening, rescreen within 2 weeks. If abnormal again, child should be referred for complete speech evaluation.

Figure 18-37   (continued).

Vocabulary Testing

Lexicon, or vocabulary, is an aspect of speech that is somewhat less understood. The development of a vocabulary seems to be related to both environment and intelligence, and intelligence tests are often heavily weighted with vocabulary subtests. In fact most verbal or written tests presuppose a certain level of vocabulary. Some specific tests do exist for evaluating the lexicon. Examples of these are the Houston Test of Language Development and subtests of the Illinois Test of Psycholinguistic Ability, the Picture Story Test, and the Peabody test (Fig. 18-26). Of these, probably only the Peabody can be considered a screening test applicable for use in a clinical situation. It may be useful for the nurse to keep in mind some of the commonly estimated sizes of vocabulary at various ages. The first word is usually said at about 14 months for boys and 3 to 6 months earlier for girls. Between 8 months and 2 years, most children acquire about 100 words; by 3 years, the estimate is usually about 900 words, and by 4 years, 1500 words. The older the child, the less exact is the estimate of vocabulary, since it is impossible to discover exactly how many words a child knows and speaks. Smith (1941) found that the average vocabulary of first graders was 23,700; by twelfth grade this had increased to 80,300 words, showing a steady increase all through the school years. This study concerned only recognition vocabulary (that is, words children could recognize when they heard them or saw them), not spoken vocabulary. Smart and Smart (1977) estimates the adult spoken vocabulary to be much less—about 20,000 words.

Syntax Testing

Syntax, that is, the way a child combines words into sentences according to certain grammatical rules that indicate meaning, is much more difficult to test, and few tests are available for this purpose. Most of those which are available have been constructed for research purposes; a very few are available for diagnostic purposes; and only one known to the authors has been specifically made for screening purposes. One difficulty is that there are so many different aspects of syntax, and little is known about the development of these specific aspects. We know something about the development of negative and interrogative sentence structures and something about certain morphological tasks like the formation of verb tenses and noun pluralization, but we know almost nothing about the development of the ability to use passive sentence structures, possessives, variations of word order, reflexive pronouns, or many other aspects of English grammar. We know even less about the learning of the grammatical rules by children speaking other languages. Probably the best known tests are the ingenious figures and nonsense words used by Berko (1958) to test for development of pluralization and tense rules. She would show a child a picture of an imaginary amoebalike figure and say to the child, "Here is a wug." Then showing a picture of two such figures, she would ask the child to fill in the missing word in the sentence "These are two _____." In this way, she could tell when a child would pluralize by adding as "s," by adding an "es," by adding an "ez," or by changing the word itself (as in the plural of "goose"—"geese"). In a similar way she would show a picture of a man doing an imaginery activity and say, "This is a man who knows to spow. He is spowing. He did the same thing yesterday. What did he do yesterday? Yesterday he _____." This test discovered much about normal development of certain morphological forms.

Attempts have been made to design other tests of syntactic development. Carrow (1968) constructed such a test although it can be used only in assessing receptive language. The Michigan Picture Language Inventory (Lerea, 1958) tests both expressive and receptive syntactical development by asking the child to supply the missing word in a sentence. In such a way, it is able to test such grammatical constructions as comparative adjectives, demonstratives, adverbs, articles, prepositions, pronouns, verb tenses, and possessives, but is unable to test structures which utilize word order such as passive sentences, negatives, questions, auxiliary verb constructions, and noun phrases. This test is sometimes used in speech clinics. The Imitation, Comprehension, Production Test (ICP) is another available test (Fraser, Bellugi, and Brown, 1963). It also tests both expressive and receptive grammatical abilities by using sentence pairs with pictures. There are no norms available for this test, however. The only test known to the authors to be constructed specifically for screening purposes is the Northwestern Syntax Screening Test (NSST), designed by Lee in 1969. This test also uses sentence pairs and stimulus pictures to elicit both receptive and expressive ability. For instance, four pictures are presented to the child: a picture of two cats playing, a picture of an adult woman holding a little boy, a picture of an adult woman and a cat, and a picture of a cat nursing a litter of kittens. The examiner then says two sentences: "This is a mother cat," and "This is mother's cat," and the child is asked to point to each of these pictures. This tests the receptive ability to understand possessive nouns. Then only two pictures are shown, the mother cat and mother's cat. The examiner again repeats the two sentences. After this each picture is shown separately and the child is asked to repeat the sentence which is appropriate to it. This is considered the test of expressive ability. The test is designed for use with children from 3 to 8 and takes approximately 15 minutes to administer. Norms are available for both receptive and expressive ability for all ages. At present, this test is used primarily in speech clinics. It is probably not worth using routinely in well-child visits, but it might be useful for the nurse to have available for children with slow language development.

LABORATORY TESTING OF BLOOD

The nurse's role varies with regard to screening and diagnostic tests for blood. With some tests, the nurse should know when to perform them, draw the specimen, test the sample, and interpret the results; with more complicated tests the nurse may be involved only in ordering the procedure and helping in the interpretation.

Normals are given for each test, but these vary widely from laboratory to laboratory, and nurses must be familiar with their particular laboratory's values.

Although this text has not been written as a laboratory manual, some general statements are made about test methods. Some of the methods discussed are the older, more laborious, methods of performing these tests. Many of the newer laboratories in large medical centers are equipped with electronic equipment that allows these tests to be done more accurately, more rapidly, and with less expense. The principle of the tests remains the same, however.

Normal Blood

Blood cells appear very early in the developing embryo. By the second month of gestation the fetal liver is producing red blood cells; by the fourth month the spleen makes additional cells; by the fifth gestational month bone marrow begins producing blood cells. Until a child is 7 years of age all the bones contain bone marrow to produce such cells. After that period, besides the spleen and the liver, only the clavicles, ribs, scapula, skull, and sternum produce cells.

Blood is composed of both fluid and solid elements. The fluid portion of blood is called *plasma* and is produced by the liver and lymphoid tissue. Plasma is a clear, watery substance which contains certain proteins: albumin, globulin, and fibrinogen. Albumin is utilized in osmotic pressure stabilization; globulins are needed for immunity; and fibrinogen is necessary for the clotting mechanism. Plasma volume remains fairly stable during health, but can change dramatically during certain diseases. Increased plasma volume is seen in rubeola, rubella, leukemia, infectious mononucleosis, and some allergies. It may decrease after severe burns, dehydration, hemorrhage, or surgery. The solid elements of blood include red blood cells, white blood cells, and platelets.

Red Blood Cells Red blood cells (erythrocytes) are biconcave disks which carry the hemoglobin used in oxygen exchange. Erythrocytic development occurs in fives stages: hemocytoblasts (or pronormoblasts) contain a large nucleus and are produced by the red bone marrow; these develop into basophils (or erythroblasts) which begin synthesizing hemoglobin, gradually becoming polychromoatophils (or erythroblasts) and later normoblasts. Normoblasts begin to lose their nuclei and to form reticulocytes (or early erythrocytes), which show only a fragment of a nucleus; gradually the nuclei disappear entirely and the mature erythrocyte appears (see Fig. 18-38).

Normally the biconcave shape of the erythrocyte changes only slightly to allow the cell to slide through the various capillaries. However, in certain diseases the cells assume peculiar shapes and make this gliding action difficult or impossible. Chronic anemias sometimes show bizarre shaped cells, obstructive jaundice is associated with pear-shaped cells, and the familiar

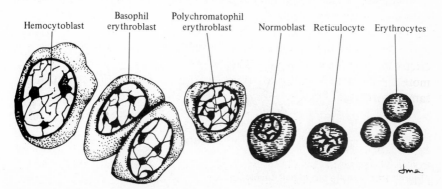

Figure 18-38 Red blood cell development.

sickle-shaped cell is seen in sickle cell disease. Uremia frequently produces cells with spiny projections. The normal erythrocyte lives from 100 to 120 days and then disintegrates within the liver. The normal total count can vary; the newborn has roughly 6 million to 8 million erythrocytes; this number falls to around 4 million to 5 million by adulthood. After childhood an erythrocytic count over 6 million can be seen in dehydration, anoxemia, cardiac disease, and bone marrow hyperplasia. Any count below 5 million is considered low and is frequently seen in anemia.

White Blood Cells White blood cells (leukocytes) are rounded, nucleated cells which protect the body by a process of phagocytosis (i.e., destruction of foreign bodies). All leukocytes develop through approximately 3 stages and 16 substages of development. The maturation process is (1) myeloblast, (2) promyelocyte, and (3) mature myelocyte with a round, rough nucleus (see Fig. 18-39).

The normal leukocyte lives from 1 to 5 days and is probably destroyed by the liver, spleen, lung, or intestinal tract. The normal leukocytic count varies with age, the newborn having 10,000 to 20,000 per cubic millimeter and the 8- to 9-year-old attaining the adult level of 5,000 to 10,000 per cubic millimeter. There are five varieties of leukocytes: neutrophils, eosinophils, basophils, monocytes, and lymphocytes. While all produce phagocytosis, each functions slightly differently. Neutrophils engulf bacteria and aid in the formation of pus. Eosinophils have less efficiency in phagocytosis but respond primarily against foreign protein, allergic reactions, and parasites. Basophils are present in the storage and release of heparin, and lymphocytes help produce globulins and antibodies. These varied leukocytes all have normal ranges which differ at certain ages (see Table 18-2).

Abnormal leukocyte values often pinpoint specific conditions. The leukocyte count may be a total of all varieties of leukocytes or tallies of specific types. Leukocytosis (increased leukocytes) can be physiological or pathological. Physiological leukocytosis occurs at birth, during the ninth

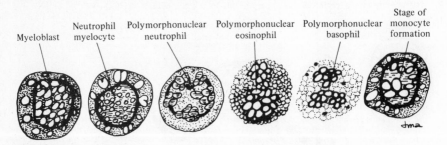

Figure 18-39 White blood cell development.

month of pregnancy, and after exposure to excessive sunlight. Pathological leukocytosis may be caused by infection, severe hemorrhage, cancer, ingestion of certain drugs (chloroform, quinine), dehydration, or leukemia. Leukopenia (decreased leukocytes) may be seen in some infections, bone marrow defects, malaria, rubeola, mumps, and aplastic anemia.

Platelets Platelets (thrombocytes) are smaller than erythrocytes, circular with rough edges and a definite nucleus, and utilized in blood coagulation. Bone marrow produces the thrombocyte, which begins as a megakaryocyte and develops through several stages to a mature cell. The normal thrombocyte lives from 3 to 5 days and is destroyed by the spleen. The normal platelet count is around 200,000 to 400,000 per cubic millimeter. There is a physiological increase in platelets during pregnancy and normal menstruation and with excessive exercise. Low platelet counts are seen in thrombocytopenia, aplastic anemia, infectious mononucleosis, and megakaryocytic thrombocytopenia. High platelet counts occur in thrombocytosis, trauma, and hemorrhage and postsplenectomy.

Table 18-2 Normal Values for Leukocytes

Age	Neutrophils, %	Eosinophils, %	Basophils, %	Monocytes, %	Lymphocytes, %
Premature infants					
0–24 hours	15.49	1.22		3.24	14.62
3 weeks	8.67	1.22			15.17
Full-term infant					
24 hours	23.3	1.32	0.08	5.28	6.10
1–7 days	22.05	2.92	0.057	5.18	14.45
7–30 days	5.8	6.0	2.5	6.8	12.1
3 months	8.1	3.9	0.1	5.0	51.0
6 months	10.6	3.2	0.2	8.0	37.2
12 months	29.25	1.9	0.0	3.4	27.6
Preschool					
2 years		2.9	0.2	6.1	21.98
4 years	13.98	5.9	0.2	7.4	24.3
6 years	14.1	3.15	0.2	6.31	24.5
School					
10 years	31.0	2.9	0.2	6.1	14.4
12 years	12.2	2.9	1.8	3.8	16.0
Adult					
18–20 years	13.9	6.5	2.2	2.9	16.1

Printed by permission of Ross Laboratory, *Children are Different,* Ross Laboratories, Columbus, Ohio, 1970, pp. 104–105.

Obtaining the Specimen

Most blood samples for screening or diagnostic testing come from capillary or venous blood.

Since the advent of microtechniques capillary blood is sufficient for a good many blood tests, and it is easily obtained. Included in the needed equipment are (1) dry cotton balls, (2) alcohol sponges, (3) lancets (or hemolets), (4) two capillary tubes or pipettes (capillary tubes are usually heparinized), (5) clay for closing one end of capillary tube, and (6) a bandage for the younger child. The choice of site varies with age. Infants usually have sufficient surface area on the large toe or lateral heel, while older children and adults usually have capillary blood drawn from the end and lateral side of the middle or index finger or sometimes from the earlobe. Blood flow is increased if the finger or toe is warm; running the extremity under warm water or asking older children to open and close the hand several times sometimes makes it easier to obtain sufficient blood.

The position of the child's extremity and the examiner's hand is important. The child's hand and finger should be at a lower level than the elbow with the arm and hand firmly on a table or the examiner's knee. The examiner's hand should rest on his or her own knee or the table for support (see Fig. 18-40).

The area should be scrubbed with cotton and alcohol and either allowed to dry or wiped dry with a dry cotton ball. The child's finger is grasped firmly between the examiner's fingers (since the pressure reduces the pain slightly), and with a swift, firm swing, the lancet is plunged through the skin. A good puncture requires that the lancet point fully

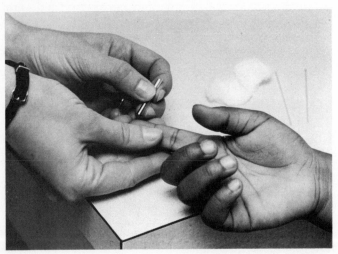

Figure 18-40   Capillary blood being drawn from a child's finger.

penetrate the skin; a slight nick will not do. The first drops of blood are removed and the capillary tube held to the site for drawing up the specimen. Two tubes are drawn for comparison and in case one tube breaks. The finger should not be "milked," since this damages the red blood cells and may give false readings. Once the specimen is drawn, a dry cotton ball is applied to the site and the child instructed to hold the cotton tightly over the site for a few minutes. Some children like a bandage to show off their bravery. This is not a painless test, and the child should be allowed to cry and should be comforted after the procedure. Before transporting, the capillary tubes must be stoppered on one end with a plug of clay. This should be done at only one end.

If more than a few drops of blood are needed, venous blood must be withdrawn. This is a more complicated procedure, but a necessity for some screening and diagnostic tests.

The equipment needed for venous samples includes (1) a blood pressure cuff or tourniquet, (2) cotton balls, dry and with alcohol, (3) a large (#20 to #23) needle and syringe or a Vacutainer, and (4) the proper collecting tubes. The choice of site for venous blood varies with age. For older children and adults the median basilic and/or median cephalic veins at the inner elbow are good sites. Newborns can have venous blood withdrawn from the jugular vein. However, nurses may wish to confine their blood punctures to the older child at the elbow area and let someone else withdraw the samples at the other sites.

The position of the child's extremity and the examiner's hand is important. Since this is a painful procedure, the child will have to be firmly restrained. The arm of the child should be relaxed and resting on a firm surface. The examiner may brace the fingers and hand against the child's arm (see Fig. 18-41).

The blood pressure cuff is inflated to a point below systolic and above diastolic, or the tourniquet is applied between the shoulder and elbow. The child can be instructed to open and close the fingers vigorously several times. It is wise to palpate the veins for location and firmness before scrubbing the area firmly with an alcohol sponge and allowing it to dry. With one hand holding the skin taut, the other hand slides the needle into the vein with the bevel facing upward and the plunger slightly withdrawn. If blood is to be drawn into the syringe, the plunger can be slowly withdrawn to the level needed. If blood is to be drawn into special collecting tubes and a Vacutainer is used, the blood will appear in the Vacutainer; the first tube can be pushed into the needle and following tubes connected carefully so as not to disturb the needle point in the vein. When a sufficient sample has been withdrawn, the tourniquet is removed, a dry cotton ball is placed over the puncture site, a slight pressure is applied, and the needle is withdrawn. Then firm pressure is put on the site to help coagulation.

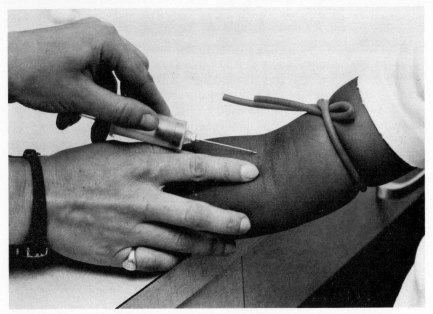

Figure 18-41   Venous blood being drawn from a child's arm.

Knowing how to perform these two procedures should enable the nurse to obtain specimens for all screening blood work and most diagnostic blood tests.

Screening Tests

Several procedures that can be considered screening tests will be described here: colorimetric G6PD, colorimetric lead, Dextrostix, galactosemia, hematocrit, hemoglobin, Sickledex, serum hexosaminidase assay, and tests for venereal disease. Each examiner must choose which of the listed tests are appropriate and needed and must ensure that follow-up can be provided for children with positive findings. For instance, a neighborhood with many black children might need routine Sickledex; the community with many Jewish descendants might benefit from the serum hexosaminidase assay; and a community filled with old, dilapidated homes might warrant the colorimetric lead screening test, etc. While all these tests are considered screening, not all are simple, easily performed tests, and the nurse may have to find a laboratory that is equipped and knowledgeable enough to run some of the tests.

Colorimetric Test for G6PD   Glucose-6-phosphate dehydrogenase (G6PD) is a deficiency of glucose metabolism within the red blood cell causing hemolytic anemia; it is present in 10 percent of the black male population. It is also found in some Caucasians, especially from the Middle Eastern countries, and in some Chinese children.

Although some laboratories are equipped to run this test on capillary blood, most require 4 ml of venous blood. The blood must be drawn into heparinized, citrated, or oxalated tubes for transporting to the laboratory. This is not a simple test, and the nurse will not usually perform it. Generally the procedure requires that the blood be centrifuged and the red packed cells watered, buffered, and mixed with several chemicals, including a brilliant cresyl blue dye. The mixture is sealed in the test tube with a layer of mineral oil and placed in the water bath. Readings are taken at specific times (at 50, 75, and 100 minutes and at 2 and 6 hours). A normal reading shows complete decolorization at 100 minutes, and an abnormal reading shows partial or no decolorization after 100 minutes. Any abnormal readings mean the specimen should be sent for the diagnostic test.

Colorimetric Lead Screening Children who eat old paint or inhale fumes from lead-containing substances have an increase in the lead levels of their blood which causes increased erythrocyte destruction and delayed hemoglobin synthesis leading to anemia. Many of these children are suspect from their living conditions—old houses which were painted many decades ago or houses situated near high-speed roadways where there are many fumes and exhausts. Some children become suspect with a history of pica—eating nonfood substances such as paint, dirt, and cigarette butts. This test is not easy to run, and the nurse will need the assistance of a laboratory and laboratory technicians.

Only capillary blood is needed, and the specimen can be drawn up in heparinized capillary tubes. The equipment needed by the laboratory includes a test tube with rubber plug, scale, burner, special filter paper, and some specific chemicals such as sulfuric acid and ammonium citrate. A 40-ml test tube is weighed, the blood sample added, and the tube reweighed. Chemicals are added and the tube is left standing for 30 minutes; then it is heated and additional chemicals added. The tube is shaken for 30 seconds, and the special filter paper is then inserted into the mixture and a reading taken. The reading is then calculated according to a formula to obtain the standard.

Interpretation is based on a microgram percent, and there is much controversy over the normal range. Some feel that any level between 60 and 100 microgram percent may be toxic with no symptoms and that any level over the 100 microgram percent will be accompanied by symptoms. Others feel that a lead level below 40 microgram percent is normal, a level between 40 and 80 microgram percent is suspect and needs referral, and any level over

80 microgram percent needs immediate care. The nurse must check with the laboratory to know how to interpret results.

Dextrostix Some children, especially newborns, are prone to changes in blood glucose, and any large changes can be damaging to the child. Dextrostix reagent strips are simple dipsticks that can be used to measure hyper- or hypoglycemia.

Because only a drop of capillary blood is needed, the heel, finger, or earlobe can be punctured with a lancet and the special filter paper held to the wound for absorption. The only equipment needed besides the puncture apparatus is a watch, running water, the special filter paper, and the standardized color chart. After placing one large drop of blood on the special filter paper, wait exactly 60 seconds, quickly wash the filter paper with running water (from tap or wash bottle) for 1 or 2 seconds and hold the filter paper against the color chart for interpretation.

Only a gross estimate of the amount of glucose present is possible with a range of 0, 25, 45, 90, 130, 175, and 250 mg/100 ml of blood. No color or a creamy yellow color is a negative normal reading; dark purple is a positive or abnormal reading and indicates that the child should be referred for more diagnostic testing.

Galactosemia Screening Galactosemia is an autosomal recessive trait causing a deficiency of galactose-1-phosphate uridyl transferase which causes the galactose to increase, resulting in galactosemia and galactosuria. If it is allowed to continue, the infant will develop cataracts, mental retardation, and hepatic failure; without treatment the disease is fatal. The only treatment is restriction of galactose intake; in order to be effective, such restriction must be instituted very early. For this reason, early detection is imperative. This is a complex test, and the nurse will need the aid of a good laboratory technician and a well-equipped laboratory. The procedure can be done on capillary blood; therefore the examiner will need to draw up blood into heparinized capillary tubes. Equipment includes a calibrated pipette, centrifuge, freezer, water bath, and certain chemicals. The blood specimens from the child and one control are mixed separately with some well-chilled chemicals and centrifuged for 5 minutes; additional chemicals are then added and this mixture is centrifuged for 10 more minutes and frozen for several days. Additional test tubes are prepared with specific reagents, and the original test tubes are removed from the freezer, dipped in a water bath for several minutes, solutions added, and the test tubes rebathed. The meniscus is then measured on all tubes, which are then incubated overnight in a water bath. A final reading of the meniscus is taken after removing the tubes from the water bath.

Interpretation is based on changes in the meniscus. A normal (negative) reading is indicated by tubes showing a lowered meniscus and an abnormal (positive) reading is indicated by tubes showing a meniscus at the same level before and after the final water bath. A positive reading needs further evaluation promptly.

Hematocrit The hematocrit is the comparison of packed red cell volume and the volume of the whole blood. It does not tell the examiner the quality of red blood cells, only the number. Generally this test is used as a screening device for nutritional anemia. A child showing a low hematocrit is given several weeks of medicinal iron and rechecked. If the anemia was nutritional the second hematocrit will be improved. If there is no improvement and the examiner is certain the child has been getting the medicinal iron, further diagnostic tests are needed to determine the cause of the anemia.

This is a very simple test that every nurse should be able to perform. Equipment needed includes two heparinized capillary tubes, puncture apparatus, a centrifuge, and a gauge for reading. Many nurses in outlying well-baby clinics draw up the blood at the clinic and transport the tubes back to the local laboratory for centrifuging and reading. Using the procedure for obtaining capillary blood described earlier, the nurse should draw up two tubes of blood. Depending on the type of reading gauge available, the nurse should fill one-half to three-quarters of the tube. One end of the tube is sealed with the clay for transporting. The capillary tubes are placed in the centrifuge with the sealed end out. The nurse should remember to balance the wheel with extra empty tubes if necessary and to tighten the screw lid before closing the top so that the tubes are held snugly in place. After centrifuging for 3 to 5 minutes, the tubes are removed and read on the gauge. There are two types of gauges: one is a small plastic card and the other a metal, multiwheeled device (see Fig. 18-42). The card is handy for traveling but difficult to read because the lines are so closely spaced. It also requires three-quarters of a tube of blood for reading. The multiwheeled device is much more precise and easier to read and can be used on less than three-quarters of a tube of blood. In either case, the capillary tube is lined up with the 100 percent mark at the top of the serum and the top of the red cells at some point below the 100 percent mark.

Remember that whole blood is 100 percent; the normal values are given in percentages since the red blood cells are a fraction of the whole. Depending on age, normal hematocrit values are usually considered to be over 32 to 35 percent and abnormal values are anything below 32 percent or over 50 percent (see Table 18-3).

Accepted norms vary from clinic to clinic and state to state, and so the nurse must be familiar with the prevailing standards.

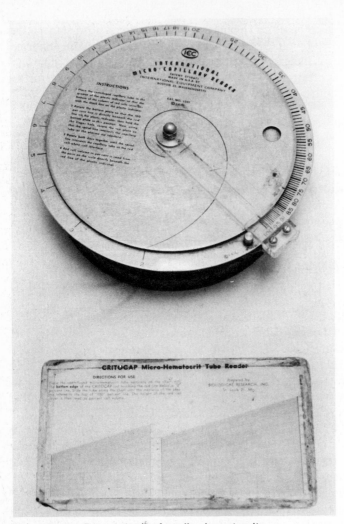

Figure 18-42   Two methods of reading hematocrits.

Hemoglobin A hemoglobin reading refers to the measurement of hemoglobin (a protein) within each red blood cell. There are at least 12 different kinds of normal hemoglobins and as many as 150 abnormal types. The abnormal hemoglobins include anemic hemoglobin and the sickle cell hemoglobin. Some children with anemia have enough red blood cells, but not enough hemoglobin in each cell. Thus it is often important to know both the hemoglobin and the hematocrit of a certain child (see Table 18-4).

This can be a very simple test, and nurses may want to include it in their routine. Many hospitals now perform the test by electrophoresis, which is much simpler and more accurate, but the older methods can be used in the

Table 18-3 Lower Limits of Hematocrit Values for Definition of Anemia

Age	Lower limit of normal, %
Birth	45
3 days to 1 month	33
1–2 months	30
2–4 months	30
4–8 months	32
8–12 months	32
12–18 months	34
18–36 months	35
3–8 years	36
8–10 years	37
11–18 years	38
Males	
14–15 years	42
16 years	44
Females	
14–15 years	38
16 years	39

Printed by permission of Dr. Burris Duncan at Colorado General Hospital.

clinical area. Several different tests are used for determining hemoglobin. The colorimetric methods include the direct matching (Tallquist and Dare) and the acid hematin methods (Sahli, Haden-Hausser, and Spencer). Iron concentration can be determined with a chemical method and specific gravity with physical methods (see Fig. 18-43).

Depending on the method being used, either capillary or venous blood is needed. If capillary blood is used, it must be drawn up into a pipette with tubing. The Tallquist method uses a kit with specific absorbent paper and a color scale. After capillary blood is collected, the first one or two drops are discarded and a large drop released onto the absorbent paper and allowed to saturate a large area. A percentage reading is obtained by comparing the blood spot with the scale provided. The other direct matching test is the Dare. This also can be performed on capillary blood drawn into a pipette. The first two drops are discarded and the remainder drawn into a pipette within the Dare hemoglobinometer. Immediately the scale is adjusted to match the specimen and a reading is taken from the standard. The test must be read in artificial light and before the blood clots.

The Sahli, Haden-Hausser, and Spencer tests change the hemoglobin to acid hematin before a reading can be obtained. The Sahli test comes in a small, compact kit containing pipettes; graduated, marked test tubes; a meter; rubber tubing; and three bottles (1% acetic acid, dilution of HCl,

Table 18-4   Normal Values for Hemoglobin and Hematocrit

	Hemoglobin, g/100 ml		Hematocrit, %	
	Full-term	Premature	Full-term	Premature
Cord	15.3–18.9		47–57	
1 day	17.3–21.5		51–65	
2–6 days	17.4–22.2	14.2–18.6	58–74	55–61
14–23 days	14.2–17.2		47–57	
24–31 days	12.2–16.0	9.8–11.4	38–52	27–37
38–50 days	10.9–14.7		36–45	
2–2$\frac{1}{2}$ months	10.3–12.5	8.5–10.4	34–43	24–32
3–3$\frac{1}{2}$ months	10.4–12.0	9.0–11.0	34–40	28–34
5–7 months	11.8–12.2	10.8–12.3	35–41	33–39
8–10 months	11.1–12.3	10.7–12.3	31–41	33–39
11–13$\frac{1}{2}$ months	11.3–12.5	11.0–12.8	37–41	34–40
1$\frac{1}{2}$–3 years	11.3–12.3	11.0–12.7	37–41	35–41
5 years	1 1.7–13.7		34–40	
10 years	12.0–14.4		36–42	
Adult				
Male	14–18		40–54	
Female	12–16		38–47	

Printed by permission of Ross Laboratory, *Children are Different,* Ross Laboratories, Columbus, Ohio, 1970, p. 110.

and Hayem's solution). Capillary blood is withdrawn into the pipette, two drops discarded, and the remainder blown into the graduated test tube which has been filled to the #10 line with HCl. This mixture is allowed to settle for 10 minutes within the special holder and is then diluted with water until the color matches the standard and can be read. The Haden-Hausser test is similar and comes in a kit containing a hemoglobinometer, white cell diluting pipette, and glass slide and cover. The slide is cleaned and slipped into the hemoglobinometer. Capillary blood is collected in the pipette and diluted with HCl. After a brief wait the acid hematin appears and the specimen can be dropped onto the slide and matched to the provided color standard. A special filter must be used for daytime readings and a different filter for artificial light readings. The Spencer test is a further modification of the same process. The kit includes the Spencer hemoglobinometer, blood chamber, cover glass, and a hemolysing solution. Capillary blood is obtained by puncturing the finger, discarding the first few drops, and then applying the blood chamber directly over the wound. The hemolysing solution is dropped on the chamber, and the cover glass placed over the mixture. The slide is inserted into the hemoglobinometer, the lighting switched on, and the specimen matched with the color standard. Because of the color-matching requirement, all these methods have the disadvantage of being somewhat subjective.

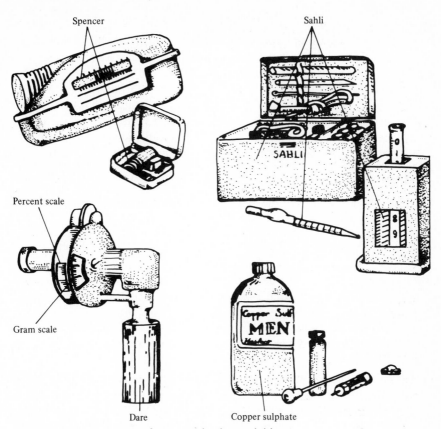

Figure 18-43 Instruments for measuring hemoglobin.

Iron concentration measurements can be obtained by using the Wong method in a laboratory setting. Capillary blood is withdrawn, and 0.5 ml of the heparinized blood is mixed in a 50-ml test tube with digestion solution. It is flamed, several chemicals are added, and the readings are calculated according to a formula to get the microgram percent of iron in the whole blood.

Specific gravity is easily measured and is used in many blood banks to determine the gross normal hemoglobin content. A stock solution of blue copper sulfate is prepared with a known specific gravity of 1.053 for women and 1.055 for men. Capillary blood is drawn into a pipette and one drop allowed to fall into the solution from 1 cm above the surface. The blood specific gravity will remain stable for 15 to 20 seconds and can be compared with the known copper sulfate specific gravity if read within that time span. Generally, the blood droplet sinks toward the bottom for 5 seconds and then suddenly rises if lighter, continues to fall if heavier, and remains stationary if at the same specific gravity as the copper sulfate. If the blood droplet goes to the bottom in 1.053 solution, this is equivalent to 12.5 g hemoglobin for women; in 1.055 solution, this signifies 15.5 g for men.

Hemoglobin values are expressed in g per 100 ml of blood. Normal values change with age, as seen in Table 18-4, being around 10 to 12 g/100 ml of blood throughout most of childhood. As with hematocrits, most clinics determine a minimum for each age; lower readings indicate a need for iron supplements. If possible, both hemoglobin and hematocrits should be done, since the comparison gives the examiner more information than either test singly.

Sickledex Sickle cell anemia is a hematological condition found in 8 to 10 percent of the black American population. It is a defect in the hemoglobin structure, in which stress or lack of oxygen will cause the cells to lose their usual rounded shape and become sickled. Sickled cells do not pass through capillaries like normal cells; instead, they become clogged, causing many clinical signs of vasoocclusion: pain, ulcers, delayed maturation, etc. Sickledex is a simple test for screening children with Hb-S—the defective hemoglobin. This is an easy procedure, and the nurse will not need laboratory help in performing it.

Two test tubes, a special holder, and two bottles of solution are needed. The two test tubes are positioned in the holder. Test tube A is filled with solution A, containing the control Hb-A working solution, and test tube B is filled with solution B. The capillary blood is drawn into a heparinized capillary tube and then blown into test tube B for 2 to 5 minutes of incubation time. A reading is taken by observing the amount of turbidity present in each of the two solutions.

A negative result is indicated by both test tubes remaining clear and a positive result is indicated by test tube A remaining clear and test tube B turning cloudy. According to one study (Loh, 1968), the Sickledex was performed on 600 patients and compared with the metabisulfite test and electrophoresis with favorable results. However, if the test is positive, the child should be referred to the medical center for a more diagnostic test. The test should be done only on black children over 6 months. It is not accurate before this time because of the amount of fetal hemoglobin still present.

Serum Hexosaminidase Assay In Tay-Sachs disease ganglioside accumulates within the blood serum, causing muscle weakness, blindness, mental retardation, and death. It is caused by an autosomal recessive gene found generally (60 to 70 percent) in the children of Ashkenazic Jewish descent. If both parents are carriers, they have a 25 percent chance of having a child with Tay-Sachs disease. It is difficult to detect this disease by symptoms alone before 6 to 12 months of age. However, there is a new test available that can detect both the disease and the carrier state—the serum hexosaminidase assay. Presently there is much controversy over whether this test is a screening test or a diagnostic test since it requires a specially equipped laboratory, specially trained technicians, and a good deal of technical time and it is fairly expensive. However, it is the only method available now, and within specific populations, on an experimental basis, it has been used as a screening tool. The nurse working within such a community should be aware of the test and know how to contact a laboratory for the information needed to do the screening.

Freezers, special ice baths, and complicated chemicals as well as the usual laboratory equipment of test tubes and centrifuges are needed. The test requires 5 ml of venous heparinized blood and takes 24 hours to run.

Interpretation is based on the percentage of hexosaminidase present; one study (O'Brien, 1970) reported the normal range to be 49 to 68 percent, the abnormal range 0 to 4 percent, with carriers showing 26 to 45 percent. These values may change with laboratories or as more studies are completed.

Because there is as yet no known cure for this disease, many authorities feel screening is useless. However, once a laboratory has been established the cost can be reduced to around $10 per couple. In some areas, rabbis are requesting couples visit the laboratory premaritally to establish a knowledge of the carrier state, and increasingly obstetricians are referring susceptible women for amniocentesis which can include such screening.

Testing for Venereal Disease   There are several tests for syphilis, but one of the more common screening tests is the flocculation test developed by the Venereal Disease Research Laboratory (VDRL) of the United States Public Health Service. There are two variations of this method, and they are named after the persons responsible for developing them: Kline and Kahn. Flocculation tests are not specific to one venereal disease. All the tests are based on precipitation caused by antigen-antibody reactions. New to the screening area are two rapid screening tests: the plasma crit (PCT) and the rapid plasma reagin (RPR); these may become more popular in the next few years.

In the older methods (VDRL, Kline, and Kahn), blood can be drawn in clinics but the tests are usually processed in a laboratory by specially trained technicians. Equipment includes a centrifuge, slides and slide holder, chemicals, and buffered solutions. After 5 ml of venous blood is taken, it is centrifuged, heated, and the serum removed. The warm serum is dropped onto a glass slide and emulsified. Antigen is then added, and the slide gently rotated and examined microscopically for clumping of short, straight, rod-shaped substances.

Interpretation is based on the clumping. No clumping is seen in a normal (negative or nonreactive) reading, and many large clumpings are seen in an abnormal (positive or reactive) reading. There is also a slightly reactive reading in which several small clumpings are seen.

Thyroid Screening From 1 to 2 percent of all mentally retarded children have diagnoses of cretinism, and this condition can be diagnosed early and treated. Several institutions (in Quebec, Pittsburgh, Denver) have begun testing for thyroid hormone deficiency at birth and in 1976 the Committee on Genetics of the American Academy of Pediatrics issued some guidelines for using the T_4 screening test for hypothyroidism in the newborn period. The T_4 (thyroxine) test has some problems with specificity and sensitivity but is the best test available at present. The cost is roughly 60¢ at this time. A blood sample is obtained from the heel prick or cord blood and blotted on special filter paper. Within a laboratory setting, the filter paper is exposed to specific reagents and procedures to determine the thyroxine level. A low blood level results in a positive test. This level must be set by each individual laboratory (one laboratory set such a level at 60). A positive test should be followed immediately with a TSH radioimmunoassay test (another screening test). The TSH test may be run from the same sample of blood—heel or cord. Positive results from this test should be followed with requests for return visits for a diagnostic workup. From birth to the results from the TSH should be no longer than $3\frac{1}{2}$ weeks for adequate treatment to be effective. There is some controversy over using the T_4 or TSH as the first step in screening. (The TSH costs $2.00 for reagents plus technician time.) The Academy is recommending that both be used before referring for follow-up.

Diagnostic Tests

The above tests are usually considered screening tests even though some of them are too complicated for the nurse to perform; however the nurse may be ordering them frequently from the laboratory and should know something about their mechanics and use. The following blood work is usually termed diagnostic and is ordered only where there is some reason to suspect a specific disease or condition. There is no reason nurses could not learn how to do some of these diagnostic tests, but in a general ambulatory clinic they would probably be responsible only for ordering them and participating in the follow-up with the pediatrician. Here again, the normals are given, but there is a wide variation from place to place; therefore nurses are encouraged to check with the laboratory for the clinical averages.

Bleeding Time A child who is suspected of having some bleeding disorder or thrombocytopenia might have a bleeding time taken. Generally the Ivy method is considered the most reliable. The blood pressure cuff is applied and elevated to 40 mm of mercury, and a 2.5-mm-deep incision is made on the forearm. Blood droplets are blotted at 30-second intervals until the bleeding stops. The normal range is 3 to 5 minutes.

Blood Smears Blood smears allow the examiner to differentiate the various types of cells present and their stage of development. Fresh blood is placed on a slide and allowed to air dry. Wright's stain is applied for 3 minutes and then a buffer is applied. The slide is left to dry for 3 to 6 minutes and then washed with clear water. The slide is slipped under the microscope and the size and shapes of the different cells are noted. Usually the red blood cells stain a light pink, the white blood cells a chrome color, and the platelets a lavender color.

Blood Typing Blood typing is a method of matching antigens and antibodies between two different sets of blood; this becomes important for newborns with hemolytic diseases, children with hemolytic anemias, and anyone with the possibility of requiring a transfusion. The blood is typed (A, B, AB, or O, and Rh positive or negative) and cross-matched (tested for compatibility with the donor blood). Blood that is compatible does not clump when mixed with the donor blood and can be safely given to that person.

Blood Urea Nitrogen (BUN) This test is done to ascertain the functioning of the kidney in producing urea and maintaining a low blood urea level. It requires 5 ml of heparinized venous blood; the blood urea is reduced to ammonia which is then titrated and measured. Many drugs (Garb, 1971) such as bacitracin, chloral hydrate, kanamycin, polymyxin B, salicylates, etc., can affect this test and result in false readings. A normal BUN is 9 to 20 mg/100 ml of blood, and any reading over 20 mg/100 ml of blood is a positive or abnormal result.

Bilirubin Hemoglobin is destroyed within the liver, and one of the by-products of this destruction is bilirubin. If something is wrong with the hemoglobin production or the liver, this balance is destroyed. Thus it is important to check bilirubin levels in children with jaundice, certain anemias, liver damage, and similar problems.

There are several ways of checking the bilirubin: direct, indirect, and total. The direct method tests for free bilirubin after the blood is allowed to clot, serum is extracted and chemicals added to produce a colored reaction that can be measured. The indirect method (van den Bergh test) tests for bilirubin which is bound to a protein. Venous blood (5 ml) is allowed to clot, the serum is extracted, and alcohol and a special reagent are added; the protein then precipitates out and the color is matched to a standard chart. With this test, the patient must be questioned about ingestion of foods and drugs, since many substances can affect the outcome, such as carrots, Vitamin A, and salicylates (Garb, 1971). Total bilirubin measures the concentration of both blood and unbound bilirubin in the serum. This test requires 5 ml of heparinized venous blood which has the serum removed and a special reagent added to produce a color that can be matched to a standardized color chart. Certain drugs and food can also alter these readings.

All three of the tests produce different normal ranges. A normal direct count should be 0.05 to 1.5 mg/100 ml of serum, an indirect count around 0.4 to 0.8 mg/100 ml of serum, and the total count 0.1 to 1.0 mg/100 ml of serum.

Clotting Time Clotting time (or coagulation time) is simply an indication of the blood's ability to clot. Using the Lee-White testing methods, 4 ml of venous blood is withdrawn and divided into four test tubes. Test tube A is tilted every 30 seconds until clotting occurs; test tube B is then tilted every 30 seconds until clotting occurs, followed by test tube C, and finally test tube D.

Interpretation is made by calculating the average time from collecting the specimen to the clotting of the blood in test tubes B, C, and D. Normal ranges are between 10 and 25 minutes.

Complete Blood Count A complete blood count is a count of all the solid elements in the blood: red blood cells, reticulocytes, white blood cells (including types of white cells), and platelets. Generally the test can be done on capillary blood, but it may be run from venous blood.

For the red blood cell (RBC) count, the blood is diluted with a special solution and the mixture channeled through a counting chamber. By using the microscope the cells are counted within the chamber and calculated for the entire sample. This formerly was done by hand, but many laboratories now utilize an electronic counter which speeds up the process considerably. A normal RBC count is usually 4 million to 6 million cells per cubic millimeter, with a higher count suggesting polycythemia and a lower count indicating anemia.

The young red blood cells, reticulocytes, are also counted, since this gives some indication of the production of red blood cells. A fresh drop of blood is placed on a slide containing dried cresyl blue dye. With the microscope and a counting chamber, the cells are then counted and calculated. This also is now being done electronically. The normal range is 0.1 to 1.5 cells per 100 red blood cells.

Total white blood cells are counted by diluting fresh blood with a special solution, channeling the mixture through the counting chamber and microscope, counting the cells, and calculating the entire number. This can also be done electronically. The normal range is 4000 to 11,000 cells per cubic millimeter. An increase generally indicates infection; a decrease may signify certain infections or blood dyscrasias.

Sometimes it is important to know the white blood cell differential, that is, the numbers of different types of white cells present. This count requires that a fresh drop of blood be spread evenly over a glass slide and allowed to dry before it is stained with a special solution and placed under the microscope. By means of a special counting chamber, 100 white cells are counted and calculated into percentages. There is a wide variation in normal range as seen from the chart on page 239 and the normal range as listed by Garb (1971).

Neutrophils, 54 to 62 percent
Eosinophils, 1 to 3 percent
Basophils, 0 to 1 percent
Lymphocytes, 25 to 33 percent
Monocytes, 0 to 9 percent

Shifts to the higher or lower percentages can sometimes signify specific disease; for instance, increased monocytes may indicate Hodgkin's disease; an increase in the number of eosinophils is usually caused by allergic reactions or parasitic infestations; measles will cause increased basophils.

Generally the platelet count is now done electronically; however, if the older method is utilized, a drop of fresh blood is diluted with a special solution, mixed into a counting chamber, and counted through the microscope. The normal range is 200,000 to 500,000 cells per cubic millimeter. A low count may indicate septicemia, and a high count is seen with broken bones, anemias, and polycythemias.

Coomb's This is a measurement of antigen-antibody levels and can be done directly or indirectly. The direct Coomb's requires 2 ml of fresh, clotted venous or umbilical cord blood. A mixture of red blood cells is dropped onto a Coomb's serum plate and observed for agglutination. Interpretation is read on a 1-to-4 scale, with a negative or normal reading indicating a complete lack of agglutination. Drugs such as penicillin, other antibiotics, and antihypertensive drugs can give false readings (Garb, 1971). An abnormal (positive) direct Coomb's is seen in erythroblastosis fetalis in the newborn. The indirect Coomb's is used to measure Rh and other blood-type factors. Fresh, clotted venous (5 ml) blood is mixed with a special serum and allowed to stand. The red blood cells are removed from the slide and rinsed, and additional serum is added. The slide is then observed for agglutination. Interpretation is again read on a 1-to-4 scale, with a normal (negative) reading indicating no agglutination and an abnormal (positive) reading indicating agglutination and indicating that the Rh factor is present.

Erythrocyte Fragility The erythrocyte fragility test (osmotic fragility test) measures the destruction rate of the red blood cells. Several milliliters of fresh blood are dropped into numerous test tubes which have different hypotonic saline solutions. The cells are then observed for rupture. A normal reading is 0.85 to 0.44 percent; an abnormal reading shows a lower rate, indicating acquired hemolytic anemias; a higher rate may suggest congenital anemias.

Fibrinogen Level The protein fibrinogen is needed for the clotting process, and one way of assessing the clotting mechanism is to measure the amount of fibrinogen present. This test requires heparinized venous blood, which is centrifuged to separate the solid from the fluid parts. Only the plasma is tested by adding sodium sulfite and observing the precipitation. The fibrinogen precipitates to the bottom and can be calculated from the biuret procedure. A normal range is 200 to 600 mg/100 ml of plasma.

Glucose The level of glucose is measured to detect certain glucose metabolic disorders such as diabetes, liver disease, and endocrine problems. The patient must fast for 12 hours prior to the test; 5 ml of venous, heparinized blood is then withdrawn. The proteins are precipitated and the glucose oxidized and the result is compared with a color chart. The normal range is 65 to 120 mg/100 ml of serum or 105 mg/100 ml of whole blood. A high level can indicate diabetes, liver disease, or endocrine problems, and a low level may suggest hypoglycemia from coma, convulsions, or endocrine problems.

Glucose Tolerance A measure of the child's reaction to a certain amount of glucose is occasionally useful when diabetes mellitus is suspected. Two tests are used: the standard test and the Exton-Rose test. For the standard test the patient is put on a 150-g carbohydrate diet for 7 days prior to the testing. For 12 hours prior to the test the patient must have no food, but can drink water. At testing time a single dose of 100 g of glucose is given at one time. There are two commercial preparations for this: Glucola and Gel-a-dex. Urine and blood samples are collected at regular intervals for the following 4 to 5 hours. For the Exton-Rose test the patient must consume a high carbohydrate diet for 3 days prior to testing, fast for several hours, and have blood and urine samples drawn. Then 50 g of glucose is given and 30 minutes later blood and urine samples are taken and a second 50 g of glucose given. Blood and urine samples are again taken after 30 minutes. The values of both these tests are shown in the Table 18-5.

Guthrie Phenylketonuria (PKU) is a metabolic disorder which develops when the enzyme phenylalanine hydroxylase is absent and the amount

Table 18-5 Normal Values for Glucose Tolerance Tests

	Standard 100-g dose				
Condition	Fasting	30 min	60 min	120 min	180 min
Normal	80	150	135	100	80
Diabetic	160	250	300	380	290
Mild diabetic	130	200	280	225	180
Hyperinsulinism	80	95	50	60	70

	Exton-Rose test			
Condition	Specimen	Fasting	30 min	60 min
Normal	Blood	80	150	160
Normal	Urine	Negative	Negative	Negative
Diabetic	Blood	130	225	250
Diabetic	Urine	Negative	Variable	Positive

Printed by permission of Ruth M. French, *The Nurse's Guide to Diagnostic Procedures*, McGraw-Hill, New York, 1971, p. 115.

of phenylalanine in the blood is increased to toxic levels, causing damage to the brain. The usual screening test for PKU is a urine (ferric chloride or Phenistex) test; however, some states use the Guthrie also as a screening test. It is performed on the third day of life and after 48 hours of ingesting any protein substance (usually milk formula). The infant's heel is pierced with a lancet and three drops of blood absorbed on a special filter paper. Once the filter paper has been autoclaved, a small sample is punched from the middle of the blood spot and placed on a specially prepared agar plate. The agar has been prepared with *Bacillus subtilis.* Interpretation is made by observing the Bacillus growth after incubation. A normal (negative) response shows no Bacillus growth near the blood spot, and an abnormal (positive) response shows Bacillus growth up to the blood spot.

Hemoglobin Electrophoresis This is a modern, electronically performed test to discover any one of the 150 different types of hemoglobin, some of which are abnormal; it is particularly useful in looking for Hb-S in sickle cell disease. The test requires heparinized, hemolyzed venous blood to which electrophoresis is applied (i.e., the solution is run through by an electric current) and which is then compared with a standard measurement. Normally the adult will show hemoglobin A and the infant will show hemoglobin A and F. Abnormal results show any of the 150 different hemoglobins present.

Heterophil This is an antigen-antibody test generally ordered to aid in the diagnosis of infectious mononucleosis, Hodgkin's disease, or serum sickness. There are three kinds of heterophils: monospot, presumptive, and diagnostic.

The monospot is really a screening test that is not very sensitive or specific. It requires 0.1 ml (2 drops) of serum which is mixed with several reagents and spread on a slide with a control smear. The slide is then observed for agglutination in the test and control areas. A positive test shows agglutination and can be a sign of mononucleosis, Hodgkin's disease, hepatitis, or lymphoma. A negative test shows no agglutination.

If the monospot is positive, the examiner must order a presumptive test. This requires 0.2 ml of unheparinized blood from which the serum is extracted, mixed with different dilutions of sheep serum, and observed for clumping. A titer of 1:56 is considered positive for mononucleosis and serum sickness and should be followed by the diagnostic test.

The diagnostic heterophil requires 5 ml of venous blood which is allowed to clot, after which the serum is withdrawn. The serum is mixed with varying dilutions of red blood cells from sheep and is then incubated and observed for agglutination. Interpretation is read as a titer. A normal (negative) result is indicated by a lack of agglutination. An abnormal (positive) is signaled by agglutination of a titer of 1:28 to 1:36 or higher. There is a wide range of what is considered diagnostic for mononucleosis, but serum sickness generally gives a titer of 1:22 to 1:56.

Lead If the screening test for lead is positive, a diagnostic test, usually including both a blood and urine test, is needed. The diagnostic test requires 10 ml of heparinized venous blood to which a series of chemicals are added, and various procedures are performed. The normal reading is 0 to 5 mg/100 ml of whole blood, and anything over 5 mg/100 ml is considered abnormal.

Prothrombin Time This is another indication of the ability of the blood to clot. This test requires 4.5 ml of venous blood which is placed in a specially prepared oxalated solution and a mixture of calcium and thromboplastin added; a stopwatch is used to time the formation of the threads of fibrin. The procedure is then repeated using normal blood. The normal range is 11 to 18 seconds. Abnormally low counts may be caused by liver diseases, vitamin K deficiencies, and certain drug ingestions; abnormally high ranges are seen in barbiturate ingestions.

Salicylate Level This test is used most frequently when children are suspected of ingesting an overdose of aspirin. Occasionally it is also used in ascertaining blood levels in rheumatic fever. It requires 5 ml of venous blood in a heparinized tube. The serum is separated and a ferric ion added before running the specimen through a colorimeter or spectrophotometer. A normal specimen shows no color. An abnormal or positive result shows a purple color. Salicylates of 35 mg/100 ml of blood are considered toxic in children.

Erythrocyte Sedimentation Rate There is some controversy about the reliability and specificity of this test, which simply measures the time it takes for the red blood cells to precipitate to the bottom of the test tube. Usually 4 ml of venous blood is withdrawn, heparinized, and placed in an upright test tube to be monitored for a period of time. The interpretation depends on the method used (Cutler, Wintrobe, or Westergren) and the sex of the patient. A normal range for the Westergren method is 0 to 15 mm/hour for men and 0 to 20 mm/hour for women.

Serological Tests for Syphilis (STS) In general there are two types of testing for syphilis: flocculation and complement-fixation methods. Flocculation includes the VDRL, Kline, and Kahn tests, which were described under screening tests. Complement-fixation methods include the basic tests (Wassermann, Reiter protein-antigen, and Kolmer), the Treponema Pallidum Immobilization Test (TPA), and the Fluorescent Treponemal Antibody Absorption Test (FTA).

The basic complement-fixation tests require 5 ml of venous blood which is allowed to coagulate with certain additives and is then observed for antigen-antibody reactions. A normal (negative) reading shows no reaction or agglutination. An abnormal (positive) reading shows agglutination and reaction. These tests can give false readings. False negatives are seen in early syphilis. False positives are seen with treated syphilis, yaws, malaria, pellagra, infectious mononucleosis, and leprosy and when equipment used to run the test was not cleaned properly.

The Treponema Pallidum Immobilization Test has a high specificity and sensitivity for syphilis and gives very few false readings. It requires 5 ml of venous blood to which live *Treponema pallidum* organisms are added and organism immobilization observed. Unfortunately it is a very complicated test to perform and not well suited for general, small laboratories. The normal result shows no organism survival, and the abnormal (positive) findings show organism immobilization.

The Fluorescent Treponemal Antibody Absorption Test is also highly specific and sensitive to syphilis and gives very few false readings. It is difficult and expensive to perform and best done by large, medical center laboratories. Venous blood (5 ml) is withdrawn and permitted to clot so that the serum can be extracted. The serum is prepared through a heating, diluting, and washing process, mixed with *T. pallidum* antigen, fluorescein-labeled antihuman globulin, and placed on a slide. The slide is then examined with a fluorescent microscope for fluorescence of the organisms. A normal (or negative) reading has weak or nonfluorescent particles and an abnormal (or positive) reading shows strong to minimal fluorescence.

Sickle Cell Smear If the Sickledex screening is positive, the child must be referred for further evaluation, including a sickle cell smear. There are several methods for performing this test, one of which is McGovern's method. Only 1 to 2 ml of capillary blood is drawn into a pipette with certain chemicals added. After three drops are discarded, one drop is positioned on a glass slide, covered, bordered with petroleum jelly, and heated to seal off oxygen. Generally the slide is examined microscopically after 2 hours for sickled cells; however, some sources feel that sickling will show immediately. A normal reading is indicated by a lack of sickled cells, and an abnormal (positive) result is indicated by sickled cells.

These are but a few of the thousands of diagnostic and screening tests available using blood. More rapid and more sensitive tests are being developed all the time, and the reader is encouraged to watch the current literature for these developments and to use a good laboratory manual when working with the different tests.

URINE TESTING

One of the most complex and highly structured systems in the human body is the urinary system. As a highly efficient and effective filtering system, it can influence the functioning of the entire body. One of the most painless but effective ways of assessing urinary tract function is to examine the by-product of the urinary tract system—urine. There are many screening tests that can be performed on urine. This chapter will list some of the screening tests and a few of the diagnostic tests most commonly used. As with blood, standards will be given, but these vary from clinic to clinic, and examiners must check the norms in their own settings.

The Renal System

Before discussing examination of the urine, it is important to review the normal anatomy and physiology of the renal system, which includes the two kidneys, two ureters, urinary bladder, and urethra. Most infants are born with two kidneys, which are rounded, firm, small, lima bean-shaped structures lying deep within the upper pelvis. These are difficult to palpate, but are best felt with deep palpation within the first few hours of life before the GI tract fills with material. Anatomically the right kidney is lower than the left kidney, and by adulthood the kidneys measure 4 to 5 in by 2 in. The kidney has a *cortex* (covering) and *medulla* (inner surface). The medulla is subdivided into 10 to 16 smaller portions called *pyramids,* which finally unite to become one ureter leading from the kidney.

The basic renal unit is the *nephron,* and there are 1 million nephrons which begin in the cortex and empty into the pyramids of the medulla. As the nephron leaves the cortex it widens into a clump of vessels (called the *glomerulus*) which are covered by Bowman's capsule. From there the nephron twists and turns, becoming the proximal tubule, the loop of Henle, the distal tubule, and finally the collecting tubule. The collecting tubule empties into the kidney pelvis.

From the kidney pelvis, the urine is drained into the ureters, which are long tubes of circular and longitudinal muscle fibers. By adulthood the ureters can be up to 14 to 16 in long. They display spontaneous contractions which are a form of peristaltic movement which keeps the urine flowing into the bladder.

The two ureters attach on the superior portion of a large hollow balloon called the *urinary bladder.* The bladder lies behind the pubis and low in the pelvic girdle and consists of a series of muscular levels allowing for both contraction and relaxation. The bladder shape and capacity vary with age, sex, health, and certain diseases.

Urine leaves the bladder through the urethra. In the adult female the urethra is a narrow, $1\frac{1}{2}$-in-long tube opening anteriorly to the vagina and used solely for the passage of urine. The urethra of the adult male is generally about 8 in long, opens at the tip of the penile shaft, and is used for the discharge of both urine and semen.

The kidneys have many functions, but one of the most important is their filtering action. Within the kidney, substances are either reabsorbed for continued use within the body or discarded as waste. Large amounts of blood plasma (about 1200 ml/minute in an adult male) are filtered through the glomerulus and into the nephron tubules. As the fluid passes through the tubules, substances are selectively reabsorbed (such as water, urea, phosphates, creatinine, vitamin C) or discretely discarded (such as sodium chloride and dextrose); the discarded substances are passed into the collecting tubules and kidney pelvis. Some substances are always discarded, and some are discarded only when the level circulating in the body reaches a certain level.

Through the peristaltic movement of the ureters the urine is continually passed from the kidney pelvis to the bladder. When 1 to 8 oz (depending on age) is collected within the bladder, the nerve endings cause the bladder to constrict and force the urine into the urethra. As Table 18-6 shows, bladder capacity changes with age.

Urine is a mixture of organic and inorganic substances; the proportions of these substances may change slightly with each voiding since the kidneys are maintaining a specific chemical level within the body. Macroscopically

Table 18-6 Normal Bladder Capacity and Voiding

Age	Number of voidings in 24 hours	Average quantity at each voiding, oz
Under 3 months	13.5	1
3–6 months	20.0	1
6–12 months	16.0	$1\frac{1}{2}$
1–2 years	12.0	2
2–6 years	8.7	3
6–8 years	7.4	5
8–11 years	7.1	7
11–13 years	7.9	$7\frac{1}{2}$
Adults	7.0	$6\frac{1}{2}$

Printed by permission of Louis Gershenfeld, *Urine and Urinalysis*, Romaine Pierson, New York, 1948, p. 35.

urine is a bright, golden, clear liquid with a distinct aromatic odor. Substances normally found in urine are listed in Table 18-7.

Specimen Collection

The method used to obtain the urine specimen depends on the age of the child and the type of test to be performed. For accurate results, it is important that the examiner collect the specimen in the proper way, at the correct time, and store or preserve it correctly.

For a single, clean-catch specimen on an older girl, the nurse need only give the patient a wide-mouthed, clean specimen bottle and instructions on how to hold the labia apart while wiping from front to back over each side of the vestibule, using a fresh cotton ball each time. Finally, with a third cotton ball, the meatus is wiped, also in a front-to-back direction, and urination is begun. The first few drops are discarded and the rest of the urine collected in a clean container. Some institutions insist on a sterile container, but this is probably not essential. Some authorities advocate special soap and sterile water but this is probably not necessary either. Urine from older boys can be collected in a similar manner.

Clean catches on infants are less reliable, but can be attempted. The genital area is cleansed with damp and dry cotton and a small plastic urine bag with adhesive is attached around the penis or between the labia majora. If the bag is applied as the child is weighed in, the infant will generally void sometime during the examination and the bag can be removed. If not, giving the infant a few ounces to drink will usually produce the desired results. Once a child is toilet-trained, a specimen can be obtained in the adult manner, but with direct supervision and help from the nurse.

Specimens may be collected as a single catch or as a total of all urine

Table 18-7 Substances Found in Urine

Substance	Amount, g	Substance	Amount, g
Water	1200.0	Chloride (as NaCl)	12.0
Solids	60.0	Sodium	4.0
Urea	30.0	Phosphate (as P)	1.1
Uric acid	0.7	Potassium	2.0
Hippuric acid	0.27	Calcium	0.2
Creatinine	1.2	Magnesium	0.15
Indican	0.01	Sulfur (as S)	1.0
Oxalic acid	0.02	Inorganic sulfur	0.8
Allantoin	0.04	Neutral sulfur	0.12
Amino acid nitrogen	0.2	Conjugated sulfates	0.08
Purine bases	0.01	Ammonia	0.7
Phenols	0.2		

Printed by permission of Ruth M. French, *The Nurse's Guide to Diagnostic Procedures*, McGraw-Hill, New York, 1971, p. 17, and B. L. Oser (ed.), *Hawk's Practical Physiological Chemistry*, 14th ed., McGraw-Hill, New York, 1965.

voided over a period of time. Single specimens are best collected and examined promptly; if that is impossible, refrigeration is necessary. Specimens collected over 24 hours need some type of preservative to prevent bacterial contamination. Some of the more commonly used chemical preservatives are toluene, glacial acetic acid, formaldehyde, and commercial preservative tablets (Urokeep). Some tests require specific preservatives: 17-ketosteroid examinations require a larger amount of glacial acetic acid, and urobilinogen examinations require sodium carbonate. Specimens may also require refrigeration. This is usually done by refrigerating a large container and bringing each new specimen to the container as it is obtained.

Urine Screening Tests

Since urine is so easily obtained, it is used for many screening tests. The majority of the tests described in this section are easily done and read by the nurse. Basically urine is screened macroscopically and chemically.

Macroscopic inspection of urine includes observation of clarity, color, and odor. All urine specimens should be observed before any testing is done. Fresh, normally voided urine should be clear and transparent. It should contain no sediment, clouding, or mucous. Cloudiness can be caused by bacteria; blood; pus; casts; a large, all-vegetable meal; or epithelial cells. Freshly voided normal urine should be some shade of yellowish-amber. Small fluid intake, vomiting, diarrhea, or excessive perspiration may show a darker, more burnt-yellow-orange color, while large fluid intake may produce dilute, pale, or colorless urine. Many drugs and diseased conditions can cause urine to change color dramatically. Povan, used in the treatment of pinworms, for instance, may turn the urine a brilliant red. The mother of the child should be warned of this occurrence before it happens. Table 18-8 shows some of the other conditions that can change urine color.

Odor is another important characteristic of urine. Due to the organic acids, fresh, normal urine has a definite aromatic smell. With time and pathological conditions, the odor can change drastically. As urine is allowed to stand and decompose, there is a strong ammoniacal aroma. Freshly voided urine that has bacteria present may have a foul, putrid odor. Acidosis caused by diabetes, severe vomiting, or prolonged fever may produce urine that smells sweet and fruity. This is due to the increased acetone present in urine. Decomposed, diabetic urine can smell acidy like vinegar or yeasty like dough. Urine smelling like a rotten egg (hydrogen sulfide) may contain cystine. Fecal contamination, from either accidental or pathological

Table 18-8 Common Causes of Urine Color Changes

Color	Cause of coloration	Pathologic condition
Nearly colorless	Dilution or diminution of normal pigments	Nervous conditions; hydruria; diabetes insipidus; granular kidney
Dark yellow to amber	Increase of normal, or occurrence of pathologic, pigments; concentrated urine	Acute febrile diseases
Milky	Fat globules; pus cells; amorphous phospate	Chyluria; purulent diseases of the urinary tract
Orange	Excreted drugs, such as santonin, chrysophanic acid, pyridine	
Red or reddish	Hematoporphyrin; hemoglobin; myoglobin; erythrocytes	Hemorrhage; hemoglobinuria; trauma
Brown to brown-black	Hematin; methemoglobin; melanin; hydroquinone; pyrocatechol	Hemorrhage; methemoglobinuria; melanotic sarcoma
Greenish-yellow or brown, approaching black	Bile pigments	Phenol poisoning; jaundice
Dirty green or blue (dark-blue surface scum, blue deposit)	Excess of indigo-forming substances; methylene blue medication	Cholera; typhus (seen especially when urine is putrefying)

Printed by permission of Ruth M. French, *The Nurse's Guide to Diagnostic Procedures*, McGraw-Hill, New York, 1971, p. 19, and B. L. Oser (ed.), *Hawk's Practical Physiological Chemistry*, 14th ed., McGraw-Hill, New York, 1965.

causes gives urine a foul, fecal odor. Some foods (e.g., onions and asparagus) give a specific, definite odor, and some strong-smelling drugs (e.g., peppermint, turpentine, and menthol) will carry their odor through the urine. Table 18-9 lists some of the odor changes found in urine.

Chemically there are several simple procedures that can be performed to gather more data about the urine specimen. When screening urine, the examiner can test for pH, specific gravity, and presence of protein, glucose, ketones, bilirubin, blood, phenylalanine, and sulfite. Many of these tests can be done simply with commercial products that require no more than a special filter paper briefly exposed to the specimen. The tests come in many varieties, and the examiner is wise to pick the test that gives the most information for the least amount of money.

pH This is a test for the amount of acid or alkaline present in the urine. The blood pH is controlled by the kidney, which filters all excessive ions into the urine. Thus pH of the urine varies according to blood levels. The pH is easily tested with the use of special filter paper, sometimes built into such tests as the Bili-Labstix. A filter paper is dipped into freshly collected urine and immediately matched with the color-coded chart for acidity or alkalinity. The standard matching is orange = pH 5, tan = pH 6, light

Table 18-9 Odor Changes Found in Urine

Disorders	Compound	Odor
Phenylketonuria	Phenylacetic acid	Musty odor
Maple syrup urine disease	Branched chain a-keto acids	Maple syrup or burned sugar
Isovaleric acidemia	Isovaleric acid	Cheesy or sweaty feet
Oasthouse disease*	a-Hydroxybutyric acid	Oasthouse or brewery
Methionine malabsorption*	a-Hydroxybutyric acid	Oasthouse
Hypermethioninemia	a-Keto-γ-methiol butyric acid	Rancid butter or rotten cabbage
Butyric/hexanoic acidemia	Butyric and hexanoic acids	Sweaty feet
Trimethylaminuria	Trimethylamine	Stale fish

*It has been suggested the methionine malabsorption syndrome and the oasthouse disease may be identical disorders.

Source: G.H. Thomas and R.R. Howell, *Selected Screening Tests for Genetic Metabolic Diseases,* Yearbook Medical Publishers, Inc., Chicago. Used by permission.

green = pH 7, dark green = pH 8, and dark blue = pH 9. A normal pH is between 4.8 and 8.0 on the scale.

Specific Gravity Specific gravity is a measure of the concentration or dilution of dissolved substances within the urine. The test can be performed by using a hydrometer (or urinometer); the newer method uses the refractometer. The hydrometer is a small, glass-enclosed tube, fat at the bottom and thin at the top. The top portion contains demarcated spaces and numbers. The hydrometer method requires 20 ml of urine, which is poured into the cylinder holding the hydrometer. The hydrometer floats free until it stabilizes, and a reading is taken at the level of the urine. The new method requires only a drop of urine, which is placed on the slide of the refractometer. This instrument looks like a small flashlight with a flapping door on one side. Once the urine is dropped on the slide, the door is held firmly in place; the examiner looks through one end while pointing the other end toward a light source. A reading is taken by observing the sharp line seen through the lens at the end of the refractometer. A normal specific gravity is 1.003 to 1.030.

Specific Elements There are many commercial products for screening for specific elements present in urine.

Bili-Labstix is probably one of the most complete; one filter paper gives six readings; pH, protein, glucose, ketones, bilirubin, and blood. The papers come in a dark bottle containing 100 reagent strips, and the standardized color chart is on the bottle. The strips must be stored at room temperature in the tightly capped bottle. Freshly voided urine is preferable for testing, but urine preserved with Urokeep or Kingsburg-Clark urine preservative tablets can also be used. Other preservatives give false readings. The reagent strip is removed from the bottle with care to avoid touching the filter areas and the strip dipped completely into the urine sample. Any excess urine is removed by gently shaking or tapping the strip. The filter portion can be matched immediately against the color-coded chart on the bottle. pH may be read immediately and should give a reading around 5 to 8. Protein may be read immediately and should be negative (a light yellow). A trace calls for a repeat test with a second urine specimen. Glucose can be read at 10 seconds and should be negative (a brilliant pink); a reading at "light" (light purple) indicates 0.25 g/100 ml of glucose present, and the test must be repeated. Ketones can be read at 15 seconds and should be negative (a light tan). Occult blood is read at 30 seconds and should be negative (a soft tan). Bilirubin is read at 20 seconds and should be negative (a light tan).

Clinitest is used to test for glucose in urine. The test comes as 100 reagent tablets in a dark brown bottle. The procedure involves setting one tablet on a dry, clean surface, placing 2 drops of urine on the tablet, adding 10 drops of water, and waiting 15 seconds for the reaction. Interpretation is based on a color chart provided with a scale of 0 to 5 percent. Thus:

Dark blue = 0 (negative)
Dirty green = trace
Olive green = 0.5 percent
Yellow-green = 1 percent
Yellow-brown = 2 percent
Yellow-tan = 3 percent
Orange = 5 percent

Clinistix is a similar product for testing urine for glucose. It consists of reagent strips which are dipped into fresh urine and read after 10 seconds. Results are interpreted according to a color chart on the bottle. Clinistix is not considered as sensitive as other tests since it will give a false negative with sugars other than glucose.

Combistix is similar to Bili-Labstix but tests for only three elements: pH, glucose, and protein. It is a special reagent filter which is dipped in fresh urine. All the tests are read immediately, with pH ranging from 5 to 9, glucose being negative, small, medium, or large, and protein being negative, trace, $1+$, $2+$, and $3+$.

Keto-Diastix is a fairly new screening test for detecting glucose and ketones in the urine. The urine must be at room temperature. The reagent strip is dipped into the urine for 2 seconds and withdrawn. Excess urine is removed and the strip is read at 15 seconds for ketones and 30 seconds for glucose. Interpretation is made according to the color chart on the side of the bottle. The color code is:

Soft-buff = negative ketones
Light pink = positive ketones (small amount)
Darker pink = positive ketones (moderate amount)
Light purple = positive ketones (large amount)
Pale blue = negative glucose
Darker blue = positive glucose (trace)
Deep blue-brown = positive glucose $(1+)$
Dark blue-brown = positive glucose $(2+)$
Brown = positive glucose $(4+)$
Dark brown = positive glucose $(4+)$

The Keto-Diastix is intended only for use as a screening tool; it can give false readings due to chilled urine, oral hypoglycemic agents, etc.

Uristix is another product which tests for glucose and protein. The reagent strip is immersed in the fresh urine specimen and immediately withdrawn. Protein is determined immediately by comparing the strip with the color chart on the bottle. Lack of color indicates no protein, and traces of color show little, moderate, or large amounts of protein. Glucose is read at 10 seconds, and by color comparison a reading of small, medium, or large is made.

All these tests are easy to administer, inexpensive, and can be very useful screening tools when used appropriately.

PKU Testing PKU is a serious disease, and many states now require some form of screening on all infants. Blood testing for PKU has already been discussed; there are also two very simple screening devices for testing urine for PKU: the Phenistix and ferric chloride test.

Phenistix reagent strips must be stored at room temperature in a dark, tightly capped bottle. The strips should be used on fresh urine or urine preserved with the Kingsbury-Clark urine preservative tablets. The procedure calls for the strip to be pressed between two areas of freshly wetted diaper (avoid diaper with fecal soiling) until the strip is well-saturated. Interpretation is made by comparing the strip with the color chart on the bottle after a 30-second interval. A negative reading shows no change in the strip colors, and a positive reading shows shades of blue-gray (meaning 15, 40, 100 mg of phenylpyruvic acid per 100 ml of urine).

The ferric chloride test can also be used to screen for PKU, histidinemia, tyrosinemia, alcaptonuria, maple sugar disease, and oasthouse disease, and for the presence of some medications (i.e., salicylates, antipyrine, isoniazid, etc.) (Thomas and Howell, 1973). A squirt bottle or eye dropper is filled with a 10% solution of ferric chloride (10 g of $FeCl_3$ in 100 ml of water). One to two drops of the solution is squirted on fresh urine (usually on the diaper) and the color observed after 30 to 60 seconds. No color change (a slight yellowing on the diaper) indicates absence of disease. A positive result shows a different color for each of the specific diseases listed. Phenylketonuria turns the diaper a dark green color and histidinemia will show a dark green, blue, or purple spot. Tyrosinemia may show no color or a transient green or blue. Alcaptonuria shows either no color or a transient blue, and maple sugar disease gives no color or a purple discoloration. A dark green spot can be the result of oasthouse disease. The drugs also give different colors: salicylate, purple; antipyrine, red; and isoniazid, yellow-green to lavender. It must be remembered that this is a screening test and should alert the examiner to more diagnostic, definitive testing.

Sulfite Screening This test is used to detect a urinary sulfite disorder which leads to damaged eye lenses, neurological defects, and mental retardation. A special reagent strip is placed in a freshly voided urine specimen and withdrawn to be read after a 10-second interval. The presence of sulfite results in a brilliant pink; its absence is indicated by a light pink.

Testrip This relatively new screening device is a VMA-sensitive reagent strip to test for neuroblastoma and pheochromocytoma. The test requires freshly voided urine in a clean container or on a clean diaper. Urine that has been preserved can be used, but must have the pH adjusted to between 5 and 7. The reagent strip is thoroughly saturated in the urine and then positioned on a clean, hard surface for 7 to 10 minutes. Interpretation is made by matching the strip to the color chart on the bottle. A negative reading shows a yellow or brown color. A positive reading shows a purple color indicating the presence of at least 20 micrograms (g) of VMA per milliliter. False readings are obtained if the child has ingested vanilla, coffee, bananas, specific fruits, and some medications within the previous 24 hours.

These are a sampling of the many urine screening devices available to the nurse. Most of them are easily run and fairly inexpensive and within certain ranges give reliable results as screening procedures.

Bactiuria Screening By far the most useful of the products available for urinary screening tests are the recently released bacteriological screening agents. These can be used to screen for urinary infections. Many tests currently available are based on the principle that bacteria will multiply on agar plates under incubated situations. Most of these tests are quite inexpensive compared with a complete urinary culture and for this reason are more practical for screening purposes. They do not, however, give all the information that a complete culture will give; they tell only whether bacteria are present in the specimen and if so, in what amounts they are present; they do not tell what specific bacteria are present, and they do not tell the antibiotic sensitivity of the bacteria that are present. Most of them consist of a small agar plate and a dipstick which is dipped into the urine and then brought in contact with the agar plate before incubation. After incubation, bacterial colonies are visible to the naked eye and are counted. A specified number is interpreted as minimal and considered to be due to skin contamination; a slightly higher number is considered suspicious, and the test should be redone; colony counts over that number are said to be infections, and a complete culture should be taken. The three most common tests available in the United States are Testuria, Quantikit, and Bac-U-Dip. Uricult is a similar product manufactured in Finland. All are well below $1.00 in cost. They do, however, have several disadvantages. The first is that although the manufacturers claim they are quite easy to read, this has not always been the authors' experience; the second is that incubation is necessary, and this may be a handicap in certain clinic situations; finally, there is the problem of obtaining clean catch in younger girls. The rate of skin contamination with this procedure in young girls is very high and can invalidate some of these screening tests. There are now several tests available which circumvent these problems. One such product is Uriglox[1] manufactured only in Sweden at the time of this writing. The Uriglox test is based on the principle that normal urine contains minute amounts of glucose in a first morning specimen (2 to 20 mg/100 ml). But if bacteria are in the bladder, they ingest the glucose, lowering the concentration to less than 2 mg/100 ml. When a paper strip is dipped into the specimen, the urine filters up to a certain spot. If the strip turns blue, the normal glucose concentration is present, indicating no infection. But if the strip remains colorless, no glucose is present, indicating a possible infection.

Bactiuria screening devices are among the most useful of the urinary screening devices currently available, and the nurse should consider using it routinely at periodic intervals for all girls.

Urine Diagnostic Tests

Once a child has been screened and there is a positive reading or some question about the results, more specific laboratory work and a more complete history and physical examination are necessary. While urine is screened macroscopically and chemically, it is diagnostically tested both microscopically and chemically. The following diagnostic urine tests are not all the tests that can be performed on the urine, but only a sampling of some of the more popular procedures.

The microscopic examination is done after the urine has been examined macroscopically for color, clarity, and odor. The specimen should be freshly voided and obtained by the clean-catch method. About 15 ml of urine is poured into a centrifuge tube and spun for 3 to 5 minutes at medium speed. The supernatant fluid is poured off the top by inverting the tube quickly and returning it to its upright position. By quickly tapping the bottom of the tube against the finger or palm, the sediment and remaining urine are mixed. One drop of this mixture is placed on a glass slide and a cover glass dropped over the specimen. The slide may be viewed under the microscope by using a low light, beginning with the 16-mm lens (or low power) for finding casts and proceeding to the 4-mm lens (or high power) for the smaller substances.

Various cells are the first substances to be observed for: epithelial (renal, transitional, squamous), glitter, neoplastic, inclusion bodies, red blood cells, and white blood cells. Epithelial cells are simply the sloughed

---

[1]Uriglox is available from: Mr. Betil Jarnhall, Ab Kabi, Fac. S-104 25, Stockholm, Sweden. A newer kit, Bac-U-Dip, which works just as well, can be obtained from Warner-Chilcott Laboratories, Morris Plains, N.J. 07950.

cells from different parts of the urinary tract. Usually the 16-mm lens is used and all types of cells are lumped together for a count of $1+$ to $4+$ or more. Renal cells are small with a large nucleus and come from the renal pelvis. These should not normally be seen. Transitional cells have large odd-shaped diameters and come from the pelvis, ureter, or bladder and are seen only in certain pathological conditions. Squamous cells show a tiny nucleus in a large, flat diameter and can be seen in normal specimens. Glitter cells require a special dye for each observation and are seen only in pyelonephritis. Neoplastic cells and inclusion body cells are seen only in certain pathological conditions and usually require special preparations of the slide for easier viewing. Red blood cells can be seen with both high and low power and appear as roughly rounded cells with no nucleus. Red blood cells should not be present in normal, voided specimens. A catheterized specimen may show a few red blood cells, but generally any presence of such cells means kidney disease or trauma. White blood cells are absent in normal urine; however, with the 4-mm lens adult male urine may show one white blood cell and the urine of adult females and all children may show one to five white blood cells and still be within normal ranges. Both red and white blood cells look the same in urine as they do in a blood smear. They should definitely be absent from multiple voidings, catheterizations, and bladder taps.

Casts are abnormal plasma-protein gel produced by the renal tubules after trauma or damage. There are several kinds of casts: hyaline, blood, and epithelial. Degeneration of an epithelial cast forms a granular cast which may be fine or coarse. Other types of casts degenerate to form fatty casts, waxy casts, and amyloid casts. Casts are usually seen with the 16-mm lens, and their presence is reportable and needs further investigation (see Fig. 18-44).

Parasites are rarely seen in urine and are never normal. Trichomonas, schistosoma, and filaria are those most likely to be observed.

Sediments are another abnormal substance to be observed for when examining the urine. Colorless, bumpy substances are amorphous phosphate sediment which can be dissolved in acetic acid and is seen in alkaline urine. Bumpy, granulated substances are calcium carbonate sediment which can also be dissolved in acetic acid. Yellow, diffuse granulated sediment is amorphous urate found in acid urine and dissolved with heating and alkali.

Crystals should not be present in freshly voided, warm urine, but they will form in normal urine as it cools. Acid urine shows calcium oxalate crystals and uric acid (or urate) crystals. Alkaline urine shows ammonio-magnesium phosphate, calcium carbonate, and ammonium biurate crystals.

Various other particles can be seen such as thread fibers from panties and cotton left from washing the area. Either external or internal contamination will show bacteria in the specimen (see Fig. 18-45).

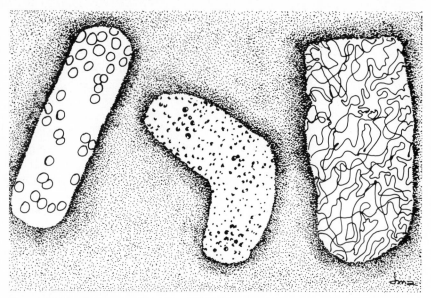

Figure 18-44   Casts seen in urine. *(a)* Blood cast. *(b)* Granular cast. *(c)* Renal cast.

Once the urine has been examined for visible particles, it can be tested chemically for the presence of other substances.

Acetone   Three types of ketone bodies are found in urine: acetone, acetoacetic acid, and beta-hydroxy-butyric acid. Ketones and incomplete ketones are formed in the metabolism of fat; when low or no carbohydrate intake occurs, fat may be used as an energy source; when this happens, the breakdown products of fat metabolism—ketones—will appear in the urine. A high production of ketones is known as ketosis and leads to acidosis, which is most often associated with uncontrolled diabetes mellitus. Ketosis is also seen after the administration of ether or after severe vomiting or starvation. If a screening test shows ketosis, a diagnostic test for acetone is indicated. Some authorities feel that the presence of acetone indicates the presence of the other two types of ketones as well. A fresh sample of urine is mixed with a solution of ammonium sulfate and nitroprusside and additional ammonia is carefully poured on the top surface to give a layered effect. A positive reading (acetone present) shows a reddish-purple ring between the layer of ammonia and the solution. A negative reading indicates absence of acetone. False positive tests can be obtained if the patient has recently taken certain drugs such as L-dopa, Levodopa, or Phenformin, (Garb, 1971) or has been exposed to bromosulfonphtalein or phenolsulfonphthalein testing.

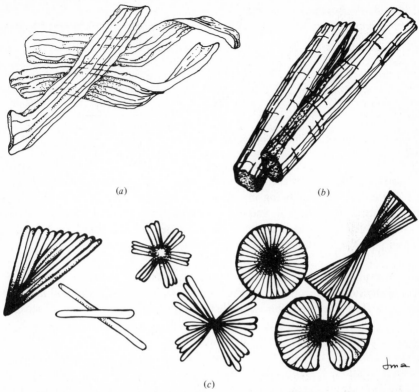

(a)　　　　(b)

(c)

Figure 18-45 Sediment found in urine. *(a)* Cotton fibers. *(b)* Hair. *(c)* Sulphonamide crystals.

Addis Test The Addis test (Table 18-10) is done to diagnose a specific kidney disease by counting the cells and casts present in the sediment. For reasons of safety, this test is not to be performed on any patient of known renal pathology. For 24 hours the patient may eat but consume no fluids. After 12 hours the patient voids one specimen, which is discarded. For the remaining 12 hours the patient collects all the urine voided (generally around 800 to 1600 ml). During the collecting period, the urine must be refrigerated. The urine is completely mixed and then centrifuged; the sediment is then examined through the microscope. The diagnosis of nephritis is based on the number of red blood cells, white blood cells, and casts present.

Amylase In some pancreatic pathology, the pancreatic digestive enzymes may ooze into surrounding tissues and serum and finally overflow into the urine. Depending on the laboratory, the test for amylase can be done with a 2-, 12-, or 24-hour collection of urine. The urine is hydrolyzed and

Table 18-10 Addis Test Values

Condition	RBC/mm^3	WBC/mm^3	Casts/mm^3
Normal	0–5,000	0–500,000	1,000,000
Acute nephritis	690,000	405,000,000	48,000,000
Chronic nephritis (active)	1,850,000	34,000,000	14,000,000
Chronic nephritis (latent)	48,000	16,000,000	2,000,000

Source: Opal Helper, *Manual of Clinical Laboratory Methods*, 4th ed., 1954. Courtesy of Charles C Thomas, Publisher, Springfield, Illinois.

observed for the development of a blue color. Interpretation is made by comparing the color of the urine with a standard color chart, with readings of 270 units per hour being in the normal range. Many drugs such as codeine, morphine, demerol, and ethyl alcohol (Garb, 1971) give false positive results. Such conditions as intestinal obstructions, mumps, and salivary gland pathology will also give false readings.

Bilirubin   If there is an increase in the destruction of red blood cells or a malfunction within the liver, the bile pigments and bilirubin will increase and overflow into the urine. A single urine specimen can be used to measure this. It is important for the patient to avoid several specific drugs such as acetophenazine, phenaxopyridine, and ethoxazene prior to the testing, since these invalidate the test results (Garb, 1971). There are several different tests (Gmelin's, Rosenbach's, Smith's, etc.); they all depend on oxidation of the bilirubin to produce a specific color, which is then compared with a standard. A negative, or normal, result indicates the absence of bilirubin or bile; a positive, or abnormal, result indicates the presence of those substances.

Hormonal Studies   There are many complicated, esoteric tests that can be done on urine for the presence of specific hormones; only two are mentioned here: 17-hydroxy-corticosteroid and 17-ketosteroid. The 17-hydroxy-corticosteroid test measures the amount of corticosteroid being produced by the adrenal cortex. The patients must be instructed in the 24-hour collection of urine. The specimen is then processed to extract the corticosteroid with butanol and buffered with a special reagent which produces some color changes which are matched to standard charts. Many drugs will give false readings—cortisone, digitoxin, estrogens, iodides, reserpine, etc. (Garb, 1971)—and the patient must be questioned closely before attempting the test.

The 17-ketosteroid test measures a specific male hormone produced by the adrenals or the testes. Again a 24-hour collection of urine is necessary, as is the avoidance of such drugs as cortisone, meprobamate, penicillin, and oral contraceptives before and during the testing period. In the laboratory, the urine is processed by adding a special chemical and measuring the depth of the red color that results. A result of 8 to 20 mg/day for men and 5 to 15 mg/day for women is considered within the normal range.

Kidney Function The normal kidney has the ability to excrete certain substances, and by measuring these substances some idea of kidney condition can be obtained.

The creatinine clearance test is a measurement of the amount of creatinine (a by-product of metabolism) excreted through the kidney; this directly reflects the adequacy of glomeruli functioning. During the test the patient may eat a normal diet omitting certain beverages (i.e., coffee and tea) and all meat, fish, and poultry. The patient saves all urine for 24 hours. Blood is drawn and tested chemically for the amount of creatinine present. A mathematical formula is then used to calculate the amount of creatinine clearance. The normal range is 100 to 140 ml/minute.

The Fishberg (or concentration) test measures the kidney's ability to dilute or concentrate urine. This is a 2-day test and requires hospitalization. Twelve hours prior to testing, the patient's food intake is restricted and fluid intake limited to 8 oz. The patient is also on limited activity. The first morning specimen is saved, as well as two additional specimens at 1-hour intervals. The patient is then allowed unlimited fluids and food. After a normal supper on the first day of testing, food and fluid is again restricted until the test is complete. The following morning, the first specimen is discarded and the patient instructed to drink 40 oz of water within a 45-minute period. Urine specimens are collected hourly for 4 hours. As each specimen is taken, the specific gravity is measured and recorded. Normally the concentration period should show a specific gravity of 1.026 or higher and the dilution period should show 1.003.

The phenolsulfonphthalein (PSP) test measures the ability of the kidney's proximal tubules to excrete a certain dye after it has been injected. There are slight variations in the test, but generally the patient must consume 16 oz of water at the beginning of the test. After 30 minutes 1 to 2 ml of phenolsulfonphthalein dye is injected. Urine specimens are collected at 15, 30, 60, and 120 minutes. The specimens are processed and each compared with a standardized color chart giving the amount of dye normally excreted within each of those time ranges. Bauer (1962) lists the range of normal as

At 15 minutes, 30 percent dye present
At 30 minutes, 15 percent dye present
At 60 minutes, 10 percent dye present
At 120 minutes, 75 to 85 percent dye present

Such drugs as penicillin, pyridium and some diuretics will give a false reading on this test (Garb, 1971).

Lead If a lead screening test is positive, the patient must be referred for a diagnostic test. After the patient has been on a low calcium diet for 3 days, a 24-hour urine specimen is collected. The lead level may be obtained by chemical or spectrographic procedures. A normal reading is less than 100 g/24 hours; anything over this is considered abnormal.

Morphine This test is used to measure the amount of morphine or heroin ingested within the preceding 24 hours. Several specific chemicals are mixed with a single voided specimen. The resultant color is matched to a color standard to determine the amount of morphine present.

Pregnancy There are many tests for pregnancy, and newer ones are constantly being developed. Most of the procedures are harmless for the mother and the infant; however, some of the more recent tests requiring the mother to ingest specific substances are still being studied for fetal effects.

The newer, more commonly used tests are of two types: the latex-inhibition slide tests (the HCG test, the Gravindex, and the Pregnosticon slide test) and the direct latex agglutination slide test (the DAP test). None of the tests are 100 percent reliable. In fact, Hobson (1969) relates that they have no more reliability than flipping a coin. Kerber's (1970) comparison shows that the Pregnosticon slide test is probably the most useful. One of the newest screening tests being advertised is the E.P.T. (Early Pregnancy Test) by Warner-Chilcott, which can be used by the woman to test her own urine within ten days of a missed period.

Porphyrins Porphyins are pigments which are formed by the destruction of red blood cells; they are excreted through the kidney. By measuring the proportion of porphyrins in the urine, the examiner can get some idea of the amount of red blood cell destruction going on in the liver. A 24-hour urine specimen is needed. The porphyrins are precipitated, dissolved, and examined spectroscopically for specific characteristics. A normal urine shows no or very slight amounts of porphyrins; the presence of even small or moderate amounts of porphyrins is abnormal. Drugs like alcohol, sulfonamides, and barbiturates will give false results (Garb, 1971).

Albumin The terms *protein* and *albumin* are frequently used interchangeably; strictly speaking, this is inaccurate, since there are several kinds of protein found in the urine (albumin, globulin, fibrinogen, etc.).

Albumin is the protein most frequently looked for in the urine; both qualitative and quantitative measurements are possible. There are at least four qualitative tests for albumin. The Heller ring test uses filtered urine which is slowly poured into 3 ml of nitric acid, allowed to stand for 3 minutes, and observed for a fine gray line between the two solutions. The amount and density of the gray ring gives a result of trace, $+1$, $+2$, or $+3$. The heat-acetic acid test requires filtered urine to be heated and observed for cloudiness. Several drops of acetic acid are added and cloudiness is again observed. The cloudiness is rated on a scale from 1 to 4. The refined heat-acetic acid test is used to rule out cloudiness caused by any substance other than albumin. The procedure is the same, but sodium chloride and glacial acetic acid are added before the first heating. The sulfosalicylic acid test requires that acetic acid be added to the urine before it is filtered and divided. Half this solution then has sulfosalicylic acid added and is observed for cloudiness; the other half is heated and is also observed for clouding. Cloudiness of either specimen indicates albumin. Such drugs as neomycin, vitamin D, and salicylates will invalidate this test (Garb, 1971).

Quantitatively, there are at least two tests for albumin. The Tsuchiya test requires a 24-hour collection of urine. The urine is diluted to a certain specific gravity, acidified, added to a special reagent, and observed for precipitation. The amount of albumin is measured by the depth of the precipitation. The Kingsbury and Clark test also needs a 24-hour urine specimen. A specific amount of filtered urine is mixed with a certain reagent and allowed to stand for 5 minutes before being compared with a commercial standard. Both of these tests can be invalidated by many drugs (e.g., bacitracin, aminophyllin, penicillin), and a thorough history of drug ingestion should be obtained before the testing (Garb, 1971).

Sugar Sugar may also be tested for quantitatively and qualitatively. If a screening test has detected the presence of sugar in the urine, a quantitative test is necessary to find out exactly how much sugar is present. One such test is Benedict's test, which requires a 24-hour urine collection. The urine must be preserved by refrigeration and Toluol. When Benedict's solution, sodium carbonate, and a pebble are added together they produce a blue color. The urine is then heated, filtered, and dropped into the Benedict's solution until all the blue color is titrated out. The results can be calculated and interpreted into percentages and g/24 hours. Steroids, penicillin, and chloral hydrate can give false positives (Garb, 1971).

Sometimes it is important to know what kind of sugar is present; in this situation, qualitative tests must be used. One such test is the fermentation sugar test. The urine from a single specimen is boiled, mixed with yeast, and incubated for 24 hours. Interpretation made is by measuring the amount of carbon dioxide gas present. If only carbon dioxide is present, the test is positive for glucose. If Benedict's test is done and is negative, the test is positive for lactose, glucose, and pentose. Further tests can be performed for additional sugars.

These are a few of the laboratory tests done on urine; there are many more, and the reader is referred to the bibliography for more details and tests. Many of these tests are now being done electronically, with a specimen fed into the computer and any number of tests run automatically, speedily, and inexpensively. Not all laboratories are so equipped, and some continue to use the older, slower, but equally accurate methods.

REFERENCES

Bauer, John D., Gelson Toro, and Philip G. Ackermann: *Bray's Clinical Laboratory Methods,* C. V. Mosby, St. Louis, 1962.

Bench, R. J., and K. P. Murphy: "The Papousek Cradle: A Device for Measuring Babies; Head Movement Responses to Auditory Stimulation," *Journal of Laryngology and Otology,* vol. 84, pp. 521–523, May 1970.

Bennett, S. M.: "A Group Test of Hearing for Six-Year-Old Children," *British Journal of Educational Psychology,* vol. 21, pp. 45–52, 1951.

Berko, J.: "The Child's Learning of the English Morphology," *Word,* vol. 14, pp. 150–177, 1958.

Botwin, Elaine D.: "Should Children Be Screened for Hypertension?" *The American Journal of Maternal-Child Nursing,* vol. 1, no. 3 (May, June, 1976), pp. 152–158.

Brown, Marie S., and Mary A. Murphy: *Ambulatory Pediatrics for Nurses,* McGraw-Hill, New York, 1975.

Carrow, Sister Mary Arthur: "The Development of Auditory Comprehension of Language Structure in Children," *Journal of Speech and Hearing Disorders,* vol. 33, no. 2, pp. 99–111, 1968.

Carter, Eunice T., and Buck McKenzie: "Prognostic Testing for Functional Articulation Disorders among Children in the First Grade," *Journal of Speech and Hearing Disorders,* vol. 33, 1958.

Clark, J. R.: "Testing the Hearing of Children with Noisemakers—A Myth," *Exceptional Children,* vol. 22, p. 323, 1956.

Downs, Marion P.: "The Familiar Sounds of Test and Other Tests for Hearing Screening in Children," *Journal of School Health,* vol. 26, pp. 77–78, 1956.

Downs, M. P. and W. G. Hemenway: "A Report on the Hearing Screening of 17,000 Newborns," *International Journal of Audiology,* vol. III, no. 1, pp. 72–76, February 1969.

Downs, Marion P. and Henry K. Silver, "The A.B.C.D's to H.E.A.R." *Clinical Pediatrics,* vol. II, no. 10 (October, 1972), pp. 563–565.

Ewing, I. R., and A. W. G. Ewing: "The Ascertainment of Deafness in Infancy and Early Childhood," *Journal of Laryngology and Otolaryngology,* vol. 59, pp. 309–338, 1944.

Fay, Thomas H., Irving Hochberg, Clarissa R. Smith, Norma S. Rees, and Harvey Halpern: "Audiologic and Otologic Screening of Disadvantaged Children," *Archives of Otolaryngology,* vol. 91, pp. 366–370, April 1970.

Fiedler, M. F., E. H. Lenneberg, U. T. Rolfe, et al: "A Speech Screening Procedure with Three-Year-Old Children," *Pediatrics,* vol. 48, pp. 268–276, August 1971.

Frankenberg, William K., Bonnie W. Kamp, and Pearl A. Van Natta: "Validity of the Denver Development Screening Test," *Child Development,* vol. 42, pp. 475-485, April 1971.

Fraser, C., U. Bellugi, and R. Brown: "Control of Grammar in Imitation, Comprehension, and Production," *Journal of Verbal Learning and Verbal Behavior,* vol. 2, pp. 121-135, 1963.

Garb, Solomon: *Laboratory Tests in Common Use,* Springer, New York, 1971.

Glorig, Aram, and H. P. House: "A New Concept in Auditory Screening," *Archives of Otolaryngology,* vol. 66, p. 228, August 1957.

Green, Morris, and Julius B. Richmond: *Pediatric Diagnosis,* Sannoles, Philadelphia and London, 1962.

Hardy, J. B., A. Dougherty, and W. F. Hardy: "Hearing Responses and Audiometric Screening in Infants," *Journal of Pediatrics,* vol. 55, pp. 382-390, 1959.

Hatfield, Elizabeth Macfarlane: "A Year's Record of Preschool Vision Screening," *The Sight-Saving Review,* vol. 36, no. 1, pp. 18-23, 1966.

Heron, T., and R. Jacobs: "Respiratory Curve Responses of the Neonate to Auditory Stimulation," *International Audiology,* vol. 8, pp. 77-84, 1969.

Hobson, B. M.: "Pregnancy Diagnosis," *Lancet,* vol. 2, p. 56, 1969.

Irwin, R. B.: "Consistency of Judgments of Articulatory Productions," *Journal of Speech and Hearing Research,* vol. 13, pp. 548-555, September 1970.

Irwin, R. B., and Barbara Willson Musselman: "A Compact Picture Articulation Test," *Journal of Speech and Hearing Disorders,* vol. 27, no. 1, pp. 36-39, February 1962.

Kerber, I. J., A. P. Inclan, E. A. Fowler, K. Davis, and S. A. Fish: "Immunologic Tests for Pregnancy: A Comparison," *Obstetrics and Gynecology,* vol. 36, p. 37, 1970.

Krupke, Sidney S., Constance A. Dunbar, and Vivian Zimmerman: "Vision Screening of Preschool Children in Mobile Clinics in Iowa," *Public Health Reports,* vol. 85, no. 1, pp. 41-45, 1970.

Lee, Laura L.: "A Screening Test for Syntax Development," *Journal of Speech and Hearing Disorders,* vol. 35, no. 2, pp. 103-112, 1969.

Lerea, I.: *The Michigan Picture Language Inventory,* University of Michigan Press, Ann Arbor, 1958.

Lieberman, Ellin: "Hypertension in Childhood and Adolescence," *Clinical Symposia,* vol. 30, no. 3 (1978), pp. 3-43.

Lippman, Otto: "Vision Screening of Young Children," *American Journal of Public Health,* vol. 61, no. 8, pp. 1598-1601, August 1971.

Loh, Wei-ping: "A New Solubility Test for Rapid Detection of Hemoglobin S," *The Journal of the Indiana State Medical Association,* vol. 61, no. 12, pp. 1651-1652, December 1968.

Miller, Maurice H., and Ira A. Polisar: *Audiological Evaluation of the Pediatric Patient,* Charles C. Thomas, Springfield, Ill., 1964.

Moghadam, Hossein K., Geoffrey C. Robinson, and Kenneth G. Cambon: "A Comparison of Two Audiometers in Screening the Hearing of School Children," *Canadian Medical Association Journal,* vol. 99, pp. 618-620, September 1968.

Moncur, J.: "Judge Reliability in Infant Testing," *Journal of Speech and Hearing Research,* vol. 11, pp. 348–357, 1968.

O'Brien, John S., Shintaro Okada, Agnes Chen, and Dorothy L. Fillerup: "Detection of Heterozygotes and Homozygotes by Serum Hemosaminidase Tay-Sachs Disease-Assay," *The New England Journal of Medicine,* vol. 283, no. 1, pp. 15–20, July 1970.

Press, Edward: "Screening of Preschool Children Ambylopia," *Journal of the American Medical Association,* vol. 204, no. 9, pp. 109–112, May 1968.

Rogers, W. B., and R. A. Rogers: "A Follow-up Study of the Preschool Readiness Experimental Screening Scale (The PRESS)," *Clinical Pediatrics,* vol. 14, no. 3, pp. 253–256, March 1975.

Sheridan, Mary D., and P. A. Gardiner: "Sheridan-Gardiner Test for Visual Acuity," *British Medical Journal,* vol. 2, pp. 108–109, April 1970.

Smart, M. S., and R. C. Smart: *Children, Development and Relationships,* Macmillan, New York, 1977.

Smith, M. K.: "Measurement of the Size of English Vocabulary Through the Elementary Grades and High School," *Genetic Psychological Monographs,* vol. 24, pp. 311–345, 1941.

Snow, K., and R. Millisen: "Spontaneous Improvement in Articulation as Related to Differential Responses to Oral and Picture Articulation Tests," *Journal of Speech and Hearing Disorders,* Monograph Supplement no. 4, pp. 45–49, 1954.

Steer, M. D., and Hazel G. Drexler: "Predicting Later Articulation Ability from Kindergarten Tests," *Journal of Speech and Hearing Disorders,* vol. 25, pp. 391–397, 1969.

Thomas, George H., and R. Rodney Howell: *Selected Screening Tests for Genetic Metabolic Diseases,* Year Book Medical Publishers, Chicago, 1973.

Trotter, Robert R., Ruth M. Phillips, and Kenneth Schaffer: "Measurement of Visual Acuity of Preschool Children by Their Parents," *The Sight-Saving Review,* vol. 36, no. 2, pp. 80–89, 1966.

Van Riper, C., and R. Erickson: "A Predictive Screening Test of Articulation," *Journal of Speech and Hearing Disorders,* vol. 34, pp. 214–219, 1969.

Book Bibliography

Abbott Laboratories: *The Use of Blood,* Abbott Laboratories, Chicago, 1971.

Adams, John C.: *Outline of Orthopaedics,* Williams & Wilkins, Baltimore, 1967.

American Academy of Pediatrics: *Standards of Child Health Care,* American Academy of Pediatrics, Evanston, Ill., 1972.

Anastasi, Anne: *Psychological Testing,* Macmillan, New York, 1974.

Anthony, Catherine P., and Norma J. Kolthoff: *Textbook of Anatomy and Physiology,* 9th ed., C. V. Mosby, St. Louis, 1975.

Barness, Lewis: *Manual of Pediatric Physical Diagnosis,* 4th ed., Year Book Medical Publishers, Chicago, 1973.

Bates, Barbara: *A Guide to Physical Examination,* J. B. Lippincott, Philadelphia, 1974.

Bauer, John D., Gelson Toro, and Philip G. Ackermann: *Bray's Clinical Laboratory Methods,* C. V. Mosby, St. Louis, 1962.

Bjorn, John, and Harold Gross: *Problem Oriented Practice,* McGraw-Hill, New York, 1970.

Blum, R. H.: *The Management of the Doctor–Patient Relationship,* McGraw-Hill, New York, 1960.

Burch, George E., and Nicholas P. DePasquale: *Primer of Clinical Measurement of Blood Pressure,* C. V. Mosby, St. Louis, 1962.

Buros, Oscar K.: *The Seventh Mental Measurements Yearbook,* Gryphon Press, Highland Park, N.J., 1974.

Cattell, P.: *The Measurement of Intelligence of Infants and Young Children,* Psychological Corporation, New York, 1940.

Chinn, Peggy, L., and Cynthia J. Leitch: *Handbook for Nursing Assessment of the Child,* University of Utah Press, Salt Lake City, 1973.

Cronbach, Lee J.: *Essentials of Psychological Testing,* Harper & Row, New York, 1970.

Dale, D. M. C.: *Applied Audiology for Children,* 2d ed., Charles C Thomas, Springfield, Ill., 1967.

De Angelis, Catherine: *Basic Pediatrics for the Primary Health Care Provider,* Little, Brown, Boston, 1975.

DeGowin, Elmer, and Richard DeGowin: *Bedside Diagnostic Examination,* Macmillan, London, 1971.

Delp, Mahlon H., and Robert Manning: *Major's Physical Diagnosis,* W. B. Saunders, Philadelphia, 1968.

DeWeese, David D., and William H. Saunders: *The Textbook of Otolaryngology,* C. V. Mosby, St. Louis, 1964.

Frankenburg, William, and Bonnie Camp: *Pediatric Screening Tests,* Charles C Thomas, Springfield, Ill., 1975.

Freeman, Frank S.: *Theory and Practice of Psychological Testing,* Holt, New York, 1962.

French, Ruth M.: *The Nurse's Guide to Diagnostic Procedures,* McGraw-Hill, New York, 1971.

Garb, Solomon: *Laboratory Tests in Common Use,* Springer, New York, 1971.

Gardner, H. L., and R. H. Kaufman: *Benign Diseases of the Vulva and Vagina,* C. V. Mosby, St. Louis, 1969.

Garrett, Annette: *Interviewing: Its Principles and Methods,* Family Service Association of American, New York, 1970.

Gellis, Sydney S., and Benjamin M. Kagan: *Current Pediatric Theory,* W. B. Saunders, Philadelphia, 1971.

Glorig, Aram: *Audiometry: Principles and Practices,* Charles C Thomas, Springfield, Ill., 1975.

Green, Morris, and Julius Richmond: *Pediatric Diagnosis,* W. B. Saunders, Philadelphia, 1962.

Gunther, John: *Inside Asia,* Harper & Row, New York, 1939.

Guyton, Arthur C.: *Basic Human Physiology,* W. B. Saunders, Philadelphia, 1971.

Harper, Paul A.: *Preventive Pediatrics: Child Health and Development,* Appleton-Century-Crofts, New York, 1962.

Hollinshead, W. Henry: *Functional Anatomy of the Limbs and Back,* W. B. Saunders, Philadelphia, 1969.

Hoppenfeld, Stanley: *Physical Examination of the Spine and Extremities,* Appleton-Century-Crofts, New York, 1976.

Huffman, J. W.: *The Gynecology of Childhood and Adolescence,* W. B. Saunders, Philadelphia, 1968.

Hughes, James G.: *Synopsis of Pediatrics,* C. V. Mosby, St. Louis, 1971.

Hurst, Willis J., and H. Kenneth Walker: *The Problem-Oriented System,* Medcom, New York, 1972.

Illingworth, R. S.: *Introduction to Development and Assessment in the First Year,* William Heinemann, London, 1966.

Jerger, James: *Modern Developments in Audiology,* Academic Press, New York, 1963.

Joint Study Committee of the American School Health Association and the National Society for the Prevention of Blindness, Inc.: *Teaching about Vision,* National Society for the Prevention of Blindness, New York, 1972.

Jolly, Hugh: *Diseases of Children,* Blackweel Scientific Publications, London, 1974.

Judge, Richard D., and George D. Zuidema: *Methods of Clinical Examination: Physiological Approach,* 3d ed., Little, Brown, Boston, 1974.

Kark, Robert M.: *A Primer of Urinalysis,* Harper & Row, New York, 1963.

Katz, Jack: *Handbook of Clinical Audiology,* Williams & Wilkins, Baltimore, 1972.

Keeney, Arthur: *Ocular Examination: Basis and Technique,* C. V. Mosby, St. Louis, 1976.

Kempe, C. Henry, Henry K. Silver, and Donough O'Brien: *Current Pediatric Diagnosis and Treatment,* 4th ed., Lange Medical Publications, Los Altos, Calif., 1976.

Kunin, Calvin M.: *Detection, Prevention and Management of Urinary Tract Infections,* Lea & Febiger, Philadelphia, 1972.

Langenbeck, Bernhard: *Textbook of Practical Audiometry,* Williams & Wilkins, Baltimore, 1972.

Leiman, Sidney: *Basic Ophthalmology,* McGraw-Hill, New York, 1966.

Liebman, Sumner D., and Sydney Gellis: *The Pediatrician's Ophthalmology,* C. V. Mosby, St. Louis, 1966.

Lippman, Richard W.: *Urine and Urinary Sediment,* Charles C Thomas, Springfield, Ill., 1957.

Mahoney, Elizabeth, Laurie Verdisco, and Lillie Shortridge, *How to Collect and Record a Health History,* J. B. Lippincott, Philadelphia, 1976.

Miller, Maurice H., and Ira A. Polisar: *Audiological Evaluation of the Pediatric Patient,* Charles C Thomas, Springfield, Ill., 1964.

Mitchell, David, S. Standish, and T. Fast: *Oral Diagnosis/Oral Medicine,* Lea & Febiger, Philadelphia, 1971.

Montagna, William: *The Structure and Function of Skin,* Academic Press, New York, 1962.

Moss, Arthur J., and Forrest H. Adams: *Problems of Blood Pressure in Childhood,* Charles C Thomas, Springfield, Ill., 1962.

Nelson, Waldo: *Textbook of Pediatrics,* 10th ed., W. B. Saunders, Philadelphia, 1975.

Northern, Jerry L., and Marion P. Downs: *Hearing in Children,* Williams & Wilkins, Baltimore, 1974.

O'Brien, Donough, and Frank A. Ibbott: *Laboratory Manual of Pediatric Micro- and Ultramicro-Biochemical Techniques,* Harper & Row, New York, 1962.

O'Neill, John J., and Herbert J. Oyer: *Applied Audiometry,* Dodd, Mead, New York, 1966.

Ophthalmologic Staff of the Hospital for Sick Children, Toronto: *The Eye in Childhood,* Year Book Medical Publishers, Chicago, 1967.

Perry, Eldon T.: *The Human Ear Canal,* Charles C Thomas, Springfield, Ill., 1957.

Portmann, Michael, and Claudine Portmann: *Clinical Audiometry,* Charles C Thomas, Springfield, Ill., 1961.

Prechtl, Heinz: *The Neurological Examination of the Full-Term Newborn Infant,* Lippincott, Philadelphia, 1977.

Prior, John, and Jack Silberstein: *Physical Diagnosis,* C. V. Mosby, St. Louis, 1969.

Proctor, Donald F.: *The Nose, Paranasal Sinuses and Ears in Childhood,* Charles C Thomas, Springfield, Ill., 1963.

Ross Laboratories: *Children Are Different,* Ross Laboratories, Columbus, Ohio, 1970.

Rudolph, Abraham, Henry Barnett, and Arnold Einhorn (eds.): *Pediatrics,* 16th ed., Appleton-Century-Crofts, New York, 1977.

Schaeffer, Alexander J., and Mary Ellen Avery: *Diseases of the Newborn,* W. B. Saunders, Philadelphia, 1977.

Schlossberg, Leon: *The Johns Hopkins Atlas of Human Functional Anatomy,* The Johns Hopkins University Press, Baltimore, 1977.

Shulman, J. L.: *Management of Emotional Disorders in Pediatric Practice,* Year Book Medical Publishers, Chicago, 1970.

Silver, Henry K., C. Henry Kempe, and Henry B. Bruyn: *Handbook of Pediatrics,* 11th ed., Lange Medical Publications, Los Altos, Calif., 1975.

Smart, M. S., and R. C. Smart: *Children, Development and Relationships,* 3d ed., Macmillan, New York, 1977.

Smith, David: *Growth and Its Disorders: Basics and Standards, Approach and Classifications, Growth Deficiency Disorders, Growth Excess Disorders, Obesity,* W. B. Saunders, Philadelphia, 1977.

Smith, David W.: *Recognizable Patterns of Human Malformation,* W. B. Saunders, Philadelphia, 1970.

Stein, Harold A., and Bernard J. Slatt: *The Ophthalmic Assistant,* C. V. Mosby, St. Louis, 1971.

Stewart, William D., Julius L. Danto, and Stuart Maddin: *Synopsis of Dermatology,* C. V. Mosby, St. Louis, 1970.

Thomas, A., and Y. Chesni: *The Neurological Examination of the Infant,* Little Clubs Clinics in Developmental Medicine, Medical Advisory Committee of NPTI Spastic Society, London, 1960.

Thomas, George H., and R. Rodney Howell: *Selected Screening Tests for Genetic Metabolic Diseases,* Year Book Medical Publishers, Chicago, 1973.

Van Allen, M. W.: *Pictorial Manual of Neurologic Tests,* Year Book Medical Publications, Chicago, 1969.

Wilson, Thomas: *Diseases of the Ear, Nose and Throat in Children,* Grune & Stratton, New York, 1962.

Winter, Chester, C.: *Practical Urology,* C.V. Mosby, St. Louis, 1969.

Wold, Robert M.: *Screening Tests to Be Used by the Classroom Teacher,* Academic Therapy Publications, San Rafael, Calif., 1970.

Ziai, Mohsen, Charles A. Janeway, and Robert E. Cooke: *Pediatrics,* 2d ed., Little, Brown, Boston, 1975.

Index

Index

Page references in *italic* indicate illustrations or tables.